Persistent Pain in Older Adults

An Interdisciplinary Guide for Treatment

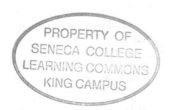

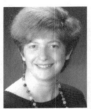

Debra K. Weiner, MD, is associate professor in the Departments of Medicine, Psychiatry, and Anesthesiology at the University of Pittsburgh School of Medicine. She is a geriatrician, rheumatologist, acupuncturist, and Director of the Older Adult Pain Management Program at the University of Pittsburgh's Pain Evaluation and Treatment Institute. She is also Medical Director of the Charles M. Morris Nursing and Rehabilitation Center in Pittsburgh. Dr. Weiner's primary areas of research include investigation of the relationship between pain and physical/psychosocial/cognitive performance, the role of radiographic pathology in older adults with chronic low-back pain, the utility of pain behavior observation as a substitute for self-report, and pain communication in nursing home residents. Dr. Weiner also teaches medical students, internal medicine residents, nurse practitioners, and geriatric medicine fellows, as well as lay groups, about comprehensive evaluation and management of persistent pain in community-dwelling and institutionalized older adults. Dr. Weiner is recognized as an expert in pain evaluation and management in the older adult. She has numerous peer-reviewed publications, and serves on the editorial board of *Pain Medicine* (the official journal of the American Academy of Pain Medicine). She has also recently spearheaded an initiative to formulate an educational agenda on pain management for medical students.

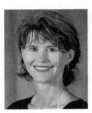

Dr. Keela Herr, PhD, RN, is Professor of Nursing at the University of Iowa College of Nursing and Adjunct Associate Director, University of Iowa Hospitals and Clinics in Iowa City. Dr. Herr is an active member of several professional organizations related to geriatric pain, including the American Society for Pain Management Nurses (ASPMN), the American Geriatric Society (AGS), the American Pain Society, and the International Association for the Study of Pain (IASP). She has been principal or coinvestigator of 14 research projects focused on the problem of geriatric pain and has numerous publications and presentations on the topic of assessing and managing pain in older adults. She is currently Coprincipal Investigator on the Robert Wood Johnson–funded project "Improving the Quality of End-of-Life Care in Iowa" and AHRQ-funded research on "Evidence-based Practice: From Book to Bedside—Acute Pain Management in the Elderly," and was recently awarded the Advancement of Science Award from the Pain Research Section of the Midwest Nursing Research Society. Dr. Herr currently serves on the editorial board for *Advances in Gerontological Nursing, Clinical Journal of Pain*, and *Pain Medicine* and the Board of Directors for ASPMN.

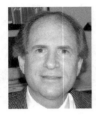

Thomas E. Rudy, PhD, is a Counseling and Quantitative Psychologist; Professor, Departments of Anesthesiology and Psychiatry, and Research Director, Pain Evaluation and Treatment Institute, University of Pittsburgh School of Medicine; and Professor, Department of Biostatistics, University of Pittsburgh School of Public Health. During the past 20 years Dr. Rudy has developed multidimensional empirical models related to biomedical, psychosocial, and behavioral measures of outcome; and psychometric innovations in pain and psychosocial measurement and test bias. Currently, he is the Project Director on a National Institutes of Health program project grant designed to develop evaluation and treatment techniques for individuals with persistent pain and spinal cord injuries or amputations, and Principal Investigator on a National Institute on Aging grant, with Dr. Debra Weiner, which is evaluating the physical/functional, psychosocial, and cognitive impact of persistent low-back pain in older adults. He has published extensively in peer-reviewed journals and has authored numerous articles and chapters on cognitive-behavioral approaches to the assessment and treatment of persistent pain conditions.

Persistent Pain in Older Adults

An Interdisciplinary Guide for Treatment

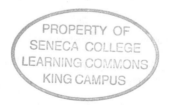

Debra K. Weiner, MD
Keela Herr, PhD, RN
Thomas E. Rudy, PhD
Editors

 Springer Publishing Company

Springer Publishing Company, Inc.
536 Broadway
New York, NY 10012-3955

Acquisitions Editor: Helvi Gold
Production Editor: J. Hurkin-Torres
Cover design by Joanne Honigman

02   03   04   05   06   /   5   4   3   2   1

Library of Congress Cataloging-in-Publication Data

Persistent pain in older adults: an interdisciplinary guide for
    treatment / Debra K. Weiner, Keela Herr, Thomas E. Rudy,
    editors.
        p. cm.
    Includes bibliographical references and index.
    ISBN 0-8261-3835-7
    1. Pain in old age.   2. Chronic pain.   I. Weiner, Debra K.
  II. Herr, Keela.   III. Rudy, Thomas E.

    RD127.P465 2002
    618.97'60472-dc21
2001057707

Printed in the United States of America by Sheridan Books

We dedicate this book to the educators of current and future generations of health care providers and to those now championing effective pain management for older adults. May you continue to teach and practice to eliminate pain sometimes, ameliorate pain often, ignore pain never.

Contents

Contributors

Robert Arnold, MD
Professor of Medicine
Leo H. Criep Chair in Patient Care
Section of Palliative Care and
    Medical Ethics
University of Pittsburgh
Pittsburgh, PA

Paula Bonino, MD, MPE
Clinical Associate Professor of
    Medicine and Epidemiology
University of Pittsburgh
Contractor Medical Director
Veritus Medicare Services
Pittsburgh, PA

Paula Breuer, PT, BS
Staff Physical Therapist
Pain Evaluation and Treatment
    Institute
University of Pittsburgh Medical
    Center
Pittsburgh, PA

Harvey Jay Cohen, MD
Professor of Medicine,
Aging Center Director and Chief
    Geriatrics Division,
Duke University Medical Center
Associate Chief of Staff for
    Geriatrics and Extended Care,
    and Director, Geriatric
    Research, Education and
    Clinical Center
Veterans Administration Medical
    Center
Durham, NC

Doris K. Cope, MS, MD
Professor and Director of Pain
    Medicine
Department of Anesthesiology
University of Pittsburgh Medical
    Center
Pittsburgh, PA

Michael J. Farrell, PhD
Research Fellow
National Aging Research Institute
Parkville, Australia

**Marie Feletar, MBBS (Hons),
    FRACP**
Center for Prognosis Studies
Toronto Western Hospital
Toronto, Ontario

Bruce Ferrell, MD
Associate Professor
UCLA School of Medicine
Division of Geriatrics
Los Angeles, CA

Perry G. Fine, MD
Professor, Department of
    Anesthesiology
University of Utah
Pain Management Center
Salt Lake City, UT

Linda A. Gerdner, PhD, RN
Assistant Professor
School of Nursing
University of Minnesota
Minneapolis, MN

Ronald M. Glick, MD
Assistant Professor of Family
    Medicine, Physical Medicine
    and Rehabilitation, and
    Psychiatry
University of Pittsburgh School of
    Medicine
Medical Director, UPMC
    Shadyside Center for
    Complementary Medicine
Pittsburgh, PA

David R. P. Guay, PharmD
Professor, Director of Education
College of Pharmacy
University of Minnesota and
    Institute for Study of Geriatric
    Pharmacotherapy
Minneapolis, MN

**Sharon M. G. Gwinn, MS, OTR/L,
    ABDA**
Research Associate
School of Health and
    Rehabilitation Sciences
University of Pittsburgh
Pittsburgh, PA

**Stephen Hall, MBBS (B Med Sci),
    FRACP**
Clinical Associate Professor of
    Medicine
Monash University
Senior Research Fellow
Institute of Rehabilitation,
    University of Melbourne
Associate Professor of Medicine
Cabrini Medical Centre
Melbourne, Australia

Joseph T. Hanlon, PharmD, MS
Professor and Director
Institute for the Study of Geriatric
    Pharmacotherapy
College of Pharmacy
University of Minnesota
Minneapolis, MN

Raymond B. Hanlon, MS
Chief Psychologist
Pain Evaluation and Treatment
    Institute
University of Pittsburgh Medical
    Center
Pittsburgh, PA

Stephen W. Harkins, PhD
Professor of Gerontology,
    Psychiatry, and Biomedical
    Engineering
Director, Psychophysiology and
    Memory Laboratory
Virginia Commonwealth
    University
Richmond, VA

John G. Hennon, EdD
Associate Director
Geriatric Education Center
University Center for Social and
    Urban Research
University of Pittsburgh
Pittsburgh, PA

Benny Katz, FRACP, FFPMANZCA
Pain Management Clinic for the
    Elderly
Melbourne Extended Care and
    Rehabilitation Service
Parkville, Victoria, Australia

Linda King, MD
Assistant Professor of Medicine
Section of Palliative Care and
    Medical Ethics
University of Pittsburgh
Pittsburgh, PA

Gary Kochersberger, MD
Assistant Professor of Medicine
University of Rochester
Rochester, NY
Medical Director
Geriatrics and Extended Care
Veterans Administration Medical
    Center
Canandaigua, NY

Thomas E. Lackner, PharmD
Professor, Director of Clinical
    Services
College of Pharmacy
University of Minnesota and
    Institute for Study of Geriatric
    Pharmacotherapy
Minneapolis, MN

Stephen P. Lordon, MD
St. Mark's Pain Management
    Center
Salt Lake City, UT

Jennifer R. Markham, PhD
Psychologist
Pain Evaluation and Treatment
    Institute
University of Pittsburgh Medical
    Center
Pittsburgh, PA

Robb McIlvried, MD
Fellow in Geriatric Medicine
University of Pittsburgh
Pittsburgh, PA

Lisa Morrow, PhD
Associate Professor of Psychiatry
Department of Psychiatry
University of Pittsburgh
Pittsburgh, PA

Max D. Neufeld, BappSc(Phty)
    GDip Manip Ther
Pain Management Clinic for the
    Elderly
Melbourne Extended Care and
    Rehabilitation Service and
    National Ageing Research
    Institute
Parkville, Victoria, Australia

Nicole L. Nisly, MD
Associate Professor Internal
    Medicine
Director, Complementary and
    Alternative Medicine
College of Medicine
University of Iowa Hospitals and
    Clinics
Iowa City, IA

Eric G. Rodriguez, MD
Associate Professor of Medicine
Division of Geriatric Medicine
University of Pittsburgh
Medical Director, Benedum
    Geriatric Center
University of Pittsburgh Medical
    Center
Pittsburgh, PA

Joan C. Rogers, PhD, OTR/L,
    ABDA
Professor, Occupational Therapy,
    Psychiatry, Nursing
Chair, Occupational Therapy
School of Health and
    Rehabilitation Sciences
University of Pittsburgh
Pittsburgh, PA

Judith Saxton, PhD
Associate Professor of Psychiatry
Department of Psychiatry
University of Pittsburgh
Pittsburgh, PA

Ann K. Williams, PT, PhD
Professor of Physical Therapy
University of Montana
Missoula, MT

Foreword

When I began my formal geriatrics fellowship training in 1987, there was little written about pain in older adults. At that time, there were very few evidence-based papers, and current geriatrics textbooks contained little discussion on the subject. Mentors with experience in both aging and pain management were few and far between. When I presented my research plan to explore pain management in older nursing home patients, I was discouraged by my advisors. They were skeptical, not only of my career development, but also of the importance of pain management compared to other issues associated with aging.

There is now ample evidence that pain is a common problem in older adults and that it is often not adequately treated. Research and experience have shown us that pain management in older adults is often very challenging. They frequently present with multiple medical problems that make diagnosis and treatment more difficult and they often experience more side effects from medications and more difficulty with some non-drug pain management strategies. Family and caregivers often take on extensive responsibilities for both drug and nondrug interventions. Many older adults may have altered goals of care, especially the very old and those near the end of life, so that more invasive or risky treatment strategies may not be desirable or justified. With these issues in perspective, clinicians often face substantial challenges to provide comfort and symptom management, especially for those patients who have a longer life expectancy.

Pain management has become quite sophisticated. More than 4,000 research papers are published each year on pain and its treatment as new and more effective drugs and interventions are introduced. Outpatient pain management is now a standard and required element in anesthesiology training. The development of training programs with defined curricula and certification processes for their graduates have raised pain medicine and palliative care to legitimate and important medical specialties. The World Health Organization, National Institutes of Health, the American Cancer Society, the Arthritis Foundation, and many others have promoted pain management as an integral part of all health care.

Over the last 10 years, pain management has reached a higher level of expectation. The development and dissemination of clinical practice guidelines, quality assurance activities, and a recent increase in litigation have brought substantial attention to uncontrolled pain and needless suffering, especially for those near the end of life. Clinical practice guidelines developed by experts for the Agency for Health Care Policy and Research, the American Pain Society, and the American Geriatrics Society have helped educate clinicians with evidence-based knowledge of appropriate principles and approaches to evaluation and treatment of many pain problems. The inclusion of pain management standards and survey criteria by the Joint Commission on Accreditation of Healthcare Organizations has helped to develop formal processes to improve pain management in many settings. And finally, several high-profile court cases have sent clear messages that individuals and health systems may be held accountable for failures to provide appropriate pain control.

In 1996, one of my fellows (Wendy Stein, MD) surveyed 102 accredited geriatric fellowship training programs in the United States and found that pain assessment and management still often receives inadequate attention in geriatrics education. The approach to health care often remains focused on functional status and disease-specific diagnosis and treatment, whereas pain is not approached as aggressively. Nearly 50% of geriatrics training programs report having no faculty with training or expertise in pain management. Although most such programs have access to settings where pain is a major focus of care, only about half require experience or rotations in pain, hospice, or palliative care services. With educational inadequacies, lack of clinical experts in geriatric pain management, and focus on other outcomes, geriatric medicine clinicians may continue to underrecognize and undertreat important pain problems.

Therefore, it is altogether fitting and proper for this book to focus specifically on pain management in older adults. Finally, in a single source, clinicians may find contemporary, evidence-based information and suggestions for treatment strategies aimed specifically at older adults. The editors, who themselves are recognized experts on this subject, have brought together writers with knowledge and skills not only in pain management but also in the care of older adults. It is important that this information be disseminated broadly to all clinicians who care for older persons. As such, I believe this work will be a valuable resource for students, clinicians, and researchers alike.

Bruce A. Ferrell, MD
Associate Professor, Division of Geriatrics
UCLA School of Medicine
Los Angeles, CA

Preface

The population in the United States and indeed around the world is aging. The fastest growing segment is the group over age 85, which will almost quadruple in the next 50 years. Aging brings with it a host of changes including physiologic declines, systems dysregulation, and the accumulation of chronic diseases. Perhaps Hippocrates said it best when he noted that "Old people, on the whole, have fewer complaints than young; but those chronic diseases which do befall them generally never leave them."

Both points are relevant to this book, which is focused on improving the lives of older adults with persistent pain. The first is that to intervene, one has to know what one is treating. Therefore, appropriate assessment is a key feature of the armamentarium. In the older patient, pain manifestations may not be as obvious as in the younger one; hence, considerable skill is required to define them properly. This book is designed to provide the practitioners the wherewithal to do so. Second, in the older adult, persistent pain may derive from one of many comorbid conditions. It is less likely to stem from a single source as may be the case in younger people. Therefore, not only does assessment require special skill but so does the application of appropriate interventions. The tools to approach these complex management issues are also well covered in this guide.

I believe that this book will be of great value to primary care practitioners, geriatricians, and subspecialists who care for older adults suffering from persistent pain. Above all, it will be of the greatest value to our senior adults and their families by increasing the pool of empathetic and knowledgeable health care providers to deal with these frustrating problems.

HARVEY JAY COHEN, MD
Professor of Medicine, Aging Center Director and
Chief, Geriatrics Division, Duke University Medical Center,
Associate Chief of Staff for Geriatrics and Extended Care, and
Director, Geriatric Research, Education and Clinical Center,
VA Medical Center, Durham, NC

Acknowledgments

The editors wish to extend their heartfelt gratitude to Ms. Christine Akers for her invaluable secretarial assistance in helping this project come to fruition. Sincere thanks also go to Mr. Gregory Turner, Dr. Lisa Rosenberg, and Dr. Evelyn Granieri for their thoughtful feedback and support.

Introduction

Persistent pain is a common and disabling problem for at least half of all community-dwelling and institutionalized older adults. There is widespread evidence that despite its prevalence and potentially devastating effects (e.g., physical, emotional, and cognitive incapacity; increased health care utilization; and compromised overall quality of life), persistent pain is vastly undertreated in those over the age of 65. This evidence comes from studies that have been conducted in older adults who live in the community as well as in the nursing home, in those with nonmalignant as well as malignant pain, and in those who struggle to derive quality from their final days or from their final years. Although numerous factors likely contribute to this unfortunate situation, knowledge deficits among health care providers regarding the assessment and treatment of persistent pain in older adults play a significant role. One of the primary purposes of this book is to provide practice recommendations, using a sound evidence base, to those working with older persons experiencing persistent pain.

Because persistent pain affects multiple spheres of life, its optimal assessment and treatment mandates input from experts who treat patients from a variety of perspectives. In compiling this book, therefore, the editors have drawn on the expertise of individuals from many disciplines—psychology, neuropsychology, traditional medicine, complementary medicine, nursing, pharmacology, physical therapy, occupational therapy, and education. The chapter authors were chosen based upon their academic accomplishments and their clinical expertise. The resulting volume, therefore, contains information that is both state of the art and clinically practical.

The opening chapter provides a framework for the entire book by addressing the question, "What is unique about the older adult's pain experience?" The remaining chapters have been organized around a unifying format, each beginning with an *Introduction* that orients the reader and articulates the chapter's purpose. The next section, *Evidence and Principles for Practice*, distills and comprehensively summarizes key relevant literature. Because geriatric pain management is in its relative infancy, evidence-based literature in any one particular area may be scant, or in rare instances, absent. In such circumstances, the authors draw upon literature from non-aged populations and supplement this information with their own clinical expertise. The next section, *Setting-Specific Considerations*, acknowledges the specific nuances involved in caring for older adults with persistent pain that are necessitated by the heterogeneity of the older adult population itself (i.e., the wide range of physical and cognitive function of older adults with persistent pain) and the uniqueness of the settings in which care is provided (e.g., hospitals, nursing homes, and outpatient clinics that are staffed by health care providers with varied educational and clinical backgrounds and experience) . A *Summary/Recommendations* section follows, highlighting the major "take home" points. Finally, actual *Case Studies* are discussed in an effort to reinforce the didactic material presented and to make it come alive in a tangible way for the practitioner.

Language directly and invariably influences thought. The use of certain terminology has contributed to misperceptions and stigmatization that interfere with positive attitudes toward aging and with the management of pain in this population. In an effort to address the challenging problem of unrelenting pain in older adults in the most positive and unbiased manner, the chapters of this book use more positive or at least neutral language, such as "older adults" (instead of "elderly"), "persistent pain" (instead of "chronic pain"), and "opioids" (instead of "narcotics").

The main target audience of this book is practitioners (e.g., physicians, nurses, physician extenders, psychologists, and physical and occupational therapists) who provide primary care for older adults in acute care settings, outpatient clinics, nursing homes, and at home. Subspecialists in medicine who provide care for older adults who suffer from persistent pain, such as rheumatologists, neurologists, oncologists, rehabilitation medicine practitioners, and pain specialists, will also find this volume valuable in their day-to-day practice. It is our hope that this guidebook will

(1) increase awareness of the complexity involved when caring for older adults with persistent pain,

(2) provide a base on which practitioners can rely for practice decisions when caring for this population,

(3) provide relevant resources that can be accessed by practitioners to facilitate their knowledge development and/or practice activities, and

(4) inform practitioners of pain specialty interventions/services to consider for the older adult with complex persistent pain problems.

The challenge of addressing the documented negative impact of undiagnosed/misdiagnosed and untreated/mistreated/undertreated pain in a rapidly growing older adult population must first be met through education of health care providers. The authors of this guidebook have provided current, practical recommendations to assist those committed to enhancing the quality of life of our seniors.

What Is Unique About the Older Adult's Pain Experience? 1

Stephen W. Harkins

> *Senescence is not universal in nature, not even common. Most creatures out in the wild die off, or are killed off, at the first loss of physical or mental power. In a real sense, aging, real aging, the continuation of living through the whole long period of senescence, is a human invention, and perhaps a relative recent one at that.*
>
> — Lewis Thomas (1984) Special Report. *Discovery*, December, pp. 24–25

Aging has come of age. Health problems and symptoms in older adults are no longer treated as expressions of the "normal" processes of growing old or as unresolved psychological issues expressed somatically. This is fortunate and reflects the increasing level of knowledge about aging and the age-related degenerative processes often observed in older adults.

Frank, in 1939, in the foreword to a seminal summary on gerontology published some threescore years ago, stated:

> From present knowledge it seems probable that much of that stubborn resistance to needed changes in the regimen of living, as well as the strong resentments, antagonisms and bitterness so frequently found among the aged, represent a lifelong accumulation of protest against experiences that have warped and twisted the individual personality. It is this very emotional resistance that frequently makes it so difficult, or sometimes impossible to help older persons. (p. xvii)

This view is certainly wrong. The idea that aging in the later years of life is associated with personality changes predisposing to neuroticism, hysteria, somatization, and nonspecific and multiple pain complaints is a disappearing example of psychobabble ageism and is unacceptable. Such views stigmatize older adults and the aging process.

One person turns 50 years of age every 60 seconds in the United States. Given the simple facts of population dynamics, it is important to understand the impact of aging on pain perception and even more so to appreciate the impact of pain on successful aging. Determination of what is unique about the older adult's pain experience requires accurate or at least commonly accepted answers to the questions: "What is older?" "What is pain?" "What is pain experience?" "What are pain behaviors?" These questions are addressed briefly here and in detail in the following chapters.

Simple demographics and concern for humanitarian care have led to increased interest in the pain problems of older adults. Traditionally, pain clinics focused on working middle-age adults and ignored older individuals with persistent pain. Some years ago a director of an interdisciplinary pain clinic commented that he preferred not to treat older adult pain patients because of their "locked-in-neuron syndrome," multiple comorbidities, and his clinical bias that they were not likely to respond favorably to interventions. There were no empirical data at that time to counter such views. This volume addresses such issues and presents strategies for pain assessment, treatment, and follow-up in the older adult. Nevertheless, persistent pain in older adults, particularly those who are frail or who have dementing illness, is at best underdiagnosed and undertreated and, at worst, ignored.

Normal life-span developmental changes are well characterized in the earliest stages of life. By the mid-teens or early third decade of life, humans make a physiologic shift from development to maintenance of structure and function. As time progresses, changes continue to occur and a transition to a gradual loss of ability to maintain systems takes place. In the sensory systems, which include nociception, these changes are frequently characterized by specific losses in sensory acuity due to both genetic and environmental factors. These changes are adverse and may lead to isolation of the individual from a normal and desired social world, decreased ability for self-care, and even depression. In the primary senses of vision and hearing, age-related changes in sensory acuities are termed *presbyopia* (*presby* = old; *opia* = vision) and *presbycusis* (*cusis* = audition), respectively. Does *presbyalgos* (*algos* = pain), a decrement in sensitivity to nociceptive stimuli, occur? Does the sense of pain decrease with normal aging in a fashion that parallels that of the other senses?

Critchley (1931), in a series of lectures on the neurology of old age that is clinically sensitive and worthy of reading to this day, pointed out that the older adult can "suffer" minor surgical procedures and even dental extractions with little or no discomfort. If true, this loss of sensitivity to normally painful events would certainly be a blessing for many older adults with persistent musculoskeletal pain. It appears, however, that unlike the other senses, the processes subserving sensitivity to, and perception of, nociceptive stimuli are not markedly obtunded with normal aging.

In this chapter, findings concerning the impact of aging on sensitivity and perception of pain are reviewed. Based on these findings it is suggested that the effects of aging on pain are less important than the effects of pain on successful aging. Table 1.1 presents several working definitions, which may not be familiar to individuals in gerontology and geriatrics.

EFFECT OF AGING ON ACUTE PAIN

There are at least six factors that might influence sensitivity to, and perception of, acute pain in the later years of life. These are loss of receptors for pain (nociceptors), changes in conduction properties of primary nociceptive afferents, changes in central mechanisms coding the sensation and perception of pain, changes in segmental nociceptive reflexes and autonomic nervous system response to nociceptive input, changes in descending modulation of pain, and psychosocial influences affecting the meaning of pain to the individual. Psychosocial influences include effects of experiences with pain over the lifetime and social history or secular change (birth cohort effects). These factors also apply to discussion of sites and mechanisms of persistent pain in the old.

Several situations exist that allow ethical study of acute pain in humans. The study of acute pain requires accurate definition of the stimulus. Situations in which the proximate physical causes of acute pain are relatively well specified include acute, procedural pain (e.g., injection), post-surgical pain, and experimental pain studied in the laboratory. To our knowledge, there are no systematic studies of age differences in procedural pain and only a few studies of the effects of aging on postsurgical pain. To date, the majority of the human studies on aging and pain have focused on acute experimental pain.

Experimental Study of Pain

A number of laboratory studies of pain sensation in older adults were summarized in 1980 by Harkins and Warner, who indicated that some studies find a decrease in pain perception with age, others show no change in pain perception with age, while still others indicate increased pain sensitivity with increasing age. Recent reviews of the literature sustain the untidy nature of findings from acute laboratory study of pain in human aging

TABLE 1.1 Important Working Definitions Involved in the Study of Human Pain

PAIN: An unpleasant sensory and emotional experience associated with actual or potential tissue damage, or described in terms of such damage. Pain is always subjective (Mersky, 1986).

NOCICEPTOR: A receptor preferentially sensitive to a noxious stimulus or to a stimulus that would become noxious if prolonged. Activity induced in the nociceptors and nociceptive pathways by a noxious stimulus is not pain, which is always a psychological state, even though we may well appreciate that pain most often has a proximate physical cause (Mersky, 1986).

ACUTE PAIN: A complex constellation of unpleasant sensory, perceptual, and emotional experiences and certain associated autonomic nervous system, psychological, emotional, and behavioral responses. Pain is provoked by noxious stimulation produced by injury and/or diseases of skin, deep somatic structures or viscera, or abnormal function of muscle or viscera. Its pathophysiology is fairly well understood; its diagnosis is usually not difficult, and with some notable exceptions, therapy is usually effective. Improper therapy can cause the acute pain to persist and the pathophysiology to increase, causing the pain to become persistent. Acute pain from superficial and deep structures may represent different forms of sensation (Bonica, 1990).

PERSISTENT PAIN: Pain lasting a month beyond the usual course of an acute disease or a reasonable time for an injury to heal, or associated with a chronic pathological process that causes continuous pain, or the pain recurs at intervals for months or years. In its persistent form, pain never has a biological function but is a malefic force that often imposes severe emotional, physical, economic, and social stresses on the patient and on the family, and is one of the most costly health problems for society (Bonica, 1990).

(Harkins, 1996, 2000). This reflects, in part, the use of different experimental procedures in the laboratory study of pain and, perhaps more critically, ambiguity in characterization of psychophysical endpoints and operational definitions of pain. The studies also differ substantially in stimuli, psychophysical methods, the age and gender of subjects, subject selection and screening criteria, as well as instructions and degree of practice on the psychophysical task.

Some evidence suggests that one aspect of acute pain may change with age (Chakour, Gibson, Bradbeer, & Helme, 1996; Harkins, Price, Bush, &

Small, 1994). Very brief thermal stimuli delivered to skin of the arms or legs can produce a sensation of two distinct pains. These pains have been associated with activity in A-delta (first pain) and C-fiber (second pain) nociceptive fibers, respectively. Under appropriate conditions first pain decreases in intensity (adaptation—a peripheral phenomenon), while second pain increases in intensity (slow temporal summation—a central nervous system phenomenon). In one study (results summarized in Figures 1.1 and 1.2), younger and older subjects rated the sensation intensity of first and second pain (Figure 1.1) to different levels of nociceptive range contact heat pulses delivered to arms and legs.

Response times to sensation onset of first and second pain (Figure 1.2) were also assessed. Age groups did not differ on pain intensity ratings of stimuli to previously unstimulated skin, a finding consistent with several studies summarized in Table 1.2. Slow temporal summation of second pain was not observed at the leg in the older group, suggesting that mechanisms subserving C-fiber mediated sensitization of second order nociceptive neurons may fail with age. Longer response times to first but not second pain in older persons suggest an age effect on myelinated (A-delta; first pain) but not unmyelinated (C-fiber; second pain) nociceptive afferents, and may represent small fiber peripheral neuropathy. These findings are consistent with the findings of Chakour et al. (1996), which indicate that older adults depend more on second than on first pain in making pain intensity judgments to near-threshold stimuli than do younger persons (Chakour et al.).

Age changes in response times are one of the better-established findings in the aging literature (Harkins, Nowlin, Ramm, et al., 1974). The observation that this may not hold for certain types of pain perception is of considerable interest in the study of age differences in peripheral and central factors that influence response slowing to other types of stimuli. It may well be one unique aspect of aging on acute superficial pain perception that behavioral response times to C-fiber mediated pain, or second pain, do not slow with normal aging. This would make pain quite different than the other senses, in which a behavioral response slowing is consistently observed across the adult life span.

In summary, laboratory study of pain has not demonstrated a generalized and systematic change in pain sensitivity in the old that parallels the well-documented age-related changes in other senses. Nonetheless, acute, referred pain may present atypically in older adults, and this may be related to the age effect on temporal summation of second pain (Figure 1.1). It is the absence of acute pain as a symptom that is most problematic in rapid identification of myocardial or mesenteric infarction in the frail older adult. However, the relationships among age, silent (painless) MI, and temporal summation of second pain have not been systematically explored.

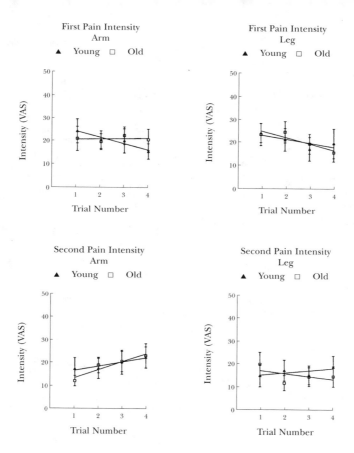

FIGURE 1.1 Psychophysical responses to very brief (0.7 seconds) contact heat pulses delivered to skin in young and older healthy volunteers. *Top panel:* Visual analogue scale (VAS) ratings of pain intensity to repeated stimuli under conditions that maximize the suppression (decreased) of first pain sensation intensity for stimuli delivered to the arm (left) and leg (right). First pain sensation is thought to be mediated by A-delta type nociceptive afferents, which are small, myelinated fibers with a conduction velocity of 8 to 14 meters/second. This type of A-delta afferent is located primarily in hairy skin. No significant age differences in the intensity ratings of first pain were observed. (Stimuli were 0.7-second heat pulses, delivered from an adapting temperature of 39°C to a target temperature of 51°C and with a stimulus rise time greater than 20°C/second. Repeated stimuli [Trial Number on X-axis] were delivered to the same location on arm or leg across trials with a 5-second interstimulus interval. At the end of each series the probe was moved to a new location in the same dermatome.) *Bottom panel:* VAS pain intensity ratings across trials under conditions that maximize the summation of second pain sensation intensity, a pain sensation thought to be mediated by polymodal C-fiber activation. These afferent fibers are small and unmyelinated with a conduction velocity of 1 to 5 m/sec. Stimuli as in top panel with the exception that interstimulus interval was shortened to 2.7 seconds. Note that the older group failed to demonstrate slow temporal summation of second pain from the leg (bottom right). These results while consistent with Chakour et al. (1996) are greatly in need of replication. (From Harkins & Scott, 1996.)

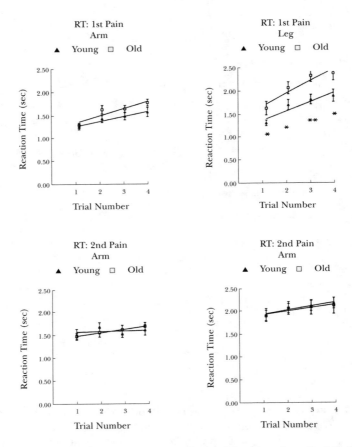

FIGURE 1.2 Behavior response times (RTs) to stimuli as described in Figure 1.1 (subjects and experimental conditions as in Figure 1.1). Note that the RTs were identical in younger and older subjects to second but not first pain. Older subjects had longer first pain RTs compared to younger subjects, and this was statistically significant for response to stimuli delivered to the leg. This is suggestive of an age-related change in conduction velocity of A-delta but not C-fibers (from Harkins & Scott, 1996).

Acute Procedural Pain

As mentioned earlier, to our knowledge there are no systematic studies of age differences in procedural pain in older adults. Procedural pain is defined here as pain resulting from a specific, limited, invasive procedure. Procedural pain has been systematically studied in evaluation of neonatal and pediatric pain (e.g., studies of reaction to heel prick in neonates or to injections in children. (See Bush and Harkins, 1992, for a detailed review of experimental and clinical study of pain in children and implications for development.) It is surprising that so little research has focused on this area in geriatric patients. There may well be age changes in hyperalgesia and allodynia, particularly in frail older adults, which would be demonstrable by well-conceived and well-conducted studies of pain in the old-old and oldest-old.

Postsurgical Pain

Available information indicates that the intensity of postsurgical pain in different adult age groups is similar in quantity and quality. Further research is sorely needed in this area and should focus on quality and quantity of procedural and postsurgical pain in relation to the later years of life.

RECURRENT AND PERSISTENT PAIN IN OLDER ADULTS

Acute pain is a sensory experience with survival value, warning of possible tissue damage. Persistent pain, in contrast, is an unpleasant experience that has outlasted its signal value. Persistent pain can be characterized as pain that is malefic, a disease in and of itself (Table 1.1).

Persistent pain has been defined as a pain that has not responded to treatment and that, according to different authorities, has lasted at least one, three, or six months. Following Bonica (1990; Harkins, 2000), persistent pain is best defined as pain that outlasts the normal healing period following tissue damage by about a month. A time of approximately one month is preferred because failure to intervene in this time period will, in some cases, result in irreversible CNS changes, increasing the likelihood that the pain will not be successfully treated. Wall (1979) points out that there are many conditions causing pain that are treatable only to a certain point.

Table 1.2 presents a summary of characteristics of presbyalgos. Presbyalgos is a general term to describe adult age-related changes and differences in pain sensitivity, pain perception, pain-related suffering or affect, and pain-related behaviors (Harkins, 1996; Harkins & Scott, 1996). It differs from terms such as presbyopia or presbycusis in that those terms are generally restricted to losses in sensory acuity and do not include the impact of these losses on daily function. Thus, presbyalgos includes sensory, cognitive, affective, and behavioral components and is not a term describing a decrease in a sensory process (sensitivity to pain) with increasing age in the later years of life. The definition of presbyalgos includes psychosocial history and thus birth cohort effects that influence the individual's interpretations of pain and the definition of socially accepted behaviors used to express the presence of pain and suffering. The ambiguities of the psychophysical studies suggest that aging in the later years of life does not have a systematic impact on nociceptive afferent traffic. Subtle age-related changes may be present (Figures 1.1 and 1.2) but a generalized decrease in sensory acuity for pain that parallels the changes observed in the other senses (see presbyopia or presbycusis) is not supported by the literature. Further, no systematic evidence yet exists for a reduction in nociceptor density with age. Such changes would likely result in a systematic reduction in pain sensitivity. While a reduction in nociceptor density might be a blessing to those older adults with persistent pain conditions, it would also confound use of the symptom of pain as a diagnostic tool.

As summarized in Table 1.2, psychosocial factors likely have a greater impact on response to pain in the older adult than do changes in physiological processes involved in pain perception and response. Further attention should be directed to the impact of pain and pain-related suffering in frail older adults. As Ferrell (1995, 1996) has pointed out, sensitivity to functional status in the face of limited potential for dramatic recovery is critical in long-term care of older adults. "Defining and treating pathologic entities [in the older adult] is often less complicated than intervening in the discomfort and disability of patients, but the latter is what truly constitutes the art of geriatric care" (Ferrell, 1996, p. 2). In this, presbyalgos differs from the other "presbys," which by their very nature produce sensory loss. Presbyalgos is more a phenomenon related to human suffering.

Pain well may be an early symptom in parkinsonian-type movement disorders. Recent population-based findings indicate that Parkinson's disease (PD) has a rate of approximately 2.3 per 100 individuals age 71 years and older, and that persistent pain is approximately twice as likely to occur in PD patients compared to older adults without PD. Persistent pain, which may be the first sign of parkinsonism in some patients, occurs in up to 40% of PD patients (Ford, 1998). Persistent pain syndromes *specifically* related to the pathophysiology of PD are poorly understood. Sources of persistent pain in PD patients can be characterized as musculoskeletal, radicular-neuropathic, dystonic, akathesic, and central in origin (Ford, Louis, Greene, & Fahn, 1998; Goetz, Tanner, Levy, Wilson, & Garron, 1986; Quinn, 1998).

Central pain has been and remains an enigma. Souques (1921) described 17 PD patients who presented with unexplained sensations of stabbing, burning, scalding, and formication—sensations now associated with neuropathic pain and with the psychophysical qualities of central

---

TABLE 1.2 Suggested Characteristics of Presbyalgos

Sensory Components: Nociception
Characteristics

Determined by stimulus intensity, location, duration, type
Sensory qualities differ for types of pain (e.g., superficial versus
deep pain)

Possible Age Effects
- Increased pain thresholds **(not likely)**
- Increased pain tolerance **(not likely)**
- Reduced ability to discriminate between pain of various intensities
  (not likely)
- Reduced ability to discriminate among different pains **(difficult
  to assess)**
- Increased frequency of atypical pain as a symptom of disease
  processes **(definitely)**
- Increased frequency of persistent pain **(definitely)**

Primary Affective Components: Stage I Pain Affect
Characteristics

Strongly related to pain intensity and autonomic nervous system arousal
Related to appraisal of the present and short-term future
Mediated by meaning and cognitive appraisal

Possible Age Effects
- Reduced unpleasantness of pain due to reduced sensory intensity of
  pain in general **(not likely)**
- Reduced unpleasantness of pain due to decreased arousal, exterocep-
  tive (sight, sound), and interoceptive (startle, autonomic) responses
  resulting in reduced segmental responses to painful injury **(no evidence
  exists for acute pain, may be true of persistent pain)**
- Reduced general aversiveness of nociceptive stimuli **(unlikely)**
- Decreased perception of threat, distress, and annoyance associated with
  the intensity of the painful sensation and its accompanying arousal
  (unlikely for acute pain)
- Differences or changes in cognitive appraisal **(likely)**

Secondary Affective Components of Pain: Stage II Pain Affect
Characteristics

Related to past and long-term future
Cognitive appraisal
Related to or representative of suffering
Not measurable in experimental studies of pain

(continued)

TABLE 1.2 *(continued)*

Stage II Pain Affect shares many properties with emotional suffering. Suffering is defined here as the state of severe distress associated with events that threaten the intactness of the person. There is confusion between persistent pain and suffering because disease models dominate thinking concerning pain.

Unameliorated pain-related suffering (Stage II Affect) requires different interventions than those traditionally used for control of the sensory intensity or the primary affective components of pain. No systematic studies exist concerning effects of age on the secondary affective component of human pain.

---

pain. Central pain may be maintained by peripheral input or by cortical reorganization following injury.

Do peripheral nociceptive changes associated with PD result in maintenance of central pain? Or does central reorganization occur resulting in development of central pain? Certainly, cortical reorganization resulting in phantom limb pain can occur following deafferentation in adult animals. The answer is likely yes and no. The fact that brachial plexus block prior to surgery (suppression of peripheral input) can eliminate both cortical reorganization and phantom limb pain suggests that peripheral processes serve to initiate central reorganization. The observation that a peripheral nerve block does not always abolish PD pain, even with relief of dystonia, also suggests a central component of pain in some PD patients (Ford, 1998; Sage, Dortis, & Sommer, 1990). A central component to PD pain is further supported by the observation that striatal or ventral tegmental lesions decrease nociceptive reflexes in rats (Saade, Atweh, Bahuth, & Jabbur, 1997). Primary parkinsonian pain may result from basal ganglia lesions enentuating in a loss of descending (and ascending?) modulation (inhibition?) of afferent nociceptive and nonnociceptive activity. This is consistent with the observations that pain tolerance (tourniquet pain test) is lower in PD patients with pain than in patients without pain (Urakami et al., 1990), and thermal pain threshold and tolerance are increased in PD patients following administration of levodopa (Battista & Wolff, 1973). These results suggest increased pain sensitivity (hyperalgesia) in some PD patients, but no controlled studies have been performed.

PD patients often present with symptoms consistent with a diagnosis of Alzheimer's disease (AD). One clinical rule of thumb is that if the earlier symptoms were movement-related, then the diagnosis is usually PD with secondary AD. If the earlier symptoms are cognitive, then a diagnosis of AD with secondary PD is considered. Interestingly, there have been no studies evaluating the nature of pain perception in patients with a joint diagnosis of AD and PD. This is important for two reasons. First, idiopathic movement disorders are frequent in AD patients and many PD patients present with a primary cognitive disorder suggestive of AD. Second, pain responses in some AD patients may be obtunded.

Given the wide range of cognitive skills lost in AD, it is not surprising to observe difficulties in some AD patients in communicating specific symptoms, including discomfort, pain, and suffering. Clinical observations, however, have suggested that fundamental defensive responses to nociceptive stimuli are lost in some patients with AD. Early reports include those of individuals with minimal response to thermal stimuli resulting in burns in the home as reported by caregivers (personal observations). Low use of analgesics in patients with AD has been reported (Scherder, 2000). The natural history of different forms of AD may well affect pain perception quite differently. Higher-order pain responses involving affect, emotion, attention, and memory may well be obtunded in patients with frontotemporal dementia.

Unfortunately, a lack of understanding of the effects of aging on pain perception has led to the undertreatment of pain in the old. Systematic education is necessary to overcome this ageist point of view. The failure to identify and, once identified, the failure to appropriately treat pain in the frail old is a major, challenging problem in geriatric medicine. Pain is the fifth vital sign. Failure to recognize this decreases compression of morbidity, increases mortality, and reduces quality of life for frail, dependent older adults.

Conditions associated with either increased pain and suffering or conditions associated with a decrease in responsiveness to nociceptive conditions should not be considered as part of presbyalgos. The following chapters discuss these important issues. They address the fact that considerable care must be exercised in evaluation and treatment of the older patient with clinically significant comorbidity, particularly the metabolically and cognitively compromised. Pain assessment is likely to remain a particular clinical challenge in the frail older individual. This is especially true in those with a dementing illness such as Alzheimer's disease. As demonstrated in the following chapters, considerable advance has occurred in pain assessment and its treatment in the older adult. It is hoped by the editors and the authors of this guidebook that humanitarian care of the dependent older adult in pain will increase exponentially in the next decade.

REFERENCES

Battista, A. F., & Wolff, B. (1973). Levodopa and induced-pain response. *Arch Intern Med, 123*, 70–74.

Bonica, J. (Ed.). (1990). *Management of pain* (2nd ed., pp. 552–559). Philadelphia: Lee & Feibiger.

Bush, J., & Harkins, S. W. (1992). *Children in pain: Clinical and research issues from a developmental perspective*. New York: Springer-Verlag.

Chakour, M. C., Gibson, S. J., Bradbeer, M., & Helme, R. O. (1996). The effect of age on A-delta and C-fiber thermal pain perception. *Pain, 64*, 143–152.

Critchley, M. (1931). Goulstonian lectures on the neurology of old age. *Lancet, 1*, 1119–1127; 1221–1230; 1331–1336.

Ferrell, B. (1996). Overview of aging and pain. In B. R. Ferrell & B. A. Ferrell (Eds.), *Pain in the elderly* (pp. 1–10). Seattle, WA: IASP Press.

Ferrell, B. A. (1995). Pain evaluation and management in the nursing home. *Ann Intern Med., 123*, 681–687.

Ford, B. (1998). Pain in Parkinson's disease. *Clinical Neuroscience, 5*, 63–72.

Ford, B., Louis, E. D., Greene, P., & Fahn, S. (1996). Oral and genital pain syndromes in Parkinson's disease. *Movement Disorders, 11*, 421–426.

Frank, L. K. (1939). Foreword. In E. V. Cowdry, *Problems of ageing: Biological and medical aspects* (pp. xiii–xviii). Baltimore: Williams & Wilkins.

Goetz, C. G., Tanner, C. M., Levy, M., Wilson, R. S., & Garron, D. C. (1986). Pain in Parkinson's. *Movement Disorders, 1*, 45–49.

Harkins, S. W. (1996). Geriatric pain: Pain perception in the old. *Clinics in Geriatric Medicine, 12*, 435–459.

Harkins, S. W. (2000). Aging and pain. In J. D. Loeser, C. R. Chapman, & S. Butler (Eds.) *Bonica's management of pain* (3rd ed., 813–823). Baltimore: Williams & Wilkins.

Harkins, S. W., Nowlin, J., & Ramm, D., et al. (1974). Effects of age, sex and time-on-watch on a brief continuous performance task. In E. Palmore (Ed.), *Normal aging II* (pp. 140–150). Durham, NC: Duke University Press.

Harkins, S. W., Price, D. D., Bush, F. M., & Small, R. (1994). Geriatric pain. In P. D. Wall, & R. Melzack (Eds.), *Textbook of pain* (pp. 769–784). Edinburgh, Scotland: Churchill Livingstone.

Harkins, S. W., & Scott, R. B. (1996). Pain and presbyalgos. In J. Birren (Ed.), *Encyclopedia of gerontology* (pp. 247–260). San Diego: Academic Press.

Harkins, S. W., & Warner, M. H. (1980). Age and pain. In C. Eisdorfer (Ed.), *Annual review of gerontology and geriatrics, 1*, (pp. 121–131). New York: Springer.

Mersky, H. (1986). Classification of chronic pain: Descriptions of chronic pain syndromes and definitions of pain terms. *Pain* (Suppl. 3), S1–S225.

Quinn, N. P. (1998). Classification of fluctuations in patients with Parkinson's disease. *Neurology, 51*(Suppl. 2), S25–S29.

Saade, N. W., Atweh, S. F., Bahuth, N. B., & Jabbur, S. J. (1997). Augmentation of nociceptive reflexes and chronic deafferentation pain by chemical lesions of either dopaminergic terminals or midbrain dopaminergic neurons. *Brain Res, 751*, 1–12.

Sage, J. I., Dortis, H. I., & Sommer, W. (1990). Evidence for the role of spinal cord systems in Parkinson's disease associated pain. *Clin Neuropharm, 13,* 171–174.

Scherder, E. J. A. (2000). Low use of analgesics in Alzheimer's disease: Possible mechanisms. *Psychiatry, 63,* 1–12.

Souques, M. A. (1921). Des douleur dans la paralysie agitante. *Rev Neurol, 37,* 629–633.

Urakami, K., Takahashi, K., Matsushima, E., Sano, K., Nishikawa, S., & Takao, T. (1990). The threshold of pain and neurotransmitter's change on pain in Parkinson's disease. *Jpn J Psychiatr Neurol, 44,* 589–593.

Wall, P. D. (1979). On the relation of injury to pain. (The first John J. Bonica lecture). *Pain, 6,* 253–264.

Comprehensive Interdisciplinary Assessment and Treatment Planning: An Integrative Overview

2

Debra K. Weiner and Keela Herr

An estimated $75–100 billion is spent each year on persistent pain problems in the United States (Weisberg & Vaillancourt, 1999). Despite these exorbitant costs, persistent pain in older adults remains significantly undertreated and is associated with physical disability, depression and anxiety, impaired cognitive function, sleep difficulty, and increased utilization of health care resources. Effective expenditure of health care dollars on persistent pain in older Americans requires appropriate targeting and tailoring of treatment that relies upon comprehensive and accurate assessment. Because the effects of persistent pain encompass a variety of interdisciplinary problems (e.g., depression, functional disablement, soft tissue injury, polypharmacy), the assessment and treatment of this potentially devastating problem may require the unique expertise of health care professionals from diverse disciplines, as exemplified by the authors of this book.

In this age of health care efficiency, practitioners may desire a streamlined and universally applicable approach to diagnosing and treating persistent pain problems. Unfortunately, because of the wide range of problems from which older adults who have persistent pain suffer, and because of the wide range of physical, mental, and economic capabilities of these patients, such an approach is not readily apparent. In this chapter, we suggest an approach to comprehensive assessment of older adults with persistent pain and introduce the wide range of treatment options that can be used to help alleviate their suffering. The chapters that follow go into considerably more depth about the issues raised in this overview. They offer the dimensionality and detail that the practitioner needs to responsibly initiate a therapeutic trial and to make thoughtful referrals to other interdisciplinary specialists for assistance with evaluation and management. We point out the unique content of each of these other chapters in this integrative overview so as to encourage the reader to take advantage of the wealth of information and wisdom that they contain.

EVIDENCE AND PRINCIPLES FOR PRACTICE

An Approach to Comprehensive Assessment: Determining the Pain Signature

The key to effective management of persistent pain lies in comprehensive assessment. In the patient with acute pain, assessment focuses on identification of the pathology responsible for the nociceptive stimulus and on assessment of pain intensity. Because older patients with persistent pain often suffer from a variety of physical, psychosocial, and cognitive pain-related consequences, however, the assessment process must incorporate a wide focus in order to formulate optimal treatment. Successful identification of the underlying physical pathologies is only one component of the evaluative process. Assessment must also include evaluation of physical function (e.g., impairment in performance of basic/instrumental/advanced activities of daily living, sleep, and appetite), psychosocial function (e.g., mood, interpersonal interactions, fear of pain-related activity), and cognitive function (e.g., acute or subacute confusion, beliefs about pain) (Weiner, 1999b). Because these functional consequences of pain can themselves modify the pain experience (e.g., depressed and/or sleep deprived individuals tolerate pain less well than others, those with fear of activity are more prone to becoming disabled, and those with cognitive dysfunction may be more difficult to treat), their specific treatment is a key element in effective management of persistent pain.

The impact of persistent pain varies from patient to patient. Some, such as the bed-bound nursing home resident with dementia, may experience pain only as increased confusion or diminished appetite and weight loss. The active, cognitively intact, community-dwelling older adult, on the other hand, may become depressed and feel frustrated by the negative impact that pain has on his or her ability to participate in advanced activities of daily living (e.g., travel, entertaining in the home). In order for the practitioner to assess the efficacy of treatment, each patient's "pain signature," that is, the unique multidimensional impact of persistent pain on the patient, must be determined.

Some possible components of the persistent pain signature are listed in Table 2.1 and are discussed in detail in other chapters of this book. A

TABLE 2.1 Assessing Functional Response to Treatment of Persistent Pain in Older Adults: Suggested Outcome Measures

Domain Functional	Parameters	Comments
Physical (see chap. 5)	Basic & instrumental activities of daily living (ADL, IADL)	Look at degree of assistance needed.
	Mobility/activity level	Decreased activity, such as diminished participation in advanced activities of daily living (AADL) in the community dweller, or decreased ability to participate in AM care in the NH resident may indicate pain.
	Sleep	Ask about pain awakening from sleep, difficulty falling asleep because of pain, time spent in bed during the day.
	Appetite	Many persistent pain patients experience appetite suppression from pain. Follow caloric intake and weight.
	Pain intensity	In NH residents, use pain thermometer, behavioral indicators of pain, and rate of prn analgesic ingestion. In community dwellers, numeric or verbal scales (see text).
Psychosocial (see chap. 3)	Mood	Anxiety and depression may coexist and worsen in patients with pain.
	Interpersonal interactions/ behavior	Reclusiveness and/or irritability/ agitation may occur. In NH residents, tone of interactions with staff, family, and other residents may be helpful.
Cognitive (see Chaps. 3 & 10)	Mental status	Consider pain as causative in the patient who experiences decline in mental status or delirium. The mini-mental state exam may not be sensitive enough to detect subtle changes.
	Beliefs and attributions	Note if the patient has changed orientation from a "fix me" mentality to a "teach me" mentality.

Note: Adapted from "Pain in Nursing Home Residents: Management Strategies," by D. K. Weiner and J. T. Hanlon, 2001, *Drugs & Aging, 18*(1), pp. 13–29. Reprinted with permission from Adis International Limited and Dr. Debra Weiner.

brief screening questionnaire that the busy practitioner might use to quickly identify key elements of the older adult's pain signature is provided in Table 2.2. The importance of determining this information cannot be overemphasized. Patients with persistent pain often respond to treatment more dramatically with respect to their function (physical, psychosocial, cognitive) than to their pain intensity (Flor, Fydrich, & Turk, 1992). Once treatment has been initiated, it is essential that the practitioner follow not only the patient's pain intensity, but also his or her physical, psychosocial, and cognitive functions. Only after the practitioner has comprehensively assessed the older adult with persistent pain, and, therefore, has determined its unique impact on each patient, will he or she be prepared to prescribe optimal treatment and determine its effectiveness.

TABLE 2.2 Brief Pain Impact Assessment for Verbal Patients

1. How strong is your pain (right now, worst/average over past week)?

2. How many days over the past week have you been unable to do what you would like to do because of your pain?

3. Over the past week, how often has pain interfered with your ability to take care of yourself, for example with bathing, eating, dressing, and going to the toilet?

4. Over the past week, how often has pain interfered with your ability to take care of your home-related chores such as going grocery shopping, preparing meals, paying bills, and driving?

5. How often do you participate in pleasurable activities such as hobbies, socializing with friends, travel? Over the past week, how often has pain interfered with these activities?

6. How often do you do some type of exercise? Over the past week, how often has pain interfered with your ability to exercise?

7. Does pain interfere with your ability to think clearly?

8. Does pain interfere with your appetite? Have you lost weight?

9. Does pain interfere with your sleep? How often over the past week?

10. Has pain interfered with your energy, mood, personality, or relationships with other people?

11. Over the past week, how often have you taken pain medications?

12. How would you rate your health at the present time?

The reader is referred to other chapters in this book for detailed guidance regarding assessment of physical, psychosocial, and cognitive function in the older adult with persistent pain. In chapter 3, Dr. Rudy and his colleagues discuss the many critical psychosocial factors that may impact the older adult's pain experience, and that the practitioner must address in order to afford optimal pain management. Dr. Feletar and her colleagues, in chapter 4, comprehensively describe a clinical approach to evaluation of musculoskeletal disorders, the most common cause of persistent pain in older adults. Tools to aid the practitioner in evaluating many aspects of physical function, both before and after treatment, are discussed by Dr. Rogers and her colleague in chapter 5. Cognitive function is a vital but ignored facet of functional assessment that should be a component of the comprehensive evaluation of every older adult with persistent pain; this is thoroughly discussed by neuropsychologist Dr. Morrow and her colleagues in chapter 10.

Physical Pathology Associated with Persistent Pain

A wide variety of pathologic conditions may underlie persistent pain in the older adult. Those most commonly encountered are discussed below. It is important for the practitioner to recognize that multiple pathologies often contribute to the older adult's persistent pain and that identification of all of these conditions is necessary in order to prescribe appropriate treatment and maximally alleviate suffering. If, after thorough evaluation, no physical pathology can be identified, the practitioner may want to consider the possibility of an underlying psychiatric disorder and refer the older adult to a mental health professional for assistance with evaluation and management. It is important also to recognize that all pain problems cannot be directly linked to specific pathology, and that even if an underlying cause cannot be identified, the practitioner is still obligated to treat the older adult's pain. That is, pain may need to be treated as a disease in and of itself.

Musculoskeletal Disorders

Osteoarthritis (OA) Osteoarthritis commonly tops the list of underlying causes of persistent pain in older adults (Andersson, Ejlertsson, Leden, & Rosenberg, 1993; Harkins, Price, Bush, & Small, 1994; Sternbach, 1986). Patients generally present with pain and stiffness in the axial skeleton (lumbosacral and cervical spine), weight-bearing joints of the appendicular skeleton (e.g., knees and hips), and/or the interphalangeal joints and first carpometacarpal joint of the hands. The wrists and elbows are infrequently involved in the setting of OA unless there is a history of antecedent trauma; thus, arthritis involving these joints should prompt the practitioner to consider arthritides other than OA, such as rheumatoid arthritis or pseudogout. If the patient complains of prolonged morning stiffness (> 30 minutes) and/or constitutional symptoms (e.g., fever, weight loss), alternate diagnoses should also be sought. Initial pharmacological management of OA should consist of regularly scheduled acetaminophen (AGS Panel on Persistent Pain in Older Persons, 2002; Bradley, Brandt, Katz, Kalasinski, & Ryan, 1991; Brandt, 1993). More potent analgesic therapy should be considered if acetaminophen is ineffective.

Certainly OA is common, if not universal, on x-rays of older adults' skeletons (Weiner et al., 1994). However, soft tissue or biomechanical abnormalities often exist in the setting of OA, and it is these disorders that may be the primary source of pain. Such disorders include paravertebral spasm, strain of the piriformis and/or tensor fasciae latae, myofascial pain, leg length discrepancy, and/or postural abnormalities in the setting of OA-associated persistent low back pain. In addition to prescribing analgesics for control of the osteoarthritis-associated pain, therefore, the soft tissue and biomechanical problems must also be addressed in order to alleviate the patient's pain optimally. It is prudent, therefore, to involve a physical therapist early on in the evaluation and treatment of most older adults with persistent pain.

Fibromyalgia Syndrome   Often the practitioner attributes generalized musculoskeletal pain in the older adult to OA when, in fact, the underlying cause is fibromyalgia syndrome (FMS). Both men and women may suffer from FMS, although the prevalence is much higher in women. A large-scale epidemiological survey revealed that as many as one in fourteen women age 60–79 may suffer from this disorder (Wolfe, Ross, Anderson, Russell, & Hebert, 1995). FMS is typically characterized by generalized pain, fatigue, nonrestorative sleep and 11 of 18 designated tender points (Leventhal, 1999; Wolfe et al., 1990). Approximately 4 kg of force should be delivered by the examiner when examining the patient for tender points, and the patient must complain of localized pain, not merely discomfort, when these points are palpated (Ang & Wilke, 1999). If fewer than 11 tender points are found but the patient's clinical presentation is consistent with FMS, he or she should be treated for FMS. Nonpharmacological modalities should always be considered in the treatment of FMS, such as learning how to balance rest and activity, effective pain coping skills, and stress management techniques (chapter 3). FMS is also discussed in chapters 4 and 8.

Treatment of FMS typically consists of aerobic exercise, nonopioid analgesics, and/or a tricyclic antidepressant (TCA) (Ang & Wilke, 1999). In the absence of clinical depression, FMS is typically treated using 30–50% of the antidepressant TCA dose. Precautions to be exercised when prescribing TCAs for the older adult are reviewed in chapter 6. Fluoxetine may be helpful in the treatment of FMS (Goldenberg, Mayskiy, Mossey, Ruthazer, & Schmid, 1996), but its very long half-life makes it an unattractive choice for most older adults. The efficacy of shorter acting selective serotonin reuptake inhibitors (e.g., citalopram, paroxetine, sertraline) in the treatment of FMS is unknown.

Myofascial Pain   Myofascial pain (MP) is common, although incompletely understood (Han & Harrison, 1997; Borg-Stein & Simons, 2002). An estimated 30–85% of patients who present to a pain clinic suffer from MP, although the prevalence of this disorder in older adults with persistent pain is unknown. MP consists of pain and/or autonomic phenomena that are referred from active myofascial trigger points. Physical examination may reveal taut bands in muscles, trigger points (i.e., radiating pain that emanates from local muscle pressure applied by the examiner), local twitch responses, and/or decreased active and passive range of motion (Finando & Finando, 1999). In contrast with FMS, in which pain is usually widespread, the pain associated with MP is typically local or regional. MP occurs most commonly in the head, neck, shoulders, extremities, and low back. Interdisciplinary treatment appears to be most beneficial and may include such modalities as trigger-point injections, dry needling, and transcutaneous electrical nerve stimulation (TENS) as discussed in chapters 4 and 7.

Low Back Pain   Recently it has been estimated that more than 17 million older adults (age ≥ 65) experienced at least one episode of low back pain during the prior year (Lawrence et al., 1998). Six million of these individuals suffer from compromised quality of life because of frequent episodes. The first step in treating persistent low back pain (PLBP) typically involves a combination of physical therapy and nonopioid analgesics such as acetaminophen and nonsteroidal anti-inflammatory drugs (NSAIDs) (van Tulder, Koes, & Bouter, 1997). Patients with refractory pain despite these frontline modalities pose a significant therapeutic challenge. While opioid analgesics are appropriate for those with refractory pain, they are not without risks in older adults, as discussed below and in chapter 6. Epidural corticosteroids have no proven efficacy in the absence of radicular pain (Deyo, 1996) and surgery may be contraindicated in the frail older adult with multiple comorbidities.

Lumbar spinal stenosis occurs not uncommonly in older adults with low back pain and lumbosacral osteoarthritis, although the precise prevalence of this condition is unknown. Patients classically present with neurogenic claudication, that is, pain that radiates to the buttocks and posterior thighs that is precipitated by prolonged standing or walking and other scenarios that cause hyperextension of the spine (e.g., walking down a hill). The discomfort is typically relieved with rest and/or spinal flexion (e.g., leaning forward, pushing a grocery cart). Differentiation of this disorder from the lower extremity pain that results from peripheral vascular disease (i.e., vasogenic claudication) is a key step in prescribing treatment. Spinal MRIs have become increasingly popular, but because of the prevalence of asymptomatic spinal stenosis, they should be ordered thoughtfully. The following questions should be answered affirmatively before an MRI is ordered:

1. Is the patient a surgical candidate?
2. In the absence of neurological compromise, have noninvasive management modalities (physical therapy, analgesics, weight loss, corsets) been aggressively pursued?
3. Is there neurological compromise or intractable pain that severely impairs quality of life?

If there is clearly an indication for surgery, then an MRI should be ordered. Because of the residual pain and disability that often persists even after surgical intervention (Johnsson, Uden, & Rosen, 1991), however, patients with lumbar spinal stenosis should be managed conservatively unless there is a clear indication for aggressive management. Exercise considerations in the patient with spinal stenosis are discussed in chapter 8, and the role of epidural corticosteroids is discussed in chapter 7. For additional diagnostic and therapeutic considerations, the reader is referred to chapter 4.

Osteoporosis In the absence of vertebral or other fractures, osteoporosis is typically not painful. Even in the presence of vertebral compression fractures, osteoporosis is often asymptomatic (Melton, 1997). Vertebral compression fractures may, however, cause significant pain, functional limitation, and depression (Gold, Shipp, & Lyles, 1998). The most effective treatment of pain associated with osteoporosis lies in its prevention, with the use of exercise, calcium and vitamin D supplementation, hormone replacement therapy, and/or other modalities. Postural abnormalities that develop as a result of accumulated thoracic compression fractures may further exacerbate pain, as discussed in chapter 4. Calcitonin has analgesic properties and should be considered in the older adult who has sustained an acute vertebral compression fracture (Maksymowych, 1998). In addition, the paravertebral spasm that may perpetuate the pain associated with vertebral compression fractures should be treated. Muscle relaxants are typically associated with prohibitive CNS side effects in the older adult. Alternative nonpharmacological modalities such as heat and massage should be considered instead.

Regional Musculoskeletal Disorders   Practitioners have often been poorly educated about the approach to diagnosing regional musculoskeletal disorders (e.g., shoulder pain, hip pain). The older adult who presents with these syndromes, therefore, often poses a diagnostic challenge. Dr. Feletar and her colleagues, in chapter 4, offer practical instruction in how to evaluate these patients.

Peripheral Neuropathy and Postherpetic Neuralgia

Neuropathic pain occurs most commonly in the lower extremities and can be caused by a wide variety of pathologic conditions including trauma, vascular insufficiency, diabetes mellitus and other metabolic disorders, hereditary neuropathies, motor neuron disease, paraproteinemia, nutritional deficiencies, connective tissue disease, toxins, and malignancies. Patients may complain of "pins and needles," "burning feet," as well as a variety of other sensations including allodynia (pain caused by a stimulus that does not normally provoke pain), dysesthesia (an unpleasant abnormal sensation), and hyperalgesia (an increased response to a stimulus that is normally painful). Typically, pain is worse at night and better with ambulating. Recently, gabapentin has been shown to be effective in treating both diabetic neuropathy and postherpetic neuralgia (Backonja et al., 1998; Rowbotham, Harden, Stacey, Bernstein, & Magnus-Miller, 1998). Because of its relatively benign side effect profile and absence of adverse interactions with other medications, gabapentin has become the drug of first choice among many pain medicine experts for the treatment of neuropathic pain. Its high cost is the major barrier to its use. Carbamazepine, tricyclic antidepressants, and opioids are also commonly used. These and other agents that may be utilized in refractory cases are discussed in chapter 6.

   Postherpetic neuralgia (PHN) is more common in older adults than in young and middle-aged individuals who develop herpes zoster (de Moragas & Keirland, 1957). Patients complain of severe burning and lancinating pain. Because of its severity, protracted nature, and refractoriness to treatment, PHN can be especially disabling, both physically and psychologically. Forty percent of PHN sufferers typically have limited or no response to treatment efforts (Watson & Loeser, 2001). PHN treatment is similar to that for peripheral neuropathic pain. Gabapentin, as discussed above, and controlled release oxycodone appear to provide superior pain relief as compared with placebo (Watson & Babul, 1998; Watson et al., 1988). Nortriptyline has been shown to provide an equivalent level of analgesia as compared with amitriptyline, and, because of fewer anticholinergic side effects, it is better tolerated in older adults. Transcutaneous electrical nerve stimulation (TENS) may be helpful (Nathan & Wall, 1974), but the role of sympathetic blocks remains controversial (Wu, Marsh, & Dworkin, 2000). Intrathecal methylprednisolone has been recently shown to have promise in the treatment of refractory PHN (Kotani et al., 2000).

Patients with refractory PHN symptoms despite the more traditional therapies discussed above should be referred to an interdisciplinary pain management program. Clearly the most effective treatment is prevention. Early initiation of antiviral therapy has been shown to decrease the incidence of PHN (Bentner, Friedman, Forszpaniak, Andersen, & Wood, 1995). It has recently been hypothesized that combining antiviral therapy with analgesic treatment as soon as possible following the onset of acute herpes zoster may diminish the risk of PHN beyond that achieved with antiviral therapy alone (Dworkin, Perkins, & Nagasako, 2000). Clinical trials designed to test the efficacy of a zoster vaccine in preventing the occurrence of herpes zoster are ongoing.

Vasogenic Claudication

Dysmobility becomes increasingly prevalent with advancing age and may be caused by a variety of pain and nonpain-related factors, such as arthritis, sarcopenia, cardiovascular disease, and dementia. Thus it may be difficult, based on clinical information alone, to distinguish vasogenic claudication (that caused by atherosclerotic peripheral vascular disease) from neurogenic claudication (that caused by lumbar spinal stenosis). Older adults with intermittent claudication related to peripheral vascular disease tend to have activity-related lower extremity pain that is relieved with rest. As opposed to individuals with lumbar spinal stenosis, spinal extension does not impact the pain of vasogenic claudication.

Noninvasive treatment of vasogenic claudication should include reduction of risk factors such as smoking, and control of hyperlipidemia, hyperglycemia, and hypertension (Boccalon, 1999). Regular exercise has been shown to decrease pain, as discussed in chapter 8. While the prescription of antiplatelet agents is indicated in those with atherosclerotic cardiovascular and cerebrovascular disease, the efficacy of these agents in the treatment of pain associated with lower extremity peripheral vascular disease is unknown. Superior long-term benefit of percutaneous angioplasty, as compared with noninvasive management, has also not been demonstrated. Open surgical revascularization, however, may be necessary.

Evaluation of Pain Intensity

Evaluation of pain intensity is an important component of comprehensive pain assessment. Although the patient's self-report of pain intensity should be obtained whenever possible, a relatively high percentage of older adults experience alterations in cognitive, sensory-perceptual, and/or motor abilities that interfere with their ability to communicate and/or quantify their pain experience. These include older adults with dementia, dysphasia, or aphasia. Clinical staff often discount complaints of pain in persons with cognitive impairment because of inconsistent pain reports (Weiner, Peterson, Ladd, McConnell, & Keefe, 1999). While findings from a number of studies suggest that verbal complaints of pain among cognitively impaired individuals are reliable and valid (Herr & Garand, 2001), the number of pain complaints decreases as cognitive impairment increases (LaChapelle, Hadjistavropoulos, & Craig, 1999; Parmelee, Katz, & Lawton, 1993). Because the ability to respond to direct questioning is impacted in cognitively impaired older adults (Porter et al., 1996), it is likely that the lower number of reports of pain is related to difficulty communicating pain presence rather than to decreased pain sensation. However, research is ongoing to examine differences in perception and interpretation of pain in patients with dementia. To further complicate assessment in older adults, pain expression sometimes takes the form of confusion, social withdrawal, or apathy in an otherwise alert and social individual. Thus, the cognitively impaired older adult is at greatest risk for underrecognition and undertreatment of pain (Parmelee, 1996; Stein & Ferrell, 1996).

Many older adults will not report pain for a variety of reasons, including belief that pain is expected and to be endured, not wanting to be a bother, expecting that the health care provider will know if pain is present and will prescribe appropriate treatment, fear of diagnostic tests and hospitalization, and fear of loss of independence (Herr & Garand, 2001). It is thus important to initiate discussions about pain. Most older adults can respond to simple screening questions about the presence of pain, making this a useful place to begin comprehensive assessment. It is not uncommon for older adults to deny pain but admit to other sensations such as discomfort, aching, or soreness (Miller et al., 1996; Sengstaken & King, 1993). The older adult's preferred description of pain should be identified and documented, communicated to other health care practitioners, and used throughout the course of treatment.

If a self-report pain measurement scale is to be used with a person known to have cognitive, sensory, or motor deficits, it is crucial to first determine the patient's ability to use the selected scale. Recent reports from ongoing work among older adults who reside in nursing homes suggest that many patients with moderate to severe cognitive impairment can report pain reliably at the moment or when prompted, although pain recall and integration of pain experience over time may be less reliable (Feldt, Ryden, & Miles, 1998; Parmelee, 1996; Porter et al., 1996; Stein & Ferrell, 1996; Weiner, Peterson, & Keefe, 1998). Further, it is extremely important to allow sufficient time for the older adult to process the task and formulate a response (Ferrell, Ferrell, & Rivera, 1995; Parmelee et al., 1993).

If the older adult demonstrates any type of sensory, motor, or cognitive impairment, the practitioner may need to adapt a particular scale to meet the individual's capabilities. The older adult should be instructed in the use of the pain tool each time it is administered. In addition, sensory assistive devices (e.g., hearing aids) should be checked to make sure that they are working properly and adjustments should be made to accommodate patients' sensory deficits (e.g., provide written and oral instruction, use enlarged type, and ensure adequate lighting) (Ferrell, 1995; Herr & Mobily, 1991).

Pain Intensity Instruments

For older adults who are cognitively intact and even those with mild to moderate cognitive impairment, a variety of tools are available to quantify pain intensity. A large proportion of older persons will not exhibit cognitive impairment and will have adapted to sensory losses with hearing aids and corrective lenses. For individuals such as these, very few adaptations may be required when measuring pain with standard scales.

The Numeric Rating Scale (NRS), commonly used with a 0–10 or 0–20 scale with wording such as "no pain" at one extreme and "worst pain possible" at the other, is a reliable and valid pain intensity scale when used among older adults (Chibnall & Tait, 2001; Herr et al., 1998; Manz, Mosier, Nusser-Gerlach, Bergstrom, & Agrawal, 2000; Weiner, Peterson, Logue, & Keefe, 1998). However, a substantial portion of older adults (both with and without cognitive impairment) have difficulty responding to this scale, particularly if administered verbally (Weiner, Perterson, Ladd, et al., 1999; Wynne, Ling, & Remsburg, 2000). Although the NRS can be oriented either vertically or horizontally, a vertical presentation may be easier for persons with alterations in abstract thinking and is often preferred by older adults (Herr & Mobily, 1993).

The Verbal Descriptor Scale (VDS), ranging through "no pain," "mild pain," "moderate pain," "severe pain," "very severe pain," to "the most intense pain imaginable," has demonstrated good reliability and validity with older adults (Herr, Mobily, Richardson, & Spratt, 1998). When compared with other pain intensity scales, the VDS is the preferred instrument for many older adults (Herr & Mobily, 1993; Herr, Mobily, Richardson, &

Spratt, 1998) and has been used successfully with cognitively impaired older individuals (Feldt, 2000). Another common VDS, the McGill Present Pain Inventory (Melzack, 1975) has also demonstrated good psychometric properties and feasibility in older adults (Gagliese & Melzack, 1997; Manz et al., 2000). The Pain Thermometer (PT), initially developed by Roland and Morris (1983), is a variation of the VDS that is preferred for patients with moderate to severe cognitive deficits or patients who have difficulty with abstract thinking and verbal communication (Herr & Mobily, 1993; Weiner, Peterson, Logue, & Keefe, 1998). A pain thermometer that has been evaluated for use with older adults is illustrated in Figure 2.1.

The Faces Pain Scale (FPS; Figure 2.2) (Bieri et al., 1990) consists of a series of progressively distressed facial expressions that represent the severity or intensity of their current pain. The FPS has received psychometric evaluation, which suggests it is a reliable and valid alternative to assess pain intensity in cognitively intact and mild to moderately impaired older adults (Chibnall & Tait, 2001; Herr, Mobily, Kohout, & Wagenaar, 1998;

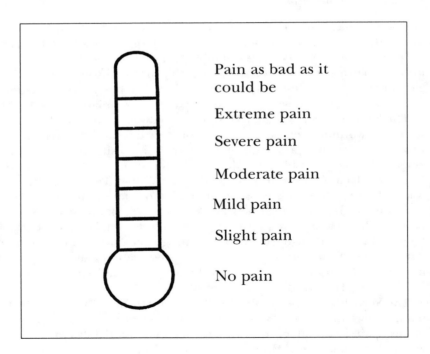

FIGURE 2.1 Pain thermometer, adapted with permission from K. Herr.

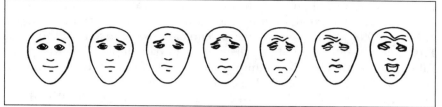

FIGURE 2.2 The Faces Pain Scale, first developed for use in children. Reprinted from "Assessing Persistent Pain in Older Adults: Practicalities and Pitfalls," by D. K. Weiner, 1999, *Analgesia, 4,* pp. 377–395. Reprinted with permission from Cognizant Comm. Corp. and Dr. Debra Weiner. Original permission from Elsevier Science and Dr. G. D. Champion.

Herr, Mobily, Richardson, & Spratt, 1998; Stuppy, 1998). The practitioner should also consider its use with the older adult who is illiterate, dyslexic, or non-English-speaking.

Verbal descriptor scales, pain thermometers, numerical rating scales, and faces pain scales have acceptable validity when used among older adults, although studies suggest that older adults prefer verbal descriptor scales and numeric rating scales (see Herr & Garand, 2001, for review). The key for practice at this time is to find an assessment tool that the patient can easily use and consistently use the same tool with each assessment. Because of its established psychometric properties, increased ability to discriminate levels of pain, and common use in clinical practice for other populations, a 0–10 NRS is a good first choice for pain intensity measurement in most older adults. For those with mild to moderate cognitive impairment, the pain thermometer or another verbal descriptor scale is recommended, followed by the Faces Pain Scale (Ferrell, Ferrell, & Rivera, 1995; Herr & Garand, 2001; Weiner, Peterson, & Keefe, 1998). If the patient has severe cognitive deficits, other methods of assessment are necessary. These are described in the section "Assessing Pain in the Nonverbal or Severely Demented Older Adult" below.

Evaluation of Pain Location

Pain location can be assessed using pain drawings, also called pain maps (Ransford, Cairns, & Mooney, 1976; Tait, Chibnall, & Margolis, 1990). The patient is asked to indicate on the drawing the areas of the body that are painful. The extent of pain can then be quantitated with a scoring template, as shown in Figure 2.3. Test-retest reliability of this tool has been shown to be quite good, even in those with dementia (Weiner, Peterson, & Keefe, 1998). Pain drawings may be clinically useful in at least two ways. First, it has been suggested that the pattern of pain depicted may be helpful in guiding therapy. For example, a widespread or bizarre pattern may suggest an underlying psychological disorder and thus the need for psychological intervention (Ransford et al., 1976; Tait et al., 1990). Pain drawings may also be useful to rotating caregivers such as those in the nursing home. A pain map placed on the wall at the head of the patient's bed, for example, could serve to remind the certified nursing assistant (CNA) who

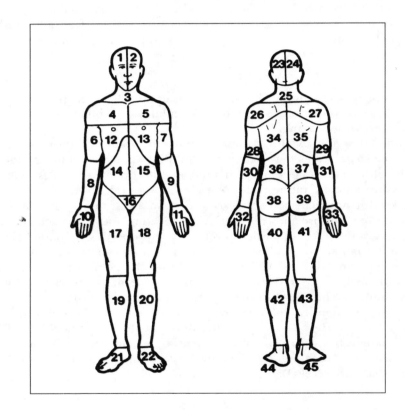

FIGURE 2.3 Pain maps and superimposed scoring template used for computation of the extent of pain (total number of areas marked). Reprinted from "Assessing Persistent Pain in Older Adults: Practicalities and Pitfalls," by D. K. Weiner, 1999, *Analgesia, 4,* pp. 377–395. Reprinted with permission from Cognizant Comm. Corp. and Dr. Debra Weiner. Original permission from Elsevier Science and Dr. R. B. Margolis.

moves the patient during personal care or transfers, about body areas that are painful. In this way the CNA, who is a critical member of the caregiver team, would be cued about pain-precipitating movements that should be altered or avoided.

Assessing Pain in the Nonverbal or Severely Demented Older Adult

The most challenging geriatric assessment patients are those with severe cognitive impairment and those unable to report their pain verbally. If the older adult is unable to use any scale to transmit information on the presence of pain, the individual must be observed for nonverbal signs. Indicators in older adults with dementia that could indicate the presence of pain include facial expressions (e.g., frown, grimace, distortion), body movements (e.g., guarding, gait/mobility changes, increased pacing/rocking), vocalizations or verbalizations (e.g., groaning, grunting, calling out, asking for help), changes in interpersonal interactions (e.g., combativeness, decreased social interactions, disruptiveness), mental status changes (e.g., increased confusion, irritability), and changes in usual activities (e.g. refusing food, increased wandering, increased sleep), (Herr & Garand, 2001). Family members or other consistent caregivers can provide valuable insight into the patient's usual behaviors and changes in behaviors or activities that might indicate the presence of pain. Because observation for pain behaviors at rest can be misleading, the older person should be observed for indicators of pain during activities such as transferring, ambulating, and repositioning (Feldt, 2000; Feldt et al., 1998; Hadjistavropoulos et al., 2000; Weiner, Pieper, McConnell, Martinez, & Keefe, 1996). In noncommunicative older adults with severe cognitive impairment, typical pain behaviors may be absent or difficult to interpret. For example, some forms of dementia tend to mute facial expression while other forms appear not to impact facial expression at all (Asplund et al., 1991).

In an effort to enhance the validity and reliability of pain behaviors for quantifying pain in older adults with severe cognitive impairment, clinically useful assessment approaches that focus on behavioral observation are being developed and evaluated. A promising instrument, the Checklist of Nonverbal Pain Indicators (CNPI), involves observation of six pain-related behaviors at rest and during movement: vocalizations, grimacing, bracing, rubbing, restlessness, and verbal complaints (Feldt, 2000). This tool addresses the unique needs of the demented population in the acute care setting, but further research is needed to validate its utility in the demented older adult with persistent pain. Because of very individualized presentations or responses to pain in individuals with cognitive impairment, a tool focused on common pain behaviors may not capture subtle and unique pain indicators. It is important to determine baseline or unusual activities and/or behaviors and monitor for changes.

If pain behaviors or activity changes are observed, the practitioner should attempt to determine if pain is the cause, as many of these non-specific behaviors (e.g., agitation, restlessness, yelling, withdrawal, pacing) could be related to other etiologies or to the disease process of dementia. Figure 2.4 presents a practical approach to evaluate this complex clinical scenario. A careful review of the patient's situation should take the following into consideration: unmet basic comfort needs (such as toileting, positioning, hunger, loneliness) and other possible causes of pain (such as infection, inflammation, distended bladder, constipation). If pain behaviors continue after other potential causes are ruled out or treated, the practitioner may want to consider an empiric analgesic trial starting with a nonopioid analgesic. If pain behaviors lessen in response to a therapeutic analgesic trial, further pain management interventions may be warranted. Preliminary research on the use of an analgesic trial as part of the protocol for assessing presence of pain in the noncommunicative older adult suggests this approach can reduce pain-related behaviors (Baker, Bowring, Brignell, & Kafford, 1996; Kovach, Weissman, Griffie, Matson, & Muchka, 1999). Further research is needed, however, in order to validate an algorithm to guide practice decisions.

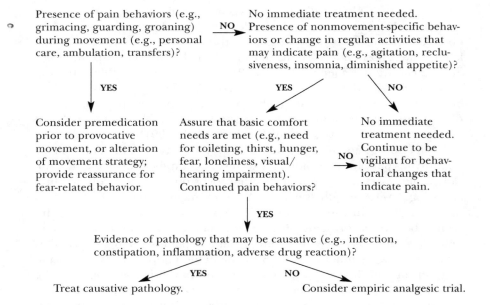

FIGURE 2.4 Algorithm for the evaluation of pain in nonverbal older patients.

Treatment Considerations

How to Communicate with the Patient

Management of persistent pain in the older adult should begin at the time of the initial encounter between the primary provider and the patient. The message that the provider conveys should be both positive and realistic, in order to instill hopefulness and a desire to comply with treatment recommendations. The provider must deliver the message that (1) help *is* available, and (2) although patients with persistent pain should not expect to become pain free, it is realistic to anticipate improvement in pain severity as well as improvement in functional ability and quality of life. It is also critical that the older adult be taught some sense of control over pain; this mind-set in and of itself has therapeutic value.

Integrative Approach and the Nurse Case Manager

Although a multidisciplinary approach to pain management (in which each discipline provides treatment without input from others) is useful for providing consultation and management of selected pain problems, the interdisciplinary model of pain management in which multiple disciplines interact as a professional team to accomplish mutual objectives in patient care can be most efficient and constructive (Ashburn, 1994; Texidor, 1998). The interdisciplinary team focused on management of persistent pain in older adults often consists of health care providers in medicine, pharmacy, psychology/mental health, social work, nursing, nutritional management, and physical and occupational therapy, all with knowledge and experience in addressing the needs of older adults. In addition, the patient and his or her caregivers should be considered integral parts of the team and should be involved in the establishment of care goals and evaluation of progress and outcomes. A pain management treatment plan can be particularly useful to define goals and outcomes, to identify specific goals to be achieved by each practitioner, and to monitor progress in achieving outcomes.

The challenges of managing the care of older adults in persistent pain, while taking advantage of the interdisciplinary team approach, require coordination and management for which the nurse case manager is particularly well prepared. This individual should be able to serve as patient advocate, educator, counselor, and provider and coordinator of care. Because nurses and CNAs often have more contact with the older adult than any other health care provider does, they can provide in-depth knowledge of the patient's unique situation and needs. This is particularly important when they work with cognitively impaired older adults who are unable to verbalize their needs. Whether the older patient in pain resides at home or in a long-term-care or assisted-living facility, the nurse case manager (or patient care coordinator) is responsible for coordinating all care issues, including educating patients and families, assisting patients and families in care provision, implementing safety precautions, administering non-pharmacologic and pharmacologic pain interventions, providing physical and psychological care, addressing insurance and finance concerns, attending to patient and family/caregiver coping needs, and coordinating care with other providers and services (Callahan, 1999). Of primary importance, the nurse case manager facilitates communication among the patient/family and the multiple care providers to ensure patient, family, and provider satisfaction.

How to Approach a Therapeutic Trial

A vast array of therapeutic modalities is available to the primary provider who treats older adults with persistent pain. Arrival at the optimal combination for a given patient should be guided by a carefully crafted, step-care approach. The practitioner should take into consideration the etiology of pain (e.g., fibromyalgia, myofascial pain, osteoarthritis, peripheral neuropathy), pain severity, the older adult's pain-related (e.g., depression, dysmobility) and nonpain-related (e.g., orthostatic hypotension, peptic ulcer disease, dementia, renal insufficiency) comorbidities, and patient preferences and ability to comply with therapeutic instructions. Ethical issues must also be carefully considered; Dr. Kochersberger offers a thoughtful discussion of the ethics of pain management in chapter 12.

Because there exists no systemic medication that is free of potential side effects, implementation of nonpharmacologic (e.g., massage, heat, cognitive behavioral therapy) and nonsystemic (e.g., topical preparations, joint and trigger point injections) pharmacologic strategies should always be considered. Depending upon the severity of the pain and its genesis, these modalities may be useful either alone or in combination with systemic medications to help enhance drug efficacy and/or limit dose and potential for adverse drug reactions. Cognitive-behavioral strategies, reviewed by Dr. Rudy and his colleagues in chapter 3, can be extremely helpful in the management of persistent pain conditions, no matter what the underlying physical pathology, or even when the underlying pathology is elusive. Similarly, exercise, as discussed by Dr. Farrell and his colleagues in chapter 8, may have a range of disease-specific and general therapeutic benefits for the older adult with persistent pain.

For many older adults with persistent pain, systemic medications will be required to optimize pain control. Because persistent pain threatens independence by causing physical inactivity, analgesics should be thought of not as an end but as a means of promoting compliance with rehabilitation efforts (e.g., physical therapy) and ultimately ameliorating disability. Analgesic prescribing for the older adult with persistent nonmalignant pain parallels that outlined by the World Health Organization (WHO) for the treatment of pain associated with malignancy (American Geriatrics Society [AGS] Panel on Persistent Pain in Older Persons, 2002; World Health Organization, 1996).

The three steps in the WHO ladder as applied to the treatment of nonmalignant pain are as follows. *Step 1 medications* consist of nonopioid analgesics and are indicated for the treatment of mild pain. Two different types are available: acetaminophen and nonsteroidal anti-inflammatory drugs. If anti-inflammatory effects are not required, acetaminophen, with its many dosage forms (tablet, liquid, and suppository), offers flexible and effective treatment for most older adults. If anti-inflammatory effects are required, the use of nonacetylated salicylates (e.g., Salsalate) and shorter half-life NSAIDs (e.g., ibuprofen) may reduce the risk of gastropathy and are less expensive than the COX-2 inhibitors. If prolonged use is anticipated, a COX-2 inhibitor should be considered, although it appears that these agents may have significant long-term toxicity, including nephrotoxicity and a prothrombotic effect (Anonymous, 2000; Perazella & Eras, 2000). *Step 2 medications* consist of weak opioid analgesics either alone (e.g., codeine, hydrocodone) or combined with a nonopioid analgesic (e.g., acetaminophen). While fixed-dose combination products that combine an opioid and a nonopioid may be convenient for treatment of moderate pain, their use is limited by the ceiling effect and potential toxicity associated with the nonopioid agent. Care must be exercised, therefore, in their titration. *Step 3 medications* consist of strong opioid analgesics, indicated for the treatment of severe pain that has been refractory to other treatment efforts. Medications in this category include morphine, fentanyl, oxycodone, hydromorphone, methadone, and so forth. For the patient with severe pain, it may be necessary to begin treatment with step 3 medications rather than first proceeding through step 1 and step 2 agents.

When deciding whether to institute opioid analgesic therapy for the older adult with persistent nonmalignant pain, the practitioner must weigh the risks and benefits. The quality-of-life benefits in terms of pain relief are inarguable, and the potential for development of drug dependence is extremely low (Porter & Jick, 1980). Potential risks about which the patient should be educated include constipation, sedation/cognitive impairment, urinary retention, and dysmobility/falls. The approaches to preventing and treating these complications are discussed in chapter 6. Sedation and mental confusion can be particularly disturbing. Sedation is usually transient when opioids are initiated in older adults who are exhausted from severe pain, but it may continue for several days. Doses should generally be reduced when sedation persists. The practitioner should also identify other medications in the resident's regimen that may be sedating, and, if possible, discontinue them, reduce their dose, and/or administer them at bedtime. While cognitive impairment may occur as a result of opioids, pain itself may impair cognition (Eccleston, 1994, 1995; Eccleston, Crombez, Aldrich, & Stannard, 1997; Lorenz, Beck, & Bromm, 1997), and it is critical that the practitioner determine whether it is the pain itself or the medication being used to treat it that is responsible for mental status changes. If uncontrolled pain is the culprit, then further titration of the opioid dose may be indicated. The use of opioids has been associated with an increased risk of falls and fractures in older adults (Hanlon, Cutson, & Ruby, 1996; Shorr, Griffin, Daugherty, & Ray, 1992; Weiner, Hanlon, & Studenski, 1998); thus, the practitioner should exercise caution when utilizing opioids in patients with dysmobility. If the risk/benefit analysis supports opioid use in these patients, a physical therapy evaluation should be considered to minimize postural instability and decrease the risk of falls.

Adjunctive agents should also be considered when treating persistent nonmalignant pain in the older adult. These medications are not primarily analgesic, but have analgesic properties. They can be instituted singly or in combination with traditional analgesics during any of the first three pain management "steps." Agents in this category include tricyclic antidepressants for the treatment of neuropathic pain and fibromyalgia, anticonvulsants, corticosteroids, calcitonin, and others. In chapter 6, Dr. Guay and his colleagues, provide a detailed discussion of the mechanisms of action, pharmacokinetics, efficacy, side effects, and drug interactions of key steps 1, 2, and 3 and adjunctive medications used to treat the older adult with persistent pain.

When the older adult with persistent pain has failed to benefit from traditional/noninvasive therapeutic interventions, interdisciplinary pain clinic referral should be considered. Depending upon the underlying disease, comorbidities, and patient preferences, interventional modalities as discussed by Dr. Lordon and his colleagues in chapter 7 may be appropriate. A wide variety of complementary and alternative modalities are also available, although most have not been subjected to rigorous research methods. Because of their overall safety, however, these therapies are worth considering as primary or adjunctive treatment. A thorough review of those modalities that may be most potentially useful in treating the older adult with persistent pain is provided by Dr. Gerdner and her colleagues in chapter 9.

In addition to prescribing pharmacologic and nonpharmacologic analgesics, treating depression, anxiety, and sleep disruption is critical in the older adult with persistent pain because these conditions reduce pain tolerance. A wide variety of pharmacological and nonpharmacological therapeutic options are available, and for individuals with refractory symptoms, psychiatric referral should be considered.

The specific components of a therapeutic trial for the older adult with persistent pain should be highly individualized. For the older adult with moderate pain associated with osteoarthritis, the therapeutic approach depends upon the extent of disease. If the patient's pain is primarily localized to the knees, joint injection may provide adequate pain relief. For the patient with more widespread disease, the practitioner may want to begin with a two-week trial of acetaminophen (see chapter 6 for details). If this treatment is ineffective, a two-week trial of an NSAID (preferably a COX-2 inhibitor if long-term use is anticipated) is warranted. If inadequate pain relief results, then an opioid such as oxycodone should be considered. Because of the potential side effects of opioids in the older adult, every effort should be made to minimize their dose. Strategies that may be helpful include the concomitant use of a step 1 or adjunctive agent (e.g., a full dose antidepressant for the patient with clinical depression, or a low dose tricyclic to promote sleep), as well as the use of nonpharmacologic pain management strategies. For the patient with fibromyalgia, an interdisciplinary approach that includes exercise and analgesic therapy should be considered at the outset. Concomitant treatment with a tricyclic antidepressant (e.g., low dose desipramine or nortriptyline) or an SSRI should be considered. For the older adult with painful peripheral neuropathy, a therapeutic trial that begins with an adjunctive agent is more appropriate; gabapentin is the drug of first choice because of its efficacy, relatively benign side effect profile, and lack of drug-drug interactions. In addition to treatment of pain, older adults nearing the end of life may require treatment of a variety of other contributors to their suffering such as dyspnea and existential angst. Drs. King and Arnold provide the practitioner with a thoughtful approach to the management of these difficult issues in chapter 11.

Prevention of Disease Exacerbation/Progression

To optimize the quality of life and function of the older adult with persistent pain, treatment should project beyond immediate pain control and include efforts to prevent progression of the pain-causing pathology. There is evidence, for example, that naturally occurring vitamin C slows the progression of knee osteoarthritis (McAlindon et al., 1996). Practitioners may want to consider supplemental vitamin C (e.g., 500 mg/day) in the older adult with osteoarthritis. Oral glucosamine and chondroitin sulfate might also be considered, as it may have analgesic effects (Towheed et al., 2001; McAlindon et al., 2000) as well as disease-modifying properties (Reginster et al., 2001). Additional research is needed before definitive recommendations can be made. The older adult with osteoporosis should also be treated aggressively, including supplemental calcium, vitamin D, and antiresorptive agents in order to prevent fractures. The older adult with peripheral neuropathy caused by diabetes mellitus should be particularly scrupulous about control of this disease. This principle also holds true for the patient with vasogenic claudication and modifiable risk factors. Addressing pain in the older adult necessitates relieving pain—to the extent possible—and treating etiologic factors. The older adult with persistent pain requires the care of a well-trained pain medicine practitioner as well as a vigilant primary care practitioner.

Because the underlying pain-causing pathology is likely to progress over time, making the older adult with persistent pain at risk for functional decline, ongoing efforts to maintain functional status are critical. For the older adult in whom pain may interfere with the performance of prescribed physical therapy exercises, the practitioner should consider administration of an analgesic 30–60 minutes prior to each physical therapy session. As discussed earlier in this chapter, because opioids have been shown to increase the risk of falls in older adults (Hanlon et al., 1996), a physical therapy consultation or, at minimum, the prescription of an assistive device should be considered for those individuals who require opioids. Aerobic exercise should also be given serious consideration, to maintain both physical function and psychological well being (see chapter 8).

Interdisciplinary Pain Management Programs

Since persistent pain is a multidimensional experience, it is not surprising that comprehensive interdisciplinary treatment programs have been shown to have superior outcomes to those that utilize a unidimensional approach (Flor et al., 1992). Because of their emphasis on nonpharmacological treatment approaches (e.g., physical therapy, occupational therapy, cognitive behavioral therapy), interdisciplinary programs have particular appeal for the frail older adult in whom analgesic-associated toxicity carries substantial morbidity. They also have particular appeal as compared with many invasive modalities. We believe that all older adults who have failed pain management by their primary practitioner should undergo assessment by an interdisciplinary team of pain specialists prior to being referred for invasive modalities. Unfortunately, the majority of studies that have examined the efficacy of comprehensive pain rehabilitation programs have excluded older adults. For the few that do include these patients, data suggest that older adults benefit from these programs as much as younger patients with persistent pain (Cutler, Fishbain, Steele-Rosomoff, & Rosomoff, 1994; Helme et al., 1996; Kung, Gibson, & Helme, 2000b; Middaugh, Levin, Kee, Barchiese, & Roberts, 1988).

At the University of Pittsburgh's Older Adult Pain Management Program (OAPMP), a clinic geared toward the treatment of older adults with persistent pain, patients are initially seen by a geriatrician/rheumatologist/acupuncturist who then makes the necessary referrals to other team members (physical therapist, occupational therapist, psychologist, anesthesiologist). Virtually every patient is seen by the physical therapist. If the patient reports ADL difficulties, an occupational therapy evaluation is scheduled. While patients may well benefit from psychological evaluation and treatment, many older adults are reluctant to proceed down this path. In addition, many insurers do not reimburse for psychological services. Therefore, it is prudent to assess the patient's willingness to proceed with psychological evaluation and the willingness of the insurance company to reimburse for these services prior to scheduling a psychological assessment.

Older adults with persistent pain are heterogeneous (Weiner, Rudy, & Gaur, 2001). One hundred older adults who presented to the OAPMP were administered the McGill Pain Questionnaire short form, the Geriatric Depression Scale, the Pittsburgh Sleep Quality Index, pain interference ratings for basic and instrumental ADLs, and frequency ratings of performing advanced ADLs. Cluster analyses indicated that three clusters, or patient profiles, existed for these measures. Patients assigned to Cluster 1 (30%) appeared to have adapted quite well to their pain, exhibiting relatively low levels of pain, depression, and sleep disruption, and high levels of activity. In contrast, Cluster 3 (28%) had more pain and were more severely disabled. Cluster 2 (42%) was mixed and showed some similarities to Clusters 1 and 3, but had its own unique profile. External validation was performed, including laboratory-based physical capacity measures, and found significant differences across patient clusters in both the performance of repetitive lifting and chair-rise tasks. This information suggests that older adult patients with persistent pain are not homogeneous in their reaction to pain.

Additional research is needed to validate such a classification system. Ultimately this type of information could be helpful in tailoring treatment and appropriately allocating health care resources. Patients who fall into Cluster 1, for example, may require medication alone, physical therapy alone, or a combination of the two in order to afford relief of pain and restoration of function. Those in Cluster 3, on the other hand, would likely require treatment by an interdisciplinary team to afford optimal results.

Quality Assurance Issues

The serious problem of underrecognition and undertreatment of pain in older adults highlights the importance of organizational commitment to recognize and address these concerns. Establishing quality assurance procedures that improve the structure and process of care delivery, monitor adequacy of relevant documentation, and identify measurable pain outcomes can assist in this process. The American Pain Society (APS) recommends that institutions perform routine quality assurance monitoring of their pain management services, in an attempt to assist organizations in improving pain practices (APS, 1995). This has led to the recognition of pain as "the fifth vital sign," meaning that routine screening for the presence of pain should accompany traditional vital sign measurement of blood pressure, pulse, respiratory rate, and temperature at appropriate intervals. Of considerable importance in the quality assurance process is the establishment of clinical documentation approaches that provide evidence of regular assessment and monitoring of the presence and relief of pain in older adults, which continues to be a challenge for many organizations (Malek & Olivieri, 1996).

In an effort to address the issue of inadequate pain treatment, clinical practice and quality assurance guidelines have been published by the Agency for Healthcare Research and Quality (AHRQ; formerly the Agency for Health Care Policy and Research, [AHCPR]) (AHCPR, 1992, 1994), the American Pain Society (APS, 1995, 1999, 2002), and the Joint Commission on Accreditation of Healthcare Organizations (JCAHO, 2000). While these guidelines are broad in scope, considerations unique to the care of older persons are limited. To address the special concerns of pain in older adults, the American Geriatrics Society has published specific clinical practice guidelines for the assessment and management of pain in older persons (AGS, 1997, 2002); and the American Medical Directors Association (AMDA) has published clinical practice guidelines for the management of pain in the long-term care setting (AMDA, 1999). These guidelines provide explicit and useful information on which to base clinical practice decisions. They are also intended to guide development of policies and procedures that enhance routine assessment, as well as pharmacologic and nonpharmacologic therapy for the older adult with persistent pain. Although early guideline recommendations were based mostly on expert consensus, the accumulation of research on assessment and treatment approaches has contributed to stronger evidence-based recommendations. However, continued research in the area of pain assessment and management in older adults is sorely needed.

Although patient satisfaction is certainly an important factor in evaluation of pain practices in an organization, a dichotomy exists between the report of high levels of satisfaction with practitioners' management of pain and the report of significant levels of unrelieved pain (Comley & DeMeyer, 2001; Ferrell, Whedon, & Rollins, 1995). Thus, this should not be the sole indicator used to monitor and evaluate pain management practices.

Education Issues

Patient education is considered an integral component of the comprehensive management of persistent pain. Evidence suggests that educational programs can be effective as an adjunctive therapy in managing persistent pain in older adults (Ettinger et al., 1997; Mazucca et al., 1997) and even alone (Ferrell, Ferrell, Ahn, & Tran, 1994; Lindroth et al., 1997). Comprehensive educational programs commonly include the following information:

1. The nature and causes of the pain (including the fact that pain is not a normal part of aging and can interfere with healing and rehabilitation)
2. Methods of pain assessment and measurement
3. Goals of treatment
4. Treatment options—pharmacologic and nonpharmacologic
5. Expectations of pain management (addressing concerns related to tolerance and management of common side effects)
6. Self-help techniques

Inclusion of the family caregiver in educational programming is very important; adherence to the treatment plan is often dependent on this individual's understanding of the purpose and process of the intervention's approach. Educational strategies should be tailored to the patient's needs and level of understanding, with teaching/learning strategies and use of written and audio materials adapted to accommodate sensory and cognitive impairments (e.g., pacing of instruction, use of repetition, use of alternative methods of communication, provision of written materials in large font and fifth-grade reading level, use of assistive devices).

Provider education is also a key component of the comprehensive management of persistent pain. Underdiagnosis and undertreatment of persistent pain in older adults is largely related to undereducation of health care professionals. In an effort to help rectify this problem, Drs. Hennon and Weiner, in chapter 13, provide guidance on how to create a well-structured educational program that targets this area of critically needed learning.

Adherence Issues

Nonadherence to medication regimens and nonpharmacologic interventions is a complex and common problem that impacts outcomes of persistent pain management approaches. For long-term disease management, adherence is frequently no better than 50%. Estimates indicate that

10–25% of older adults do not take their prescription medication, while others adjust their medication regimen, including skipping doses and under- or overdosing (Durso, 2001). Numerous factors are thought to impact the high nonadherence rate among older adults, such as complex medication regimens, severity of age-related disease and disability, cognitive impairment, visual/auditory/manual deficits, poor understanding of medication use, beliefs about their illness, financial factors, environmental factors, lack of use of external aids, fear of drug side effects, fear of addiction/tolerance/dependence, inability to access medications, and inadequate patient-provider communication. Surprisingly, studies focusing on improving medication compliance have shown that older adults are often better than younger patients at managing medications and adhering to a medication regimen (Park et al., 1999; Viller et al., 1999). Thus, efforts to address factors that impact adherence should be encouraged in this population.

Approaches that can be used with the older adult persistent pain sufferer to help ameliorate medication nonadherence include

1. Patient education regarding the nature and purpose of analgesics
2. Careful education on the medication regimen
3. Debunking the misbeliefs regarding addiction, tolerance, and dependence
4. Prescribing simpler drug regimens (such as use of sustained release analgesics, rather than short-acting agents)
5. Use of a medication organizer or electronic pill dispenser (with instructions on loading procedure)
6. Use of an external prompting device (such as a beeping wristwatch)

New technologies, including instrumented medication vials, beeping key chains, programmed watches, and telecommunications devices such as pagers and personal data systems, are under investigation as strategies to promote medication adherence (Durso, 2001; Fulmer et al., 1999).

Reimbursement Issues

Even in the face of a perfectly designed pain management program that takes into consideration all of the issues raised in this chapter, fiscal constraints may limit the extent to which such a program can be implemented. In chapter 14, Drs. McIlvried and Bonino discuss these issues and provide suggestions to guide the practitioner in tackling this not uncommon and frustrating problem.

SETTING-SPECIFIC CONSIDERATIONS

The challenges of addressing persistent pain problems exist in all settings in which older adults reside. The cognitive and physical condition of the older adult also substantively impacts the approach to assessment and management of pain. Each setting has unique complexities that must be considered when choosing intervention strategies.

Practitioners must carefully evaluate older adults' understanding of any intervention (whether pharmacologic or nonpharmacologic) that they or their significant others will be expected to carry out. Practitioners must also evaluate patients' access to resources required to implement the recommended intervention. For example, the older adult in the community may have difficulty with physical access to pharmacies. Additionally, unavailability of opioids is a considerable problem, not only in less populated rural settings but in inner city pharmacies reluctant to stock these medications (Paice & Fine, 2001). Also, resources for rehabilitation and nonpharmacologic interventions may be limited. Whereas community-dwelling older adults with persistent pain can often be effectively managed through their primary care provider (Cook & Thomas, 1994), there is a significant proportion that requires additional services to improve pain management. Outcome studies suggest that although many older adults can benefit from interdisciplinary pain programs (Helme et al., 1996), accessibility and cost are significant barriers to the use of these services (Kung, Gibson, & Helme, 2000a). Community-based programs that provide a choice of interventions at lower costs are being evaluated as an alternative to pain clinic approaches (Kung et al., 2000a).

Older adults who reside in nursing homes are at particular risk for underdiagnosed and undertreated pain. The barriers to effective pain management in this setting are many. The two major concerns are the challenge of recognizing pain in the severely cognitively impaired and the rapid turnover of unlicensed personnel who provide most direct care. Establishing an institutional training program should be a priority in every nursing facility. These programs should instruct staff in verbal and nonverbal pain assessment skills that can be applied to every resident. Use of the best evidence available to guide the screening process for residents who may be experiencing pain is an important step. As discussed earlier in this chapter, a rational approach to assessing and monitoring for the presence of pain in older adults is suggested, and each institution should establish pain evaluation and management as a high priority.

SUMMARY/RECOMMENDATIONS

1. Persistent pain is underdiagnosed and undertreated across all settings in which providers care for older adults.

2. Effective treatment of persistent pain depends on comprehensive assessment, with attention to diagnosis of the underlying pathologies as well as the often accompanying physical, psychosocial, and cognitive dysfunctions that also require treatment.

3. Osteoarthritis is cited as the most common cause of persistent pain in older adults, but accompanying soft tissue pathology (e.g., muscle strain and spasm, myofascial pain, fibromyalgia) may be an important, if not the major, contributor. A physical therapist, therefore, should be involved early on in the evaluation and management of most older adults with persistent pain.

4. Patients' self-reported pain intensity should be sought using tools appropriate for older adults. Behavioral observation and monitoring for changes in activities are necessary for those unable to report pain.

5. An integrated approach to evaluation and management of persistent pain in older adults is an effective strategy. The nurse case manager is important in the coordination and implementation of an interdisciplinary treatment approach.

6. Pharmacologic and nonpharmacologic analgesic modalities play a central role in treating the older adult with persistent pain. They should be viewed, however, not as an end in themselves, but as a means to promote rehabilitation and, therefore, maintenance of independence.

7. Interdisciplinary pain management clinics play a useful role in treating the older adult with persistent pain and physical, psychosocial, and cognitive comorbidities. The primary practitioner should refer patients to these clinics before considering invasive modalities.

8. Establishment and monitoring of processes to improve pain management are needed to reduce underrecognized and undertreated pain in older adults.

9. Patient education should be an integral component of the comprehensive management of persistent pain. Health care provider education also is essential to improve the practice of pain management in the older adult population.

10. Strategies for promoting adherence to medication and nonpharmacologic interventions should be included in the pain treatment plan.

CASE STUDIES

Case 1

A 68-year-old woman presented to the pain clinic with a chief complaint of severe pain in her left buttock described as "someone sticking a hot poker into me." She also complained of sleep disturbance, depressed mood, and inability to participate in her favorite advanced activity of daily living (AADL), dancing. Physical examination revealed severe tenderness of the left piriformis, which reproduced her "hot poker" pain, and physical therapy was prescribed. Her insurance carrier, however, would no longer cover noninvasive treatment of this "same problem." Piriformis strain had, in fact, never been diagnosed or properly treated. She had been treated for presumptive osteoarthritis (OA). She eventually had a series of injections of the piriformis with marked reduction of her pain, resolution of her sleep disturbance, and return of her ability to participate in her treasured AADL.

Discussion

This case illustrates several important points. First, while OA is common in older adults, there are other important sources of pathology that often underlie pain. Musculoskeletal pain may be caused by a wide variety of sources that are described in chapter 4 of this book. The older adult with persistent musculoskeletal pain deserves a comprehensive physical examination. Only with correct identification of the underlying problem can correct treatment be prescribed. Purported lack of response may be caused by treatment of an incorrectly identified problem. Second, this patient's inability to participate in her favorite AADL significantly disrupted her quality of life. With the highly functioning community-dwelling older adult with persistent pain, it is important to take a history not only about how pain interferes with performance of basic and instrumental activities of daily living, but also with participation in high-level physical and social activities, that is, AADLs. This patient would likely fall into "Cluster 1" described above. Third, systemic medications may not be necessary for the treatment of a localized musculoskeletal problem. In this patient with piriformis strain, physical therapy was the initial treatment of choice. Because of the constraints of her insurance, however, she could not receive additional physical therapy. A more invasive but reimbursable treatment was therefore prescribed. Piriformis injection resulted in substantial symptomatic relief.

Case 2

A 68-year-old man presented to the pain clinic with complaints of severe low back pain and trouble taking care of himself. Lumbar spinal stenosis had been diagnosed in 1973. At that time, he underwent decompressive laminectomy that resulted in relief of severe low back pain, allowing him to return to work in the steel mills for 20 years. Recurrent pain resulted in two series of epidural steroid injections over the course of two years, each time with temporary improvement, but then he failed to respond. He consulted a neurosurgeon, who suggested a spinal cord stimulator, which the patient refused. His history was notable for intractable low back and left leg pain, severe AADL, IADL, and ADL impairment, and fear of activity. Physical examination was notable for tensor fasciae latae strain with an antalgic gait favoring the affected extremity, and clinical depression. He had previously been on multiple nonsteroidal anti-inflammatory medications. Current medications included naproxen 500 mg bid and amitriptyline 25 mg at bedtime. He was treated with physical therapy, occupational therapy, and cognitive-behavioral therapy (see chapter 3). Because of concern about anticholinergic side effects, amitriptyline was discontinued. Regularly scheduled oxycodone and citalopram were initiated, which resulted in significant improvement in ADL, IADL, and AADL performance, remission of depression, and 60% reduction in pain within two months.

Discussion

This case illustrates the multidimensional impact of persistent pain on the lives of older adults and the benefits of an interdisciplinary pain clinic for comprehensive assessment and management. The contributors to this man's pain included lumbar spinal stenosis, tensor fasciae latae strain, depression, and fear of activity. He was treated with oxycodone to treat his back pain and leg pain, citalopram to treat his clinical depression, physical therapy for his pain (back and tensor fasciae latae) as well as his overall deconditioning, occupational therapy for his ADL impairment, and psychology for his psychosocial disruption (depression, fear, marital strain related to his caregiver's burden). Both his pain intensity and his quality of life substantially improved as a result of this treatment. This patient would likely fall into "Cluster 3" described above. Because of severe physical and psychosocial disability, interdisciplinary team treatment was clearly warranted.

Case 3

A 75-year-old nursing home resident with severe dementia exhibited escalation of her baseline combative behavior. Because of profound cognitive impairment, she was unable to give a meaningful history, and her combativeness precluded the performance of a thorough physical examination. Titration of antipsychotics did not impact her behavior, however, after empirically instituting a series of nonopioid analgesics without improvement; initiation of a fentanyl patch resulted in return to her behavioral baseline.

Discussion

For the practitioner who cares for nursing home residents, this case may echo a familiar question: How is it possible to treat pain in the individual whose profound cognitive impairment prevents adequate assessment? The answer may be arrived at only indirectly, as in this case. The nursing home staff initially thought this woman's behavioral deterioration was related to worsening of her dementia. The analgesic trial was initiated empirically, and only after its success was pain ascribed as the cause of her deterioration. Pain should always be included in the differential diagnostic list for the demented nursing home resident whose behavior worsens. Because adverse drug reactions and infections are the most common causes of delirium in this population, these possibilities should be excluded before pain is presumed to be the underlying cause. Agitation without delirium may also be caused by a wide variety of factors. Because pain occurs commonly in nursing home residents, however, the practitioner is obligated to consider pain as a potential contributor to behavioral deterioration in these individuals. When pain is established or suspected as the cause of behavioral changes, it is important to perform a realistic assessment of the benefits and risks of opioid therapy prior to empirically prescribing them. In the case presented, their use clearly resulted in improved quality of life.

Case 4

A 73-year-old nursing home resident with psychotic depression who was treated with sertraline, lithium, perphenazine, and bupropion, experienced an escalation of her baseline anxiety and depressive symptoms at the same time that she experienced worsening neck pain associated with severe cervical osteoarthritis and paracervical spasm. Her pain had been previously unresponsive to nonopioid analgesics. She was treated with physical therapy and regularly scheduled oxycodone as well as ongoing psychiatric follow-up. Within two weeks, her anxiety had nearly abated without change in her psychiatric drug regimen.

Discussion

As in case 3, this patient's physical pathology (i.e., neck pain caused by OA-associated muscle spasm) contributed to worsening of her psychiatric condition. She clearly benefited from interdisciplinary management, including care administered by a geriatrician, a psychiatrist, and a physical therapist. Because persistent pain may have multidimensional impacts, delivery of treatment by an interdisciplinary team is appropriate. An additional benefit of such an approach includes the limitation of administration of potentially toxic medications. Physical therapy techniques such as stretching, massage, heat and ice, and cognitive-behavioral interventions such as biofeedback and distraction therapy may be highly beneficial in the treatment of persistent pain, and may limit the need for systemic medication. The nursing home environment provides ready access to an interdisciplinary team of therapists, as illustrated by this case.

Case 5

An 83-year-old woman presented to the pain clinic with a three-year history of left buttock pain requiring several hospitalizations because during flares of the pain, she "couldn't move." The patient reported constant pain that was generally tolerable; she did not notice the pain at all when she went dancing. Over the past three years she had, according to her son, displayed worsening signs of dementia and had recently stopped dancing (her favorite AADL). She had a history of depression that was currently under good control with medication. When she experienced pain, she stated that she felt very afraid that she may have to undergo "another hip replacement." Prior evaluation of the pain had been extensive, including multiple radiographs and MRIs that were unrevealing except for osteoarthritic changes of the lumbosacral spine. Inpatient treatment had included a combination of bed rest and opioid analgesics with eventual improvement in her symptoms. Physical examination at the time of presentation to the clinic was notable for mild scoliosis and significant tenderness of the soft tissues between the left ischial tuberosity and coccyx, as well as diminished flexibility of the lumbar spine and right hip, but no pain with passive range of motion. She demonstrated severe short-term memory impairment, but had no focal neurological findings.

Discussion

The working diagnoses in this patient were (1) myofascial pain and (2) paralyzing fear secondary to dementia. The patient had no musculoskeletal or neurological evidence of weakness or biomechanical instability that would explain her episodic inability to move. When distracted by dancing, she was pain free. With pain flares, she literally became paralyzed because she was overwhelmed by the fear of not knowing what effect her pain would ultimately have. Because of her dementia, she had lost the ability to put her pain in an appropriate social context. This case illustrates the importance of considering the effects of fear when trying to determine the influence of pain itself on apparent pain behaviors (in this case, inability to move) in cognitively impaired older adults. In such cases, therefore, it is critically important to consider simple cognitive-behavioral strategies (see chapter 3) in the therapeutic armamentarium in order to modify the pain experience; analgesics alone are inadequate. This patient was referred for interdisciplinary team evaluation and management; treatment is ongoing.

REFERENCES

Agency for Health Care Policy and Research, Acute Pain Management Guideline Panel. (1992). *Acute pain management: Operative or medical procedures and trauma. Clinical practice guidelines*. Rockville, MD: U.S. Department of Health and Human Services.

Agency for Health Care Policy and Research. (1994). *Management of cancer pain: Clinical practice guideline no. 9*. Rockville, MD: Public Health Services, U.S. Department of Health and Human Services.

American Geriatrics Society Clinical Practice Committee. (1997). Management of cancer pain in older patients. *J Am Geriatr Soc, 45*, 1273–1276.

American Geriatrics Society Panel on Persistent Pain in Older Persons. (2002). Management of persistent pain in older persons. American Geriatrics Society. *J Am Geriatr Soc, 50*(6), 1–20.

American Medical Directors Association. (1999). *Chronic pain management in the long-term care setting*. San Diego: Author.

American Pain Society (2002). Guideline for the management of pain in osteoarthritis, rheumatoid arthritis, and juvenile chronic arthritis. *Clinical practice guideline*, no. 2. Glenview, IL: American Pain Society.

American Pain Society. (1995). Quality improvement guidelines for the treatment of acute pain and cancer pain. *JAMA, 274*, 1874–1880.

American Pain Society. (1999). *Principles of analgesic use in the treatment of acute pain and chronic cancer pain* (4th ed.). Glenview, IL: Author.

Andersson, H. I., Ejlertsson, G., Leden, I., & Rosenberg, C. (1993). Chronic pain in a geographically defined general population: Studies of differences in age, gender, social class, and pain localization. *Clinical Journal of Pain, 9,* 174–182.

Ang, D., & Wilke, W. S. (1999). Diagnosis, etiology, and therapy of fibromyalgia. *Comp Ther, 25,* 221–227.

Anonymous. (2000). Drugs for rheumatoid arthritis. *Medical Letter on Drugs and Therapeutics, 42*(1082), 57–64.

Ashburn, M. (1994). Interdisciplinary chronic pain management programs. *Journal of Pharmaceutical Care in Pain and Symptom Control, 2*(3), 7–24.

Asplund, K., Norberg, A., Adolfsson, R., et al. (1991). Facial expressions in severely demented patients: A stimulus-response study of four patients with dementia of the Alzheimer's type. *International Journal of Geriatric Psychiatry, 6,* 599–606.

Backonja, M., Beydoun, A., Edwards, K. R., Schwartz, S. L., Fonseca, V., Hes, M., LaMoreaux, L., & Garofalo, E. (1998). Gabapentin for the symptomatic treatment of painful neuropathy in patients with diabetes mellitus: A randomized controlled trial. *JAMA, 280,* 1831–1836.

Baker, A., Bowring, L., Brignell, A., & Kafford, D. (1996). Chronic pain management in cognitively impaired patients: A preliminary research report. *Perspectives, 20,* 4–8.

Bentner, K. R., Friedman, D. J., Forszpaniak, C., Andersen, P. L., & Wood, M. J. (1995). Valacyclovir compared with acyclovir for improved therapy for herpes zoster in immunocompetent adults. *Antimicrob Agents Chemother, 39,* 1546–1553.

Bieri, D., Reeve, R. A., Champion, G. D., Addicoat, L., & Ziegler, J. B. (1990). The Faces Pain Scale for the self-assessment of the severity of pain experienced by children: Development, initial validation, and preliminary investigation for ratio scale properties. *Pain, 41*(2), 139–150.

Boccalon, H. (1999). Intermittent claudication in older patients—Practical treatment guidelines. *Drugs and Aging, 14,* 247–259.

Borg-Stein, J., & Simons, D. G. (2002). Myofascial pain. *Arch Phys Med Rehabil, 83,* (Suppl. 1), S40–S47.

Bradley, J. D., Brandt, K. D., Katz, B. P., Kalasinski, L. A., & Ryan, S. I. (1991). Comparison of an anti-inflammatory dose of ibuprofen, and acetaminophen in the treatment of patients with osteoarthritis of the knee. *New England Journal of Medicine, 325,* 87–91.

Brandt, K. D. (1993). Should osteoarthritis be treated with nonsteroidal anti-inflammatory drugs? *Rheumatic Disease Clinics of North America, 19,* 697–712.

Callahan, R. (1999). Patient care coordination of adult oncology patients in home health. *Home Health Care Management and Practice, 11*(3), 33–40.

Chibnall, J., & Tait, R. (2001). Pain assessment in cognitively impaired and unimpaired older adults: A comparison of four scales. *Pain, 92,* 173–186.

Comley, A., & DeMeyer, E. (2001). Assessing patient satisfaction with pain management through a continuous quality improvement effort. *Journal of Pain and Symptom Management, 21*(1), 27–40.

Cook, A., & Thomas, M. (1994). Pain and the use of health services among the elderly. *Journal of Aging and Health, 6,* 155–172.

Cutler, R. B., Fishbain, D. A., Steele-Rosomoff, R., & Rosomoff, H. L. (1994). Outcomes in treatment of pain in geriatric and younger age groups. *Archives of Physical Medicine and Rehabilitation, 75,* 457–464.

de Moragas, J. M., & Keirland, R. R. (1957). The outcome of patients with herpes zoster. *Archives of Dermatology, 75,* 193–196.

Deyo, R. A. (1996). Drug therapy of back pain: Which drugs help which patients? *Spine, 21,* 2840–2849.

Durso, S. (2001). Technological advances for improving medication adherence in the elderly. *Annals of Long-Term Care, 9*(4), 43–48.

Dworkin, R. H., Perkins, F. M., & Nagasako, E. M. (2000). Prospects for the prevention of postherpetic neuralgia in herpes zoster patients. *Clinical Journal of Pain, 16*(Suppl. 2), S90–S100.

Eccleston, C. (1994). Chronic pain and attention: A cognitive approach. *British Journal of Clinical Psychology, 33,* 535–547.

Eccleston, C. (1995). Chronic pain and distraction: An experimental investigation into the role of sustained and shifting attention in the processing of chronic persistent pain. *Behavioral Research and Therapy, 33,* 391–405.

Eccleston, C., Crombez, G., Aldrich, S., & Stannard, C. (1997). Attention and somatic awareness in chronic pain. *Pain, 72,* 209–215.

Ettinger, W. H., Jr., Burns, R., Messier, S. P., Applegate, W., Rejeski, W. J., Morgan, T., Shumaker, S., Berry, M. J., O'Toole, M., Monu, J., & Craven, T. (1997). A randomized trial comparing aerobic exercise and resistance exercise with a health education program in older adults with knee osteoarthritis. The fitness arthritis and seniors trial (FAST). *JAMA, 277,* 25–31.

Feldt, K. S. (2000). The checklist of nonverbal pain indicators (CNPI). *Pain Management Nursing, 1,* 13–21.

Feldt, K. S., Ryden, M. B., & Miles, S. (1998). Treatment of pain in cognitively impaired compared with cognitively intact older patients with hip fracture. *J Am Geriatr Soc, 46,* 1079–1085.

Ferrell, B., Whedon, M., & Rollins, B. (1995). Pain and quality assessment/improvement. *Journal of Nursing Care Quality, 9*(3), 69–85.

Ferrell, B. A. (1995). Pain evaluation and management in the nursing home. *Ann Intern Med, 123,* 681–687.

Ferrell, B. A., Ferrell, B. R., & Rivera, L. (1995). Pain in cognitively impaired nursing home patients. *J Pain Symptom Manage, 10,* 591–598.

Ferrell, B. R., Ferrell, B. A., Ahn, C., & Tran, K. (1994). Pain management for elderly people with cancer at home. *Cancer, 74,* 2139–2146.

Finando, D., & Finando, S. (1999). *Informed touch—A clinician's guide to the evaluation and treatment of myofascial disorders.* Rochester, VT: Healing Arts Press.

Flor, H., Fydrich, T., & Turk, D. C. (1992). Efficacy of multidisciplinary pain treatment centers: A meta-analytic review. *Pain, 49,* 221–230.

Fulmer, T. T., Feldman, P. H., Kim, T. S., Carty, B., Beers, M., Molina, M., & Putnam, M. (1999). An intervention study to enhance medication compliance in community-dwelling elderly individuals. *Journal of Gerontological Nursing, 25*(8), 6–14.

Gagliese, L., & Melzack, R. (1997). Age differences in the quality of chronic pain: A preliminary study. *Pain Research and Management, 2*(3), 157–162.

Gold, D. T., Shipp, K. M., & Lyles, K. W. (1998). Managing patients with complications of osteoporosis. *Endocrinology and Metabolism Clinics of North America, 27,*
485–496.
Goldenberg, D., Mayskiy, M., Mossey, C., Ruthazer, R., & Schmid, C. (1996). A randomized, double-blind crossover trial of fluoxetine and amitriptyline in the
treatment of fibromyalgia. *Arthritis and Rheumatism, 39,* 1852–1859.
Hadjistavropoulos, T., LaChapelle, D. L., MacLeod, F. K., Snider, B., & Craig, K.
D. (2000). Measuring movement-exacerbated pain in cognitively impaired frail
elders. *Clinical Journal of Pain, 16,* 54–63.
Han, S. C., & Harrison, P. (1997). Myofascial pain syndrome and trigger-point
management. *Regional Anesthesia, 22*(1), 89–101.
Hanlon, J. T., Cutson, T., & Ruby, C. M. (1996). Drug-related falls in the elderly.
Top Geriatr Rehabil, 11(3), 38–54.
Harkins, S. W., Price, D. D., Bush, F. M., & Small, R. E. (1994). Geriatric pain. In
P. D. Wall and R. Melzack (Eds.), *Textbook of pain* (pp. 769–784). New York:
Churchill Livingstone.
Helme, R., Katz, B., Gibson, S., Bradbeer, M., Farrell, M., Neufeld, M., & Corran,
T. (1996). Multidisciplinary pain clinics for older people. Do they have a role?
Clinics in Geriatric Medicine, 12, 563–582.
Herr, K., & Garand, L. (2001). Assessment and measurement of pain in older
adults. *Clinics in Geriatric Medicine, 17*(3), 457–478.
Herr, K., & Mobily, P. (1991). Complexities of pain assessment in the elderly:
Practical considerations. *J Gerontol Nurs, 17,* 12–19.
Herr, K., & Mobily, P. R. (1993). Comparison of selected pain assessment tools for
use with the elderly. *Applied Nursing Research, 6,* 39–46.
Herr, K. A., Mobily, P. R., Kohout, F. J., & Wagenaar, D. (1998). Evaluation of the
Faces Pain Scale for use with the elderly. *Clin J Pain, 14,* 29–38.
Herr, K., Mobily, P., Richardson, G., & Spratt, K. (1998). Use of experimental pain
to compare psychometric properties and usability of pain scales in the adult
and older adult populations [Abstract]. Annual Meeting of the American Society
for Pain Management in Nursing, Orlando, FL.
Johnsson, K.-E., Uden, A., & Rosen, I. (1991). The effect of decompression on the
natural course of spinal stenosis—A comparison of surgically treated and
untreated patients. *Spine, 16,* 615–619.
Joint Commission on Accredition of Healthcare Organizations. (2000). Pain man-
agement standards. [Online]. http://www.jcaho.org.
Kotani, N., Kushikata, T., Hashimoto, H., Kimura, F., Muraoka, M., Yodono, M.,
Asai, M., & Matsuki, A. (2000). Intrathecal methylprednisolone for intractable
postherpetic neuralgia. *New England Journal of Medicine, 343,* 1514–1519.
Kovach, C. R., Weissman, D. E., Griffie, J., Matson, S., & Muchka, S. (1999).
Assessment and treatment of discomfort for people with late-stage dementia.
J Pain Symptom Manage, 18, 412–419.
Kung, F., Gibson, S., & Helme, R. (2000a). A community-based program that pro-
vides free choice of intervention for old people with chronic pain. *Journal of
Pain, 1,* 293–308.
Kung, F., Gibson, S., & Helme, R. (2000b). Comparison of chronic pain experi-
ence between pain clinic and community samples. *Pain Clinic, 12,* 193–203.

LaChapelle, D. L., Hadjistavropoulos, T., & Craig, K. D. (1999). Pain measurement in persons with intellectual disabilities. *Clin J Pain, 15,* 13–23.

Lawrence, R. C., Helmick, C. G., Arnett, F. C., Deyo, R. A., Felson, D. T., Giannini, E. H., Heyse, S. P., Hirsch, R., Hochberg, M. C., Hunder, G. G., Liang, M. H., Pillemer, S. R., Steen, V. D., & Wolfe, F. (1998). Estimates of the prevalence of arthritis and selected musculoskeletal disorders in the United States. *Arthritis and Rheumatism, 41*(5), 778–799.

Leventhal, L. J. (1999). Management of fibromyalgia. *Ann Intern Med, 131*(11), 850–858.

Lindroth, Y., Brattstrom, M., Bellman, I., Ekestaf, G., Olofsson, Y., Strombeck, B., Stenshed, B., Wikstrom, I., Nilsson, J., & Wollheim, F. (1997). A problem-based education program for patients with rheumatoid arthritis: Evaluation after three and twelve months. *Arthritis Care and Research, 10,* 325–332.

Lorenz, J., Beck, H., & Bromm, B. (1997). Cognitive performance, mood and experimental pain before and during morphine-induced analgesia in patients with chronic non-malignant pain. *Pain, 73,* 369–375.

Maksymowych, W. P. (1998). Managing acute osteoporotic vertebral fractures with calcitonin. *Canadian Family Physician, 44,* 2160–2166.

Malek, C., & Olivieri, R. (1996). Pain management—Documenting the decision making process. *Nursing Case Management, 1*(2), 64–74.

Manz, B., Mosier, R., Nusser-Gerlach, M., Bergstrom, N., & Agrawal, S. (2000). Pain assessment in the cognitively impaired and unimpaired elderly. *Pain Management Nursing, 1*(4), 106–115.

Mazzuca, S., Brandt, K., Katz, B., Chambers, M., Byrd, D., & Hanna, M. (1997). Effects of self-care education of the health status of inner-city patients with osteoarthritis of the knee. *Arthritis and Rheumatism, 40,* 1466–1474.

McAlindon, T. E., Jacques, P., Zhang, Y., and Hannan, M. T., Aliabadi, P., Weissman, B., Rush, D., Levy, D., & Felson, D. T. (1996). Do antioxidant micronutrients protect against the development and progression of knee osteoarthritis? *Arthritis and Rheumatism, 39,* 648–656.

McAlindon, T. E., La Valley, M. P., Gulin, J. P., & Felson, D. T. (2000). Glucosamine and chondroitin for treatment of osteoarthritis. A systematic quality assessment and meta-analysis. *JAMA, 283,* 1469–1475.

Melton, L. J. (1997). Epidemiology of spinal osteoporosis. *Spine, 22*(Suppl. 24), 2S–11S.

Melzack, R. (1975). The McGill Pain Questionnaire: Major properties and scoring methods. *Pain, 1,* 277–299.

Middaugh, S. J., Levin, R. B., Kee, W. G., Barchiese, R. D., & Roberts, J. M. (1988). Chronic pain: Its treatment in geriatric and younger patients. *Archives of Physical Medicine and Rehabilitation, 69,* 1021–1025.

Miller, J., Neelon, V., Dalton, J., Ng'andu, N., Bailey, D., Jr., Layman, E., & Hosfeld, A. (1996). The assessment of discomfort in elderly confused patients: A preliminary study. *J Neurosci Nurs, 28,* 175–182.

Nathan, P. W., & Wall, P. D. (1974). Treatment of postherpetic neuralgia by prolonged electrical stimulation. *British Medical Journal, 3,* 645–647.

Paice, J., & Fine, P. (2001). Pain at the end of life. In B. R. Ferrell & N. Coyle (Eds.), *Textbook of palliative nursing* (pp. 76–90). London: Oxford University Press.

Park, D., Hertzog, C., Leventhal, H., Morrell, R., Leventhal, E., Birchmore, D., Martin, M., & Bennett, J. (1999). Medication adherence in rheumatoid arthritis patients: Older is wiser. *JAGS, 47*, 172–183.

Parmelee, P. A. (1996). Pain in cognitively impaired older persons. *Clin Geriatr Med, 12*, 473–487.

Parmelee, P. A., Katz, I. R., & Lawton, M. P. (1993). Pain complaints and cognitive status among elderly institution residents. *J Am Geriatr Soc, 41*, 395–465.

Perazella, M. A., & Eras, J. (2000). Are selective COX-2 inhibitors nephrotoxic? *American Journal of Kidney Diseases, 35*(5), 937–940.

Porter, F. L., Malhotra, K. M., Wolf, C. M., Morris, J. C., Miller, J. P., & Smith, M. C. (1996). Dementia and response to pain in the elderly. *Pain, 68*, 413–421.

Porter, J., & Jick, H. (1980). Addiction rare in patients treated with narcotics. *New England Journal of Medicine, 302*(2), 123.

Ransford, A. O., Cairns, D., & Mooney, V. (1976). The pain drawing as an aid to the psychologic evaluation of patients with low back pain. *Spine, 1*, 127–134.

Reginster, J. Y., Deroisy, R., Rovati, L. C., Lee, R. L., Lejeune, E., Bruyere, O., Giacovelli, G., Henrotin, Y., Dacre, J. E., & Gossett, C. (2001). Long-term effects of glucosamine sulphate on osteoarthritis progression: A randomised, placebo-controlled clinical trial. *Lancet, 357*, 251–256.

Roland, M., & Morris, R. (1983). A study of the natural history of back pain—part 1: Development of a reliable and sensitive measure of disability in low-back pain. *Spine, 8*, 141–144.

Rowbotham, M., Harden, N., Stacey, B., Bernstein, P., & Magnus-Miller, L. (1998). Gabapentin for the treatment of postherpetic neuralgia: A randomized controlled trial. *JAMA, 280*(21), 1837–1842.

Sengstaken, E. A., & King, S. A. (1993). The problems of pain and its detection among geriatric nursing home residents. *J Am Geriatr Soc, 41*, 541–544.

Shorr, R. I., Griffin, M. R., Daugherty, J. R., & Ray, W. A. (1992). Opioid analgesics and the risk of hip fracture in the elderly: Codeine and propoxyphene. *J Gerontol, 47*, M111–M115.

Stein, W. M., & Ferrell, B. A. (1996). Pain in the nursing home. *Clin Geriatr Med, 12*, 601–613.

Sternbach, R. A. (1986). Survey of pain in the United States: The Nuprin pain report. *Clinical Journal of Pain, 2*, 49–53.

Stuppy, D. J. (1998). The Faces of Pain Scale: Reliability and validity with mature adults. *Applied Nursing Research, 11*, 84–89.

Tait, R. C., Chibnall, J. T., & Margolis, R. B. (1990). Pain extent: Relations with psychological state, pain severity, pain history, and disability. *Pain, 41*, 295–301.

Texidor, M. (1998). The nonpharmacologic management of chronic pain via the interdisciplinary approach. In *Pain management. A practical guide for clinicians* (5th ed., pp. 123–135.) Boca Raton, FL: CRC Press LLC.

Towheed, T. E., Anastassiades, T. P., Shea, B., Houpt, J., Welch, V., & Hochberg, M. C. (2001). Glucosamine therapy for treating osteoarthritis (Cochrane Review). *Cochrane Database Syst Rev, 1*, CD002946.

van Tulder, M. W., Koes, B. W., & Bouter, L. M. (1997). Conservative treatment of acute and chronic nonspecific low back pain: A systematic review of randomized controlled trials of the most common interventions. *Spine, 22*(18), 2128–2156.

Viller, F., Guillemin, F., Briancon, S., Moum, T., Suurmeijer, T., & van den Heuvel, W. (1999). Compliance to drug teratment of patients with rheumatoid arthrits: A 3 year longitudinal study. *Journal of Rheumatology, 26*(10), 2114–2122.

Watson, C. P. N., & Babul, N. (1998). Oxycodone relieves neuropathic pain: A randomized trial in postherpetic neuralgia. *Neurology, 50,* 1837–1841.

Watson, C. P. N., Evans, R. J., Watt, V. R., et al. (1988). Postherpetic neuralgia: 208 cases. *Pain, 35,* 289–297.

Watson, C. P. N., & Loeser, J. D. (2001). Herpes zoster and postherpetic neuralgia. In J. D. Loeser (Ed.), *Bonica's management of pain* (3rd ed.), pp. 424–432. Philadelphia: Lippincott Williams & Wilkins.

Weiner, D., Hanlon, J. T., & Studenski, S. (1998). CNS drug-related falls liability in community dwelling elderly. *Gerontology, 44,* 217–221.

Weiner, D., Peterson, B., & Keefe, F. (1998). Evaluating persistent pain in long term care residents: What role for pain maps? *Pain, 76,* 249–257.

Weiner, D., Peterson, B., Ladd, K., McConnell, E., & Keefe, F. (1999). Pain in nursing home residents: An exploration of prevalence, staff perspectives, and practical aspects of measurement. *Clinical Journal of Pain, 15,* 92–101.

Weiner, D., Pieper, C., McConnell, E., Martinez, S., & Keefe, F. (1996). Pain measurement in elders with chronic low back pain: Traditional and alternative approaches. *Pain, 67,* 461–467.

Weiner, D. K. (1999). Assessing persistent pain in older adults: Practicalities and pitfalls. *Analgesia, 4,* 377–395.

Weiner, D. K., Distell, B., Studenski, S., Martinez, S., Lomasney, L., & Bongiorni, D. (1994). Does radiographic osteoarthritis correlate with flexibility of the lumbar spine? *Journal of the American Geriatrics Society, 42,* 257–263.

Weiner, D. K., Peterson, B. L., Logue, P., & Keefe, F. J. (1998). Predictors of pain self-report in nursing home residents. *Aging, 10,* 411–420.

Weiner, D. K., Rudy, T. E., & Gaur, S. (2001). Are all older adults with persistent pain created equal? Preliminary evidence for a multiaxial taxonomy. *Pain Research and Management, 6*(3), 133–141.

Weisberg, J. N., & Vaillancourt, P. D. (1999). Personality factors and disorders in chronic pain. *Seminars in Clinical Neuropsychiatry, 4,* 155–166.

Wolfe, F., Ross, K., Anderson, J., Russell, I. J., & Hebert, L. (1995). The prevalence and characteristics of fibromyalgia in the general population. *Arthritis and Rheumatism, 38,* 19–28.

Wolfe, F., Smythe, H. A., Yunus, M. B., Bennett, R. M., Bombardier, C., Goldenberg, D. L., Tugwell, P., Campbell, S. M., Abeles, M., & Clark, P. (1990). The American College of Rheumatology 1990 criteria for the classification of fibromyalgia— Report of the multicenter criteria committee. *Arthritis and Rheumatism, 33,* 160–172.

World Health Organization. (1996). *Cancer pain relief* (2nd ed.). Geneva, Switzerland: Author.

Wu, C. L., Marsh, A., & Dworkin, R. H. (2000). The role of sympathetic nerve blocks in herpes zoster and postherpetic neuralgia. *Pain, 87*(2), 121–129.

Wynne, C. F., Ling, S. M., & Remsburg, R. (2000). Comparison of pain assessment instruments in cognitively intact and cognitively impaired nursing home residents. *Geriatr Nurs, 21,* 20–23.

Psychosocial Issues and Cognitive-Behavioral Therapy: From Theory to Practice

3

Thomas E. Rudy, Raymond B. Hanlon, and Jennifer R. Markham

Pain is one of the most complex of human experiences. It has been the focus of philosophical speculation and scientific attention for centuries, yet it remains one of the most challenging problems for sufferers, health care providers, and society. Individuals experiencing persistent pain frequently engage in a continual pursuit of relief, which often is elusive and leads to feelings of anger, helplessness, demoralization, and an incalculable amount of emotional suffering. Health care providers frequently share similar feelings of frustration, as patients continue to report pain despite the health care provider's best efforts. At a societal level, pain is a major health problem that affects millions of people in the United States and costs society billions of dollars in health care and loss of productivity. Additionally, third-party insurance payers are confronted with escalating medical costs, disability payments, and frustration when pain patients remain disabled despite extensive treatment and rehabilitation efforts.

As described throughout this volume, the process of aging adds complexity to our understanding of persistent pain. Persistent pain in the older adult frequently is underdiagnosed and undertreated (see chapter 2). Additionally, certain neuropsychological functional limitations, particularly dementia, further complicate the evaluation and treatment of persistent pain in older adults (see chapter 10). Perhaps even less understood and appreciated in the older adult with persistent pain is the role played by psychosocial factors and the importance of evaluating and treating these factors as part of the pain management process. At present, treatment of persistent pain in the older adult appears to largely ignore psychosocial factors and related therapeutic approaches, but rather relies almost exclusively on pharmacological interventions. This reliance on pain medications is particularly disturbing, given the fact that older patients are more sensitive to pain medications and are also more susceptible to side effects and problems resulting from drug interactions (see chapters 2 and 6).

In this chapter we will (1) provide a description of conceptualizations of pain; (2) highlight some inadequacies of unidimensional models of pain, particularly of persistent pain; (3) discuss several multidimensional models of pain, with special emphasis on psychosocial factors and the cognitive-behavioral perspective; (4) review some of the supporting evidence for the cognitive-behavioral conceptualization, with special reference to older adults; (5) outline some of the cognitive-behavioral treatment assumptions and strategies; and (6) present several case studies that illustrate the application of cognitive-behavioral principles in the diagnosis and treatment of older adults with persistent pain. Due to space limitations, we will only be able to highlight these very complex topics and related issues.

EVIDENCE AND PRINCIPLES FOR PRACTICE

Before beginning our discussion of psychological and psychosocial factors relevant to understanding persistent pain, it is important to emphasize that understanding psychological and psychosocial aspects of the pain experience is *essential* to the diagnosis and treatment of *all* pain patients. All too frequently, an artificial and erroneous distinction is made between structural or physical influences related to patients' pain conditions and factors that are labeled as "psychological" or "psychosocial." It is important for the reader to recognize that "psychosocial factors" are far broader than "psychopathology." That is, understanding patients' attributions or beliefs about their condition (e.g., what patients think causes their pain and how to treat it), the role of the spouse or other family members as allies or barriers to rehabilitation efforts, and so forth, are crucial to successful diagnosis and treatment, regardless of patients' degree of physical pathology. Thus, the cognitive-behavioral model or perspective of persistent pain described below should not be confused with "psychogenic" or psychopathological conceptualizations, which we believe create an overly simplistic and unhelpful mind-body dualism.

Conceptualizations or Models of Pain

Historically, pain has been viewed by medical investigators and practitioners as primarily a sensory-physiological phenomenon. From this perspective, patients' reports of pain are believed to be associated directly with the extent of tissue damage or organ pathology. Advanced diagnostic imaging and laboratory procedures have been developed to evaluate the extent of tissue damage in the hope that locating the area and extent of the damage will explain patients' reports of pain and thereby suggest appropriate therapeutic intervention. Therapeutic interventions for patients with persistent pain derived from variations of the sensory-physiological model have led to the development of surgical procedures to ablate the pain pathways from the periphery to the central nervous system and the synthesis of potent analgesic agents to block the transmission of signals along these pathways.

Over the past two decades, there has been increasing dissatisfaction with the purely sensory view of pain. Clinicians have frequently noted that patients with ostensibly the same degree of tissue damage react very differently to identical therapeutic modalities and that patients with similar diagnoses and organic findings respond quite differently to their condition (Osterweis, Kleinman, & Mechanic, 1987). Moreover, despite rapid advances in neuroanatomy, physiology, and pharmacology, there continue to be a large number of patients and many pain syndromes for which no physical intervention consistently and permanently eliminates pain. Conversely, many individuals with extensive physical pathology are asymptomatic and report no pain.

The Psychogenic Model

The inability to identify specific organic pathology in many patients with persistent pain, continued reports of pain following correction of pathological conditions, and continued complaints of pain following the expected period of resolution of an injury has led to two very different psychologically oriented approaches to conceptualizing persistent pain patients: a psychogenic model and a behavioral model. The psychogenic model of persistent pain suggests that pain reports in the absence of objective medical data can be explained by personality characteristics of the patient or the presence of a psychiatric disorder.

Empirical attempts to identify patient subgroups based on personality characteristics or psychiatric diagnoses have evolved from the psychogenic perspective (Blumer & Heilbronn, 1982). Findings from these research efforts, along with the results of sensory-based assessment approaches, have led to a frequently used and often abused dichotomy: the cause of a patient's pain complaints is classified as either "organic" or if not, ipso facto, "psychogenic." That is, if a physical basis can be found for a patient's subjective pain reports, the pain is considered "real." However, if organic findings are absent or the patient's pain complaints appear to be disproportionate to the amount of tissue damage, the patient's pain is categorized as "functional" or "psychogenic." In the latter case, the basis for the patient's reports of pain is believed to be emotionally or motivationally, rather than physically, determined.

The organic-psychogenic distinction makes several unwarranted assumptions. First, it assumes that there are adequate means for reliably measuring the amount of pain experienced and that normative data are available for various pain syndromes against which to compare an individual's reports of pain to determine whether they are "excessive." However, as noted, it is recognized by many clinicians that people with very similar objective medical findings show diverse responses. Additionally, this dichotomy assumes that current medical and diagnostic procedures can identify *all* sources of pathology likely to cause the pain reported by the patient. However, the predictive power of medical examinations and diagnostic tests (their sensitivity and specificity) are generally low for patients with persistent pain (Haldeman, Shouka, & Robboy, 1988). For example, physical examination, laboratory tests, and imaging procedures can be expected to lead to a definitive diagnosis in only 5–10% of patients with persistent low back pain (PLBP) (White & Gordon, 1982). Does this mean that 90–95% of back pain patients have psychogenic pain? This dichotomy further assumes that there are no individual differences other than psychopathological ones that influence pain perceptions (e.g., differences in sensory sensitivity). There appear to be well-documented and considerable individual differences in older adults with respect to sensory processes and pain perception (see chapter 1). Finally, the organic-psychogenic dichotomy makes the implicit assumption that a psychiatric problem and a pain disorder cannot co-occur in the same individual, or that a psychiatric problem cannot result from a chronic physical disorder.

The Operant Behavioral Model

Behavioral psychologists have emphasized that pain is a subjective phenomenon and, consequently, all that can be observed are behaviors emitted in response to the subjective experience of pain. Thus, behavioral manifestations are viewed as the means by which patients communicate pain and suffering and, especially in the case of persistent pain, it is these behaviors that should be assessed and treated, rather than pain per se. In other words, behavioral models of pain distinguish nociception, pain, suffering, and pain behavior. The first three are viewed as the "private" experience of pain, whereas the latter is directly observable, quantifiable, and capable of eliciting responses that serve to perpetuate pain behaviors even in the absence of nociception.

According to Fordyce (1976), behavioral operationalizations of pain—"pain behaviors"—include (a) verbal complaints of pain and suffering, (b) nonlanguage sounds (e.g., moans, sighs), (c) body posturing and gesturing (e.g., limping, rubbing a painful body part or area), and (d) displays of functional limitations or disability (e.g., reclining for excessive periods of time). It has been suggested that pain behaviors may provide a more objective means of assessing responses inferred to be pain-related than patients' self-reports, which may be biased or purposely distorted. Thus, subjective self-reports are suspect. Also, from an operant theory of behavior, if pain is considered to be composed of observable behaviors, then we can think of the production and maintenance of those behaviors as being under environmental control through selective contingencies of reinforcement.

To illustrate the consequence of environmental factors on reports of pain: significant others in the patient's environment, whether family, friends, or health care providers, respond to the patient's overt behavior. They may reinforce these behavioral manifestations by providing attention or permitting the patient to avoid the performance of undesirable functions (e.g., physical activities), and thereby unwittingly contribute to the maintenance of these behaviors. Additionally, financial subsidies from such systems as workers' compensation and disability payers may positively reinforce the expression of pain behaviors and dysfunctional conduct in response to pain. Thus, although secondary gain factors may be involved in some patients, it is important for the reader to recognize that behavioral conceptualizations of pain are far more comprehensive than simply understanding behaviors that may reflect secondary gain.

The operant behavioral approach to pain becomes particularly relevant for pain that extends over long periods of time. At an acute level, behavioral responses to injury and nociceptive stimulation may be appropriate in that they serve protective functions. However, when pain behaviors persist over extended periods of time they can become problems in their own right. The behavioral responses of inactivity, limping, guarding, bracing, and so forth, for a patient with PLBP leads to altered body mechanics and generalized deconditioning (e.g., reduction in muscle strength, mass, and flexibility; easy fatiguability). Additionally, continuation of pain behaviors can lead to the reduction of previously enjoyed activities and the increase of psychological distress (e.g., depressed mood). In essence, a vicious cycle may be initiated and perpetuated by the unwitting reinforcement of pain behaviors.

Although pain behaviors are important to consider, it is equally important to acknowledge that, like physical pathology, they are unidimensional (Turk & Flor, 1987). Pain behaviors should be viewed within the broader context that also includes cognitive, affective, psychosocial, and other behavioral factors (e.g., activities of daily living), as well as physiological factors, all of which contribute to the experience of pain.

The Gate Control Model

A dramatic shift from pain as a purely sensory phenomenon to pain as a perceptual event was given its greatest impetus in the mid-1960s by Melzack and his colleagues (Melzack & Casey, 1968; Melzack & Wall, 1965). They proposed a new conceptual model of pain, the gate control model, designed to deal with the inconsistencies manifested by different sensory models of pain and to incorporate clinical experience.

According to this model, pain is not solely an automatic sensory phenomenon, but a highly personal, variable experience influenced by cultural learning, the meaning of the situation, attention, and other cognitive activities. The gate control model proposed that besides the traditionally recognized dimension of nociception (the sensory-discriminative component of the gate control model), there also existed motivational-affective and cognitive-evaluative components. In other words, Melzack and colleagues postulated that the perception of pain was the result of the simultaneous integration of motivational-affective, cognitive-evaluative, and sensory-discriminative factors.

This view of pain differed greatly from traditional sensory views which, when they considered psychological factors at all, relegated them to reactions to pain and, consequently, nuisance variables or at best epiphenomena. The gate control model did not give priority to sensory input nor did it treat the sensory input as isomorphic with pain. Rather, pain was postulated to be the result of the integration and interpretation of sensory and psychological processes, and therefore qualified as a perceptual process.

The gate control model also claimed that there were important physiological pathways that are capable of augmenting or diminishing the subjective experience of pain. In addition to afferent pathways, some of the proposed pathways involved "top down" processing, that is, the neurophysiological influence of emotions and cognitive phenomena presumably travel down the spinal cord from the brain and can modulate sensory information traveling up the spinal cord toward the brain. Thus, the notion of a "gating" type action in the dorsal horn was proposed.

Although the gate control model has not been without its critics, particularly regarding the physical basis of the proposed gating mechanism (Nathan, 1976), it has been hailed as a resilient theory of pain with reasonable explanatory and heuristic value. Because it attributes the perception of pain to more than simply sensory stimulation, the gate control model provides some explanations as to why the surgical, electrical, or neurolytic ablation of pain pathways has not always been effective in eliminating pain. A natural consequence of the gate control model is that successful treatment of persistent pain patients will require attention to all three components of the pain experience—sensory-discriminative, motivational-affective, and cognitive-evaluative.

The Cognitive-Behavioral (C-B) Model

Although both the operant behavioral and gate control models depart significantly from sensory models of pain, each has a somewhat limited view and is inadequate to explain persistent pain by itself. The operant behavioral model fails to consider the contribution of cognitive appraisals of the patients as they influence patients' perceptions and responses to their physical problems. As pain persists, the gate control model does not consider the interaction of environmental influences, physical factors, and pain perceptions as they extend over prolonged periods of time.

An alternate model that emphasizes both the importance of environmental factors underscored by the operant approach and the psychological contributions inherent in the gate control model has been formulated by Turk and his colleagues (Turk, Meichenbaum, & Genest, 1983; Turk & Rudy, 1989), and labeled a C-B perspective on pain. A comprehensive intervention model based on the C-B conceptualization has been developed and used with a diversity of pain syndromes, for example, headaches (Holroyd, Nash, Pingel, Cordingley, & Jerome, 1991), temporomandibular pain disorders (Turk, Rudy, Kubinski, Zaki, & Greco, 1996), arthritis (Keefe et al., 1990), back pain (Hazard, Benedix, & Genwich, 1991), cancer-related pain (Fishman, 1992), and heterogeneous pain syndromes (Nicholas, 1992). Moreover, this approach has been applied to children (Richter et al., 1986), adolescents (Lascelles, Cunningham, McGrath, & Sullivan, 1989), and older adult pain populations (Puder, 1988; Sorkin, Rudy, Hanlon, Turk, & Stieg, 1990).

Like the gate control model, the C-B perspective of pain is multidimensional in that it makes an important distinction between nociception, that is, activation of sensory transduction in the nerves that convey information about tissue damage capable of being experienced as pain, and *pain* per se. The C-B perspective places strong emphasis on the longitudinal impact of cognitive factors as they affect perception and behavioral responses to nociception (Turk et al., 1983; Turk & Rudy, 1994). It is hypothesized that people who experience persistent or recurrent nociception develop negative expectations about their ability to perform physical activities without pain, adopt a negative cognitive set about pain and how pain will affect their lives, and appraise their situation as one in which there is little they can do to cope with the nociception.

Another central tenet of the C-B perspective is that patients' interpretations of nociception, their coping resources, and their situation and condition in general can have both direct and indirect effects on both physiological and psychological processes that may maintain and exacerbate pain. It is important to recognize that people not only respond to available stimuli and observe the consequences of their behavior, but also actively select from the information present and transform and categorize stimuli in idiosyncratic fashions, thereby partially determining some of the stimuli that impinge upon them. Additionally, patients may have belief systems, some of which may be irrational, that determine or guide their responses to their condition. For example, patients may believe that they "should" be able to do tasks at preinjury levels or that they "must" try to engage in a strenuous task out of bravado, guilt, desperation, or because they believe that they are "cured." In these cases, patients will engage in a cycle of overactivity and flare-up, followed by pain and inactivity. Finally, cognitive processes may have a direct effect on physiological parameters associated with pain perception, such as autonomic nervous system activation (Flor, Turk, & Birbaumer, 1985) and facilitation of the production of enkephalins (Bandura, O'Leary, Taylor, Gauthier, & Gossard, 1987).

The C-B perspective also recognizes that cognitive processes reciprocally determine and redefine perception and patients' reports of unremitting pain. Because the experience of pain, and subsequently the fear of pain, is aversive, patients' expectations of the occurrence of pain in and of themselves become strong motivators for avoidance of situations or behaviors that are *expected* to produce nociception. Moreover, the belief that pain signals harm further reinforces avoidance of activities believed to cause pain and increase physical damage. The persistence of avoidance will reduce physical activity and, consequently, the opportunities for experiencing disconfirmations. Moreover, avoidance of activity will contribute to further physical deconditioning, including reduction of muscle strength and flexibility.

To summarize, the C-B model adopts a broad perspective on pain that focuses on the patient and not just the symptom. That is, persistent pain, like any chronic disease, extends over time and affects all domains of the patient's life. Rather than focusing on cognitive and affective contributions to the perception of pain in a static fashion, as in the gate control model, or exclusively on behavioral responses and environmental reinforcement contingencies and physical pathology, the C-B model entails a transactional view that emphasizes the ongoing reciprocal relationships among physical, cognitive, affective, and behavioral factors.

Research Support for the Cognitive-Behavioral Perspective of Persistent Pain

An increasing body of literature has emerged that supports many of the assumptions of the C-B formulation of the pain experience. Space limitations do not permit a comprehensive review of this literature. However, we will present illustrative research that demonstrates the important contribution of C-B factors in the maintenance and exacerbation of recurrent and persistent pain problems and in the facilitation of disability, particularly in older adults.

The Contribution of Cognitive Factors

A number of studies have been conducted to examine the contribution of the cognitive components of the pain experience (Turk & Rudy, 1992). These studies have focused on acute and laboratory pain research models, as well as the role of maladaptive cognitions in clinical pain. For example, Flor and Turk (1989) examined the association between general and situation-specific pain-related thoughts, convictions of personal control, pain severity, and disability levels in persistent low back pain (PLBP) patients and those with rheumatoid arthritis. The general and situation-specific cognitive variables were more highly related to reports of pain and disability than were disease-related variables for both samples. Moreover, these cognitive variables explained a significantly greater proportion of the variance in treatment outcome than did demographic or medical status variables.

Coping

Many of the variables that influence pain and disability fall under the construct of coping, and many models of pain and illness give coping responses an important, if not central, role in understanding and predicting adjustment to pain and illness (Turk et al., 1983). Jensen, Turner, Romano, and Karoly (1991), in their review of the coping literature, concluded that (1) the use of coping strategies categorized as "active" (e.g., exercise, ignoring pain) may be associated with better psychological and physical functioning, whereas the use of passive coping strategies (e.g., withdrawal, medication use) predicts poorer performance; (2) the coping strategy of wishful thinking is associated with lower levels of positive affect and physical performance; and (3) although other coping strategies may play an important role in adjustment to persistent pain, the limited number of studies and the paucity of true experimental designs make it difficult to draw specific conclusions regarding their relative importance.

A great deal of recent research confirms a consistent association between catastrophizing responses and adjustment to persistent pain. Catastrophizing has been found to be associated with higher levels of psychological distress (Geisser, Robinson, Keefe, & Weiner, 1994), higher rates of analgesic use (Jacobsen & Butler, 1996), poorer physical performance and disability (Hill, Niven, & Knussen, 1995; Robinson et al., 1997), higher ratings of pain intensity (Geisser et al., 1994; Hill et al., 1995), more reports of pain interference in daily activities (Geisser et al., 1994; Robinson et al., 1997), lower levels of general activity (Robinson et al., 1997), and higher rates of psychosocial dysfunction (Hill et al., 1995). The majority of these studies, however, have not addressed the role of coping in older adults with persistent pain.

How people cope specifically with nociception also may have an indirect effect on pain through the influence on mood and behavior as well as a direct effect on nociception through the influence on the autonomic nervous system and the production and inhibition of select neurotransmitters. In a comprehensive meta-analysis of 46 laboratory studies, Fernandez and Turk (1989) concluded that cognitive strategies do appear to have a major influence on pain perception or subjects' response to noxious stimulation. They further concluded that the effects of cognitive coping strategies are significantly greater than those effects displayed by placebo and expectancy control groups. In fact, subjects trained to use one or more cognitive strategies were able to tolerate higher levels of noxious stimulation than 80% of subjects not provided with specific coping strategies. Several studies with clinical samples have demonstrated the important role of coping strategies in the maintenance of pain disability and response to treatment (Jensen, Turner, & Romano, 1991; Ressor & Craig, 1988).

Self-Efficacy

A central construct in the C-B model of persistent pain is self-efficacy. Self-efficacy refers to personal judgments of performance capabilities in a given activity domain (Bandura, 1977). An individual's self-efficacy beliefs may determine whether a specific behavior is initiated, how much effort will be expended, and how long that effort will be sustained in the face of obstacles and aversive experiences, such as pain sensations. In younger patients with PLBP, self-efficacy expectancies have been found to correlate significantly with posttreatment pain ratings, tolerance for physical activities, performance on isokinetic endurance tasks, use of pain medication, and work status (Dolce, 1987; Dolce, Cracker, Moletteire, & Doleys, 1986; Kores, Murphy, Rosenthal, Elias, & North, 1990; O'Leary, Shoor, Lorig, & Holman, 1988). The overall impact of self-efficacy on physical performance is particularly notable in older adults. Recent research into the field of self-efficacy and aging indicates that older adults tend to have lower self-efficacy and physical performance than younger adults resulting from their minimizing their abilities (Clark, 1996; Grembowski et al., 1993; Woodard & Wallston, 1987). Davis-Berman (1990) also found that reduced self-efficacy for physical activities was a strong predictor of depressive symptoms in older adults.

Depression

Clinical depression frequently is seen in individuals with persistent pain conditions. The presence of depression not only adversely affects an individual's ability to cope with pain problems, but also negatively affects physical and social functioning and overall reported quality of life. It has been shown that depression is a major, independent contributor to disability (Parker & Wright, 1995) and that the presence of even minor depression is associated with significant functional disability in younger adults (Jaffe, Froom, & Galambos, 1994).

The association between disability and depression also has undergone considerable investigation in older adults. Rozzini et. al. (1997) conducted a study of 549 community dwellers and found that a reported loss of basic and instrumental ADL functions was associated with cognitive decline and depression. However, no association was found between the psychosocial measures and physical performance measures. Conversely, Pennix and colleagues (Pennix et al., 1998) administered the Center for Epidemiologic Studies Depression Scale (CESD) and three performance measures to 1,286 persons >70 years of age twice in a 4-year period and found increasing levels of depression were predictive of a greater decline in physical performance. In a recent study by Kempen and Ormel (1998), motor impairments (measured by performance tasks) and depressive symptoms were found to act independently of one another as main effects on self-reported disability. The degree of impact of depression on self-reported disability also was found to be significant by Kivinen, Sulkava, Halonen, & Nissinen, (1998) and Cho et al. (1998). However, the degree of correlation between depression and disability has been somewhat dependent upon the measurement instruments, and previous studies have not addressed the role of persistent pain in the association between depression and physical functioning.

Fear-induced avoidance of activities

This problem has also received increased attention and is a central construct in C-B models of pain (Rudy & Turk, 1991). Several investigations have evaluated the role that the fear of pain plays in pain-related avoidance of activity and subsequent disability. These investigations have resulted in a variety of cognitively based models. Phillips (1987) theorizes that avoidance is determined by a desire to minimize discomfort and pain, plus thoughts and beliefs that reexposure to certain situations will produce both pain and suffering. More specific in theory are the Fear Avoidance Model of Exaggerated Pain Perception (Slade, Troup, Lethem, & Bentley, 1983) and the recent studies conducted by Vlaeyen, Kole-Snijders, Boeren, & van Eek (1995) that have examined the relationship between fear of movement and (re)injury in PLBP patients. The study by Klenerman and colleagues (1995) of 300 patients with acute low back pain suggests that fear-avoidance variables were the most successful in predicting outcome. Similar observations were made by Keen et al. (1999), who found that fear of pain and avoidance of physical activity were two main factors associated with changes in activity level. To date, however, studies of fear in the older adult population have largely been focused on fear of falling and the associated inactivity (Bhala, O'Donnell, & Thoppil, 1982; Murphy & Isaacs, 1982). To our knowledge, no controlled studies have investigated the fear of pain and its association with physical functioning and related disability in older adult persistent pain sufferers.

Physical Effects of Cognitive Factors

Evidence for the importance of the direct effect of cognitive factors on physical parameters in persistent pain is apparent in several psychophysiological experiments. For example, Flor, Turk, and Birbaumer (1985) examined the association of paraspinal lumbar EMG reactivity of PLBP patients, non-LBP patients, and healthy controls. All subjects participated in a psychophysiological assessment that included four counterbalanced trials (discussion of personal stress, discussion of pain, performance of mental arithmetic, and a control condition [reciting of the alphabet]). Bilateral paraspinal and frontalis EMG, heart rate, and skin conductance levels were recorded continuously. The results indicated that LBP patients displayed elevations and delayed recovery *only* in their paravertebral musculature and *only* when discussing personally relevant stress (the pain and stress trials). Neither of the other two groups displayed paravertebral hyperreactivity or delayed recovery. The extent of abnormal muscular reactivity was best predicted by depression and cognitive coping style, rather than pain demographic variables (e.g., number of surgeries, duration of pain).

In sum, the results of these illustrative studies of self-efficacy, cognitive coping strategies, depression, fear-induced avoidance, and psychophysiology underscore the important role of cognitive factors in disability maintenance of persistent pain and response to treatment. Moreover, these studies demonstrate that these cognitive factors may affect patients' reports of pain and use of the health care system, as well as directly affect physiological parameters believed to be associated with nociception.

Cognitive-Behavioral Treatment for Persistent Pain

Overview

To understand the C-B approach to the treatment of persistent pain patients it is important to understand that the techniques actually used are viewed as significantly less important than the more general philosophy and orientation. By the time patients are referred for treatment of their persistent pain, they usually have received multiple evaluations and a range of common medical treatment modalities. A shared feature across all patients, regardless of diagnosis, is that an array of interventions has failed to adequately alleviate their suffering. Thus, it is not surprising that by the time these patients are seen by a pain specialist they are quite demoralized, feel frustrated, believe their situation is hopeless, and yet still seek *the* cure for their suffering.

The general goal of a C-B pain treatment program is to assist patients to reconceptualize their view of their situation and their pain. Patients frequently view pain as an all-encompassing, entirely medical problem over which they have little or no control. The C-B approach emphasizes both the effectiveness of the rehabilitation approach and the *patient's ability* to alleviate much of his or her pain and suffering, provided he or she is willing to work as an *active member* of the treatment team. In other words, the C-B treatment approach relies heavily on active patient participation and emphasizes a mutual problem-solving approach among the treatment team, the patient, and the significant others in the patient's environment.

Evaluation

Before embarking on specific C-B intervention techniques, it is critical for the therapist (a licensed psychologist or social worker trained in C-B techniques) who will be implementing these techniques to conduct a detailed evaluation. During an evaluation interview, it is important to enter the patient's perspective (Table 3.1). Regardless of whether an organic basis for the pain can be documented or whether psychosocial problems preceded or resulted from the pain, the evaluation process can be helpful in identifying how biomedical, psychological, and social factors interact to influence the nature, severity, and persistence of pain and disability. From a C-B perspective, emotional distress, depression, beliefs about the etiology of the pain, and social reinforcement of pain behaviors all need to be addressed. These and other factors to target during the assessment process are outlined in Table 3.2.

To summarize, the primary purposes of the cognitive-behavioral evaluation are to (1) determine specific psychological and behavioral contributors to pain behaviors, impairment in functioning, and suffering; (2) determine appropriate treatment targets and intervention strategies; and (3) provide pertinent information to the treatment team about aspects of a patient's psychosocial history and current situation that may have a bearing on responses to persistent pain.

Interdisciplinary Team

We believe the most effective approach to treating persistent pain patients is in the context of an interdisciplinary team. The core of the team is composed of representatives from a variety of health care disciplines, including medicine, nursing, psychology, physical therapy, and occupational therapy. The specialty of the physician member of the team is less important than the commitment and dedication to working with pain patients.

TABLE 3.1 Entering the Patient's Perspective

- Why do you think your pain started when it did?

- What do you think is wrong with you?

- What do you think is happening to your body?

- What do you think of the reasons or explanations for your pain that were given to you by the other health care professionals you have consulted?

- Do you understand the reasons or explanations for your pain others have given you?

- Do you have any fears or worries about your pain?

- What are the main problems that your pain has caused you?

- What do your family and friends think about your pain?

- How do you think your pain problem should be treated?

- What do you hope happens as a result of treatment?

- If your pain isn't entirely relieved by the treatment, what will you do?

TABLE 3.2 Content Areas Covered in Cognitive-Behavioral Evaluation Interviews

- Secondary problems that have arisen because of persistent pain (e.g., familial, financial)
- Situational fluctuation of pain intensity, duration, and/or frequency
- How the patient expresses pain
- How others respond to the patient's complaints of pain and disability
- Behavioral manifestations of pain—pain behaviors (e.g., moaning, distorted ambulation or posture)
- What effect the patient believes the pain is having on others
- Whether the patient derives any benefits or secondary gains from having pain
- How the patient thinks about the pain and associated problems
- Pattern of medication use and substance abuse (current and previous)
- Current mood, evidence of affective distress, sleep and appetite disturbances
- What the patient has tried to do to alleviate pain
- When appropriate, patient's work history (frequency of changes, satisfaction, does the patient have a job to which he or she can/ plans to return)
- Patient's expectancies from health care professionals and treatment
- Patient's views of previous health care professionals and treatments
- Prior history of pain problems of patient or family members
- Prior and current stressful life events
- Family (marital) relations (current and past)

Additionally, we believe that it is essential for the treatment team to share a common philosophy so that patients are treated consistently regardless of the disciplines or techniques used by the various team members.

Although the therapeutic team is often conceptualized as composed of professional members only, we believe that the team definition needs to be extended to include the patient and significant others as well, who need to be alerted to their important collaborative roles as part of the treatment team. Too often the treatment team forgets about the importance of the family. However, persistent pain, by virtue of extending over long periods of time, impacts on all aspects of the patient's life, including family life. Failure to include family members is likely to contribute to the problems of maintenance and generalization of treatment gains. At a minimum, families need to be aware of the nature and logic of the treatment goals and modalities used. Some families may require additional involvement or family counseling if there is to be any hope for treatment success.

Essential Components of Cognitive-Behavioral Treatment

Following assessment, which should be an ongoing process throughout treatment, we believe that treatment should be composed of at least four interrelated components: (1) education, (2) skills acquisition, (3) cognitive and behavioral rehearsal, and (4) generalization and maintenance. Due to space limitations, we will provide only a brief overview of each of these components; see Turk & Rudy (1994) for more complete descriptions.

Education

Presentation of the C-B perspective on pain and its control (e.g., the role of thoughts, feelings, behavior, environment, and physical factors) should begin at the outset of treatment and continue throughout. C-B concepts need to be presented in a simple, direct way with numerous examples that are customized to the specific patient and in a vocabulary that he or she can understand. We believe that when exploring with patients the C-B factors that may be associated with their pain condition, a collaborative rather than a didactic approach is more effective. It is important to avoid the more traditional directive medical approach used in many settings, and communicate with patients in a manner that encourages them to begin to assume equal responsibility for their treatment. The approach is designed to be authoritative without being authoritarian.

The educational component of treatment also needs to address the unspoken fears that many patients have about their condition (e.g., fear of reinjury if they engage in certain exercises, fear that their condition is progressive, fear that health care providers do not believe their pain is real, etc.). This effort must be interdisciplinary in nature and needs to include a review and lay-oriented discussion of the evaluation findings of the treatment team that incorporates biomedical, psychosocial, and behavioral results. During this process, it is important for the team, professional as well as patient, to identify patients' idiosyncratic beliefs and inaccurate understanding of the information presented. This information then can be used to begin the process of reconceptualization.

Skills Acquisition

Cognitive and behavioral treatment techniques consist of a range of modalities and procedures that are designed to bring alterations in patients' perceptions of their situation and thus their ability to monitor and modify cognitions and behavior. A number of papers and texts have described these techniques in detail and the interested reader should consult them (see Gatchel & Turk, 1996; Holzman & Turk, 1986). We will only briefly highlight some of the most commonly used techniques. To restate, we believe that the mastery of the technical aspects of these techniques is less important than the manner in which they are presented and taught to patients. These techniques need to be individualized to the specific patient and described and taught in a way that increases the patient's perceptions of self-control and intrinsic motivation. Toward this goal, we prefer inclusion of techniques or skills that can be broadly categorized as self-management (e.g., stress management, coping skills training, problem solving).

Two general skill sets have been found to be helpful in the psychological management of persistent pain in older adults. The first set is relaxation and biofeedback techniques, which teach patients a variety of relaxation methods, including diaphragmatic breathing, progressive muscle relaxation, visualization, autogenic suggestion, and mental distraction techniques. We find that exposure to a variety of available techniques allows patients to identify the specific combinations of procedures that they find personally useful and enjoyable. The rationale for these techniques is discussed with patients, with particular emphasis on their ability to modify undesirable physiological experience, decrease tension and distress, increase a sense of personal control, and temporarily provide distraction from nociception. Each technique is then demonstrated and practiced in vivo, with guidance and training from the therapist. Finally, a concrete practice strategy is mutually agreed upon to be systematically carried through via homework assignment and monitoring in follow-up sessions.

Generally, biofeedback-assisted relaxation in not routinely used in our clinic, but is reserved for patients who have particular difficulty with awareness of physiological sensations that are the focus of relaxation efforts (e.g., breathing, muscle relaxation, and mental focus). Difficulty with awareness of such processes often can be overcome with the application of electronic biofeedback technology, which can provide immediate information to the patient via sensor recording and monitoring of muscle tension or thermal physiological responses. These responses are interpreted and fed back via the biofeedback instrument, with both visual and auditory cues. Thus, patients can observe, assimilate, and then modify their physiological responses. We find that most older adults can easily be guided to be aware of such physiological processes so that relaxation techniques can be mastered without the use of biofeedback technology, which can be both cumbersome and time-consuming to apply.

The second basic set of skills is cognitive modification. The objective of cognitive modification interventions is to help patients sort through their accumulated perceptions (thoughts) associated with all aspects of their pain experience in order to identify those that are distorted, maladaptive, and thus counterproductive to effective coping, and to reinforce those that are helpful or constructive. First, an appropriate foundation of information is provided on the rationale of cognitive intervention for persistent pain, emphasizing and demonstrating the relationships among perception, cognitions, emotions, behavior, nociception, and the experience of pain. Second, discussion that explores patients' cognitions about all aspects of their pain response is used, so that thoughts, emotions, and behaviors to be modified can be identified in a manner consistent with factual information and realistic responses to the pain condition. Finally, patients are taught a self-directed systematic paper-and-pencil procedure to identify and modify targeted thoughts, emotions, and behaviors in order to decrease distress and improve adaptive coping. These procedures are rehearsed through homework assignments and reviewed in follow-up sessions until the patient establishes confidence in self-directed use of these techniques.

Cognitive and Behavioral Rehearsal

Teaching patients strategies and techniques to manage their pain and increase their level of functioning is of little value if they do not learn to apply them regularly in their home environments. The rehearsal component of C-B treatment emphasizes the importance of practicing and consolidating the skills that patients learn during the skills acquisition phase. Rehearsal techniques can include mental practice, role playing, and role reversal. We find role reversal particularly effective in evaluating what the patient has learned. This technique simply involves the patient and therapist switching roles, with the patient "teaching" skills to the therapist, who assumes the role of a new patient. Specific details of these rehearsals are described in Holzman and Turk (1986).

Homework

A closely related component of rehearsal is the assignment of specific homework tasks to patients so that they can practice skills learned during treatment sessions and report their results at the next session. We believe that the inclusion of significant others, whenever possible, can help to increase the effectiveness and the information obtained from homework assignments. Homework assignments should be geared toward observable and manageable tasks, that is, tasks that are readily achievable, and then progress to more difficult ones. Additionally, the goals and homework assignments should be customized to the particular condition, lifestyle, and unique assessment findings of each patient. Turk et al. (1983) have described the general purposes of homework tasks between treatment sessions, and these are outlined in Table 3.3.

TABLE 3.3 Purposes of Homework Assignments

- To assess various areas of the patient's and significant others' lives and how these influence and are affected by the pain problem

- To assess the typical responses of significant others and the patient to pain and pain behaviors

- To make the patient and significant others more aware of the factors that exacerbate and alleviate suffering

- To help the patient and significant others identify maladaptive responses to pain and pain behaviors

- To consolidate the use of coping procedures and physical exercises discussed during therapy sessions

- To increase physical activity levels

- To illustrate to the patient and significant others that progress can be made in living with pain but with less suffering

- To serve as reinforcers and as enhancers of self-efficacy as the patient achieves his or her goals

- To assist the therapeutic team, including the patient and significant others, in evaluating progress and in modifying goals and treatment strategies

---

Generalization and Maintenance

Despite our best efforts and strategies, relapse remains a significant problem in persistent pain treatment (Turk & Rudy, 1991). To maximize the likelihood of maintenance and generalization of treatment gains, C-B therapists focus upon the cognitive activity of patients as they are confronted with problems throughout treatment (e.g., failure to achieve specified goals, plateaus in progress on physical exercises, recurrent stresses). These events are used as opportunities to assist patients to learn how to handle such inevitable setbacks and lapses that will occur once treatment is terminated. Rehabilitation is often not a cure.

In the final stage of treatment, discussion focuses on possible ways of predicting and avoiding or dealing with pain and pain-related problems following termination. We have found it helpful to assist patients to anticipate future problems, stress, and pain-exacerbating events and to plan coping and response techniques before these problems occur. It is important to note that all possible problematic circumstances cannot be anticipated. Rather the goal during this phase, as it is for the entire treatment strategy, is to enable patients to develop a problem-solving perspective where they believe that they have the skills and competencies within their repertoires to respond in an appropriate way to problems as they arise. Attempts are made to help patients learn to anticipate future difficulties, develop plans for adaptive responding, and adjust their behavior accordingly.

The generalization and maintenance phase serves at least two purposes: (1) it encourages the patient to anticipate and plan for the posttreatment period when symptoms are greatly improved but not totally removed; and (2) it focuses on the necessary conditions for long-term success. More specifically, this phase gives the patient the understanding that minor setbacks are to be expected, but that they do not signal total failure. Rather, these setbacks should be viewed as cues to use the coping skills at which they have become proficient. It is important for the patient not to think of his or her responsibility as ending at termination of treatment, but as entering a different phase of maintenance. Emphasis is placed upon the importance of adherence to recommendations on an ongoing basis.

Research Support for Cognitive-Behavioral Treatment of Older Adults with Persistent Pain

Considerable evidence exists in the literature for the efficacy of C-B treatment for younger persistent pain patients with numerous persistent pain conditions. As noted earlier in this chapter, it is disconcerting that treatment of the older adult with persistent pain has relied rather exclusively on pharmacological treatments, when nonpharmacological interventions such as C-B treatment may have some distinct advantages, particularly for those patients with adverse drug reactions, or those for whom drugs do not yield acceptable pain relief. Although considerably more research is needed, fortunately it appears that when older patients are offered C-B type therapies, they are as likely as younger patients to accept and to benefit from these types of treatments (Sorkin et al., 1990).

A number of studies have used prospective experimental designs to evaluate the effectiveness of C-B therapies in relatively homogeneous groups of older pain patients, particularly those with osteoarthritis. Keefe et al. (1990) evaluated pain-coping skills treatment strategies for older patients with persistent pain resulting from osteoarthritis of the knee. Subjects had a mean age of 64 years and were randomized to one of three treatment conditions: (1) a pain-coping skills training group, (2) an arthritis education control group, and (3) a treatment control condition that only received routine medical care. Following 10 weekly sessions, the pain-coping skills group had significantly less pain and less psychological disability, but not less physical disability, than the other two groups. A study by Fry and Wong (1991) also supports the effectiveness of coping skills training for reducing pain and emotional distress in homebound older adults (aged 63–82) with persistent knee pain. It is not surprising that C-B interventions that used coping skills training were as effective with older as they are with younger adults, based on the findings by Keefe and Williams (1990). Keefe and Williams compared four age groups, including an older adults group with a mean age of 72 years, on the Coping Skills Questionnaire (Rosenstiel & Keefe, 1983), which measures the use and the perceived effectiveness of common cognitive and behavioral strategies for coping with pain. All subjects had persistent nonmalignant pain, primarily cervical, low back, and headache. No significant age differences were found, and the authors concluded that individuals who are coping with a similar life event adopt similar coping strategies, regardless of age.

The literature on the effectiveness of biofeedback and other physiological self-regulation therapies in older pain patients also provides important insights into the treatment of the older adult. For example, a number of studies have examined treatment outcomes in headache patients aged 60 years or older. Arena and colleagues found clinical improvements (a 50% reduction in headache activity) in 70% of 18 tension headache patients aged 62–80 years who were treated with progressive muscle relaxation procedures (Arena, Hightower, & Chang, 1988) or frontal EMG biofeedback procedures (Arena, Hannah, Bruno, & Meador, 1991). Similar to other C-B treatment approaches, an educational component and a homework component were included in both studies, and special techniques were used to ensure that these older patients heard and understood the treatment rationale and instructions (e.g., talking slowly, simplifying instructions, avoiding jargon).

In two studies by Middaugh and colleagues (Middaugh, Kee, Peters, & Herman, 1992; Middaugh, Woods, Kee, Harden, & Peters, 1991), the performances of older (55–78 years of age) and younger (29–48 years of age) patients with persistent, nonmalignant pain were compared. All patients were taught biofeedback and other physiological self-regulations skills as part of an interdisciplinary persistent-pain rehabilitation program (PPRP). The majority of patients (70%) were diagnosed with musculoskeletal problems, primarily cervical and low back disorders. In both studies, older pain patients were found to be able to learn the physiological self-regulation skills as taught in the biofeedback protocol. Both age groups displayed significant and similar increases in digital skin temperature and decreases in respiration rate. Both age groups also showed similar improvements on measure of muscle control, and older patients achieved significant reductions in pain severity ratings that equaled or exceeded those of younger patients.

A number of studies from interdisciplinary PPRPs also demonstrate that older adults receive good benefits when offered these programs. For example, Sorkin et al. (1990) compared older and younger pain patients referred to their interdisciplinary PPRP on pretreatment physical and psychological variables, as well as on rates of treatment admission and treatment completion. Neuropathic pain was the most frequent diagnosis in the older group (35%), and myofascial pain was most frequent (42%) for younger patients. Older and younger patients were very similar in the proportion who were offered interdisciplinary treatment, the proportion who accepted treatment, and the number who completed treatment. Although the older group had a significantly higher rate of abnormal physical findings on medical examinations, particularly for neurological symptoms, no age-related differences were found on psychological examination. Sorkin et al. used the Multidimensional Pain Inventory (Kerns, Turk, & Rudy, 1985) and found no significant age-related differences for self-reported measures of pain severity, emotional distress, disability attributed to pain, and general activity levels. This study provides important evidence that older pain patients will accept and complete an interdisciplinary PPRP as often as younger pain patients, *when this treatment is offered.*

Other studies conducted with older patients in a PPRP setting that report treatment outcome data include those by Cutler, Fishbain, Steel-Rosomoff, and Rosomoff (1994) and Middaugh, Levin, Kee, Barchiese, and Roberts (1988). Both of these studies included comprehensive rehabilitation-oriented treatments that were composed of physical therapy, occupational therapy, psychology, vocational counseling, and medication management. In the Cutler et al. (1994) study, 153 patients aged 65–79 years participated in either a 4-week interdisciplinary inpatient or outpatient treatment program. Older patients showed treatment improvements comparable to those of younger patients, with the exception that they displayed less improvement in their ability to stand without pain and in their ability to perform several simple trunk movements. On the other hand, they demonstrated greater improvement on measures of compliance with the exercise programs. Middaugh et al. (1988) compared pretreatment status and treatment outcome for 17 consecutive older patients versus 20 consecutive younger patients. Comparisons between the two age groups indicated that the older patients had a higher level of health care utilization and averaged almost four times as many physician visits, emergency room visits, and hospital days in the previous year than the younger group. Nonetheless, both groups displayed positive and comparable successes on major outcome measures, including reduction in pain intensity, decreased use of pain-related medications, increased "uptime" (time spent out of a reclining position), and increased walking tolerance.

Taken together, these studies indicate that older adults with persistent pain respond well to nonpharmacological pain management approaches in general, and C-B treatment strategies in particular. Like younger adults with persistent pain problems, older adults appear to experience the best results when the application of C-B treatment techniques is conducted within the framework of a comprehensive, interdisciplinary team approach. More studies are needed to determine under what conditions or clinical diagnoses C-B techniques may not generalize to older adults, but research results to date appear quite promising and suggest that older adults receive positive outcomes similar to those that have been found for younger adults with persistent pain.

SETTING-SPECIFIC CONSIDERATIONS

Many clinicians still harbor misconceptions of older adult patients that may undermine these patients' opportunities to fully benefit from C-B interventions. Not only are older adults with persistent pain underdiagnosed and undertreated, it appears that nonpharmacological measures such as C-B treatments are underutilized. This is unfortunate; our experience indicates that older adult patients tend to be at least as compliant and enthusiastic about these treatments, if not more so, than younger adults. We find that in general, older adult patients approach their therapeutic alliance with more straightforward expectations than do younger persistent pain patients. That is, they want to know what we can offer them, how it will help them, and what they need to accomplish in order to benefit from this help. We find that they desire less socialization to the treatment process and are less threatened by, and more open to, psychological help. The older adult patient tends to be more focused, specific, and task oriented. This orientation lends itself nicely to the C-B interventions discussed earlier in this chapter. Additionally, the more concise the concepts and rationales regarding the treatment, the more easily they are assimilated by the older adult patient.

Unlike some younger patient cohorts, older adult patients do not typically find it necessary to critically analyze every dimension of a concept in determining its appropriateness or applicability. It appears that older adult patients have a greater basic trust in heath care professionals, and perhaps more confidence and experience in their own ability to select and accept from the ideas and information provided. There also tend to be fewer obstacles or distractions to the process of treatment. This, in part, may be due to the stage of their life and the reduced prospect of secondary gains from their environment. Overall, successful treatment with the older adult patient tends to be more brief and efficient in terms of the straightforwardness of the path toward treatment objectives and goals.

The C-B treatment techniques that we have reviewed in this chapter were designed primarily by clinical psychologists, who are also most frequently the professionals implementing these treatments. This is not to say, however, that other health care professionals cannot make use of some of these techniques. For example, other health care professionals with appropriate training, such as nurses practicing in nursing home settings, could implement abbreviated C-B treatment protocols that are composed of basic relaxation skills training and cognitive distraction and restructuring techniques. Similarly, social workers can and should use C-B assessment and education techniques when working with family members to identify and modify their well-intentioned but detrimental reinforcement of the patient's pain behaviors.

Finally, in addition to who can and should administer C-B treatments, there is an additional layer of complexity when using these techniques with older adults—the interaction between cognitive status and C-B techniques. Cognitive status or functioning should be a standard component of the psychological evaluations of persistent pain patients of all ages (see chapter 10). The results of this assessment are important in treatment planning and in the selection and presentation of C-B techniques. Unfortunately, studies currently do not exist that can aid the clinician in determining how and which types of cognitive impairments limit the utility of which types of C-B techniques, and to what degree. Certainly the greater the level of cognitive impairment, the less useful will be the more abstract C-B techniques (e.g., cognitive restructuring or cognitive modification).

Nonetheless, techniques such as cognitive distraction and relaxation training still may be effective despite the presence of cognitive impairment. These techniques may, in fact, be particularly important in cognitively impaired older adults who are fearful of pain because they no longer have the capacity to put it in proper social context. Treatment of fear in these patients may be as or more important than treatment of the pain itself.

The success of C-B therapy lies, in part, with the ability of the therapist to present strategies in a simple, concrete format. For example, modified or simplified cognitive distraction strategies may be given to the patient as a specific list of things to do under specific environmental situations or behavioral cues. Similarly, relaxation can be taught concretely by providing patients with specific directions (e.g., instead of teaching about shoulder muscles and the need to relax these muscles under stress conditions, the therapist could simply tell the patient to "drop your shoulders when you feel upset"). Therapists need to make certain that they talk slowly, simplify all instructions, and avoid jargon. Comprehension can be checked by having patients repeat the instructions aloud. Increased repetition throughout the treatment sessions also should be used. Additionally, whenever possible and available, the social support system should be used to help increase the likelihood that cognitively impaired patients will practice and use the strategies in their home environments.

SUMMARY/RECOMMENDATIONS

1. Persistent pain is a complex, multidimensional experience, and traditional unidimensional models are inadequate to understand and treat it.
2. A cognitive-behavioral (C-B) model of persistent pain was described that integrates physical/functional, psychosocial, and behavioral/environmental aspects of the persistent pain experience, with a particular emphasis on the dynamic, cognitive aspects of persistent pain.
3. The C-B perspective recognizes that persistent pain, like any chronic disease, extends over time and affects all domains of the patient's life—vocational, familial, marital, social, psychological, as well as physical.
4. Clinicians frequently ignore psychosocial factors that are important in evaluating and treating the older adult with persistent pain. Cognitive factors including coping skills, self-efficacy, depression, and fear-induced avoidance of activities were reviewed and numerous studies were presented to demonstrate the central role of psychosocial factors in the older adult persistent pain patient.

5. Numerous clinical trials that use treatment approaches based on the C-B model have demonstrated the efficacy of clinical methods with younger adult persistent pain patients.
6. Evidence was presented demonstrating that many of the C-B treatment approaches are just as efficacious with older adults. Unfortunately, these treatments are currently underutilized with older adults.
7. Essential components of C-B treatment were reviewed, including education, skills acquisition, cognitive and behavioral rehearsal, homework, and generalization and maintenance.

CASE STUDIES

Case 1

Ms. C is a 69-year-old single woman who is retired after 35 years of doing marketing and considerable traveling for her job with a large corporation. For the latter third of this career, Ms. C worked with extensive pain. At initial evaluation, she described a 35-year history of back pain that gradually worsened and became more debilitating after lumbar fusion surgery, approximately eight years ago. She had undergone many types of intervention, including nerve blocks, medication trials, and physical therapy, all of which she described as unhelpful. In particular, she was fearful of addiction to opioids and declined the offer of such treatment. She even engaged the help of a personal trainer to assist with exercises but determined that this only made her pain worse. Over time, the pain spread to other joints, particularly her right knee, and eventually evolved into a diffuse pattern of pain diagnosed as fibromyalgia. Because of pain and limited functional capacity, Ms. C became increasingly more sedentary.

Ms. C never married. After retirement, she moved from her long-time residence to the Pittsburgh area in order to be closer to her sister and niece, her remaining family. Because of the early death of her father and her mother's long-standing bipolar depression, family life was difficult and lacked many positive memories. Ms. C coped by learning to fend for herself via a task-focused and independent lifestyle. Her social life predominantly consisted of work relationships and related activities. At the time of evaluation, she had very few friends besides her sister and niece. Recently, much of Ms. C's time has been focused on seeking medical consultation for her pain.

Psychosocial Assessment

As part of the multidisciplinary assessment, Ms. C was provided with psychological evaluation in addition to medical, physical therapy, and occupational therapy evaluations. Her chief complaints to the psychologist included frustration regarding decreased functional capacity, even walking; fear of increasing pain and further loss of independence; increasing tension; decreasing capacity to enjoy pleasurable activities; poor sleep; and general sense of poor physical health. Ms. C also described feelings of nearly lifelong depression, at least from the time of early adolescence. She recognized depression to be a problem, but only once sought professional consultation that did not get beyond the initial meeting because she thought that the therapist was not interested in her. Ms. C reported growing difficulty with overcoming inertia. She associated this with increasing diffuse pain and decreasing physical capacity. She described increasing irritability and anger at herself for not being able to do things because of pain. Ms. C denied panic and anxiety, appetite disturbance, helplessness and hopelessness, social withdrawal, interpersonal conflicts, obsessions and compulsions, and suicidal ideation. Finally, she stated that she tends to be rigid and inflexible about her thoughts, beliefs, and behavior. She implied that she was not readily open to help that is not self-determined and elaborated on how she has coped over these many years simply by attempting to deny pain and other symptoms as a means to continue forward progress. She found this style of coping to be increasingly more difficult since her retirement and intensifying pain symptoms.

In addition to the clinical interview, a psychometric assessment of pain included administration of the Multidimensional Pain Inventory (MPI) (Kerns et al., 1985), Pain Experience Scale (PES) (Turk & Rudy, 1985), and the Center for Epidemiological Studies Depression Scale (CES-D) (Radloff, 1977). These measures were administered at the time of the initial evaluation and again at posttreatment. Table 3.4 displays pre- and posttreatment T scores ($M = 50$ and $SD = 10$) for the subscales of the MPI, PES, and CES-D measures.

Treatment

The interdisciplinary evaluation team determined that Ms. C met criteria for participating in the fibromyalgia treatment program. This program consists of nine days of structured multidisciplinary treatment conducted in a small group format three days per week over a three-week period, with all patients in the group meeting criteria for fibromyalgia diagnosis. The psychology treatment consists of one hour per day in a group format that provides information, discussion, and interventions for topics such as the cognitive, affective, and behavioral nature of pain experience; stress

TABLE 3.4 Pre- and Posttreatment *T* Scores ($M = 50$, $SD = 10$) for Case 1

Measure	Pretreatment	Posttreatment
Multidimensional Pain Inventory		
Pain Severity	37.14	43.57
Pain-Related Interference	45.87	33.26
Life Control	39.72	56.53
Affective Distress	45.33	47.74
Household Chores	33.11	50.36
Outdoor Work	41.74	41.74
Activities Away From Home	47.67	37.54
Social Activities	60.79	39.66
Pain Experience Scale		
Emotional Reactions	54.57	43.43
Worry Reactions	63.72	57.59
CES-D (Depression)		
Raw Score	27.00	23.00
T Score	53.85	50.45

management coping skills, such as relaxation techniques; and emotion/mood management coping skills, such as cognitive restructuring. Treatment goals for Ms. C emphasized clarification and validation of the pain (fibromyalgia), so that constructive and adaptive coping skills could be used, with demonstrative improvement in function as alternatives to denial and pushing herself forward. It was hypothesized that the small group format would facilitate motivation for Ms. C to explore and open herself to new coping ideas and provide support for application of more adaptive coping skills.

Discussion

Ms. C participated fully in all aspects of the treatment. She was an inquisitive consumer of information and demonstrated a need to explore new concepts thoroughly before adopting them into her perspective. This behavior was consistent with her self-reliant personality style. By the end of the program, Ms. C had benefited by incorporating new skills and behaviors into a coping program that allowed her to acknowledge, rather than deny, her pain and her related limitations. Her acceptance of new information, acquisition of coping skills, and assimilation of feedback from other patients with persistent pain made it possible for validation of the pain problem, with improved psychosocial response to the life experience of persistent pain.

The pre- and posttreatment measures (Table 3.4) support Ms. C's progress in important ways. On the MPI, the Pain Severity score actually increased slightly at posttreatment, but remained well below average. The low pretreatment *T* score of 37 may represent Ms. C's tendency to deny pain. The posttreatment score of 43 suggests her increased acknowledgment of pain, particularly in light of the positive changes observed for many of the other scale scores. For example, the Pain-Related Interference scale score decreased considerably at posttreatment (Table 3.4), and the Life Control score showed significant increases following treatment. This combination of score changes is consistent with her improved confidence and her ability to better understand and manage her pain in such a way that following treatment, usual obstacles to accomplishing tasks with pain were seen to create less interference.

The activity scales of the MPI, that is, Household Chores, Outdoor Work, Activities Away From Home, and Social Activities, provided additional evidence for changes that also were consistent with changes in other scores. As displayed in Table 3.4, Ms. C reported considerable increases in completing Household Chores at posttreatment, and substantial decreases in measures of Activities Away From Home and Social Activities, which suggest a major shift in her pretreatment tendency to deny pain and push forward as her primary mechanism of coping. These posttreatment scores likely indicate an acceptance of pain and a willingness to deal with it in a more immediate and personal context, presumably with more effective coping and self-pacing skills.

Finally, the Pain Experience Scale also showed changes consistent with Ms. C's shift in coping orientation. The Emotional Reactions scale decreased considerably at posttreatment, as did the Worry Reactions scale, but to a lesser degree. These changes suggest a softening of negative affect in response to pain, which is consistent with the other positive changes observed on the MPI. The CES-D Depression Scale indicates only a slight decrease in depression symptoms at posttreatment. These pre- and posttreatment CES-D scores are within the average range for this population and, in this particular case, are not likely to change dramatically because of Ms. C's long-standing and enduring depression.

Case 2

Ms. J is a 78-year-old widowed woman who lives alone. She has a 10+-year history of diffuse pain, with low back and leg pain her worst complaints. She has been diagnosed with fibromyalgia, diffuse osteoarthritis, scoliosis, and spinal stenosis. She reports being unable to stand for more than 5–10 minutes before experiencing severe back pain and muscle spasms in her legs, which are relieved when she sits down. She generally ambulates with a wheelchair whenever she leaves her house. At her home, she receives outside assistance with laundry, cleaning, and meal preparation. Her siblings and her children are described as providing a great deal of social support.

At the time of the psychosocial evaluation, Ms. J described experiencing significant anxiety in response to her pain, as well as generally being a "worrier." At night, she would often awaken to the pain of severe muscle spasms in her legs. This would trigger her anxiety and a feeling of being overwhelmed and not knowing what to do to manage the situation. Additionally, she had numerous general worries about her pain and her health. At the time of evaluation, she also endorsed becoming increasingly passive and sedentary, avoiding activities that she feared would trigger or exacerbate her pain. Other symptoms included long-standing difficulty falling asleep, restless sleep, occasional anhedonia associated with her pain, and occasional irritability. She was diagnosed with Pain Disorder Associated with both Psychological Factors and a General Medical Condition, and Anxiety Disorder, Not Otherwise Specified. Her goals for treatment were to better cope with her pain and, more specifically, to decrease the anxiety she experienced in association with her pain.

Ms. J was seen for eight individual psychological treatment sessions. She was provided with information to help her better understand how the anxiety triggered by her pain also could exacerbate her pain via increased muscle tension, opening the pain gate, and increasing her focus on pain. She then was provided with training in a number of relaxation skills and instructed to practice these skills on a daily basis. The relaxation techniques included the following: diaphragmatic breathing (i.e., slow, deep breathing designed to reduce heart rate, muscle tension, and other physiological signs of anxiety), progressive muscle relaxation (i.e., progressively tensing and then releasing the major muscle groups throughout her body), guided visualization (i.e., developing a multisensory image of a peaceful and relaxing place), and a passive muscle relaxation technique (i.e., learning to let go of tension throughout her muscles by imagining warm water flowing over her body bringing warmth, heaviness, and relaxation). Next, she was provided with information about how her cognitions contributed to her anxiety (e.g., "What if this pain flare does not go away?"), and with training on how to talk herself through her anxiety and pain in a more productive way (e.g., "The other flares have resolved. I can get through this one too.").

Next, she was guided to use her relaxation and cognitive coping skills at times of increased anxiety or pain. For instance, upon awakening in the middle of the night with increased pain and subsequent feelings of being anxious and overwhelmed, she was guided to "talk" to herself in a calm and productive manner. This enabled her to sufficiently reduce the immediate paralyzing anxiety to allow her to think more clearly and put her other coping skills to use (e.g., relaxation skills, and skills she was learning in concurrent physical and occupational therapy sessions). Before ending treatment, Ms. J and her therapist created a written list of coping skills to serve as a reminder of what she could do herself to gain better control over her pain and her anxiety. By the end of treatment, Ms. J reported that she was much less anxious about her pain and that she was generally worrying less. Additionally, she reported a decrease in the intensity of her pain.

Discussion

The approach to Ms. J's treatment was largely a cognitive-behavioral, coping-skills training approach, which is the standard for the psychological treatment of persistent pain. Through training and practice in relaxation techniques, Ms. J was able to effect positive change in both the physical and emotional elements of her distress. She was able to gain increased personal control over her anxiety, as well as her pain. This helped to break the vicious cycle of pain triggering anxiety and loss of control, which then led to increased muscle tension and more intense pain. The format of the cognitive component of Ms. J's treatment was somewhat less structured and formal, however, than it might otherwise be. Through simple conversation about the anxiety she experienced, she was assisted in becoming aware of the thoughts and worries she was having at those times. Because her anxiety tended to be overwhelming and paralyzing, she was assisted in identifying and realistically altering the thoughts that intensified it and placed barriers to more productive management of the anxiety and the pain flares that triggered it. Ms. J then realized that she did have some control over her anxiety. As she replaced her unproductive worries with more helpful and encouraging thoughts, she was able to calm herself down enough to put to use the skills and exercises from all of her treatment (i.e., psychological, physical therapy, and occupational therapy) and bring about improvement in her pain.

Case 3

Ms. A is a 72-year-old widowed woman who lives with one of her adult sons. She has a long history of persistent low back pain that radiates to her legs. She had surgery for spinal stenosis, but reports that her pain has been worse in the several years since her surgery. Her pain is associated only with standing or ambulating, and she has no pain sitting or lying down. She is able to conduct basic home and self-care activities, but at the time of evaluation she reported anxiety about the activities that she could not perform and for which she had to wait for the help of her children. She said that her family described her as "hard to get along with" and that they implied that her pain complaints were "in her head." Because of her pain, she became more isolated and engaged in mostly solitary seated activities at home. Furthermore, she was experiencing additional distress related to one son's severe illness and another son's alcohol problem.

Psychological symptoms included the following: anxiety, worry, and nervousness associated with activities that she was no longer able to complete independently and with family stressors; depressed mood; extreme frustration regarding limits on her activities because of pain; decreased appetite and slow steady weight loss over the past two years; and restlessness. Testing scores on the Affective Distress scale of the Multidimensional Pain Inventory were consistent with clinical impressions from the interview and suggested significantly higher than average affective distress associated with her pain. Additional test scores also suggested that she responded to severe pain episodes with significant worry and further increases in negative affect. She was diagnosed with Adjustment Disorder with Mixed Anxiety and Depressed Mood. Her goal for psychological treatment was to decrease her emotional distress.

Ms. A was seen for eight sessions of individual psychological treatment. After initial training in several simple relaxation techniques (e.g., diaphragmatic breathing and visualization), the majority of the sessions focused on providing support and encouragement for Ms. A's ability to cope with her pain and stress. Ms. A responded quickly to treatment. She found the relaxation skills gave her some control over her "nervousness," but she also began to change her outlook about her pain and her family stressors. She became more assertive with family members in situations where she had previously been distressed but passive. She began attending more social functions and keeping busy in her garden in spite of her persistent pain. Her thoughts about her pain shifted from a focus on relief to a focus on coping, and she even found ways of adapting tasks so that she could complete them independently.

As these changes occurred, she began to experience more joy and pleasure in her life, less isolation, and diminished anxiety. She was observed to smile more often in treatment sessions. Throughout, the primary interventions of the psychologist were designed to provide encouragement and a great deal of verbal reinforcement for the adaptive coping steps she was taking. At the end of treatment, Ms. A stated that her mood was significantly improved, that she was coping better with her pain and stress, and that she was surprised at how helpful "talking" could be.

Discussion

Generally, psychological intervention for the management of persistent pain involves a C-B, coping-skills training approach. In the case of Ms. A, this approach was first implemented by providing her with initial training in several relaxation skills. Overall, this was a relatively small portion of her treatment, however, and Ms. A did not engage in formal cognitive therapy. Most of the intervention took the form of support and encouragement. In the end, her thoughts and attitudes about her pain and other psychosocial stressors did change. Rather than occurring via formal cognitive modification training, however, her thoughts were altered by the support that was provided and the subsequent changes she made in her responses to pain and stressors. The support was important for her because she presented with a perceived lack of support from her family, as well as increasing isolation from her friends as she reduced her activities to avoid pain. Through the support and positive reinforcement provided by treatment, she was able to rely more on her own internal coping resources and find ways of reconnecting with her social support network and some of the activities she enjoyed. As a result, the quality of her life improved despite the fact that she did not endorse any significant decrease in her pain.

REFERENCES

Arena, J., Hannah, S. L., Bruno, G. M., & Meador, K. (1991). Electromyographic biofeedback training for tension headache in the elderly: A prospective study. *Biofeedback and Self-Regulation, 16*, 379–390.

Arena, J., Hightower, N., & Chang, G. (1988). Relaxation therapy for tension headache in the elderly: A prospective study. *Psychology and Aging, 3*, 96–98.

Bandura, A. (1977). Self-efficacy: Toward a unifying theory of behavioral change. *Psychological Review, 84*, 191–215.

Bandura, A., O'Leary, A., Taylor, C. B., Gauthier, J., & Gossard, D. (1987). Perceived self-efficacy and pain control—opioid and nonopioid mechanisms. *Journal of Personality and Social Psychology, 53*, 563–571.

Bhala, R. P., O'Donnell, J., & Thoppil, E. (1982). Phobic fear of falling and its clinical management. *Physical Therapy, 62*, 187–190.

Blumer, D., & Heilbronn, M. (1982). Chronic pain as a variant of depressive disease: The pain-prone disorder. *Journal of Nervous and Mental Disease, 170,* 381–406.

Cho, C., Alessi, C. A., Cho, M., Aronow, H. U., Stuck, A. E., Rubenstein, L. Z., & Beck, J. C. (1998). The association between chronic illness and functional change among participants in a comprehensive geriatric assessment program. *Journal of the American Geriatrics Society, 46,* 677–682.

Clark, D. (1996). Age, socioeconomic status, and exercise self-efficacy. *Gerontologist, 36,* 157–164.

Cutler, R. B., Fishbain, D. A., Steele-Rosomoff, R., & Rosomoff, H. L. (1994). Outcomes in treatment of pain in geriatric and younger age groups. *Archives of Physical Medicine and Rehabilitation, 75,* 457–464.

Davis-Berman, J. (1990). Physical self-efficacy, perceived physical status, and depressive symptomatology in older adults. *Journal of Psychology, 124,* 207–215.

Dolce, J. J. (1987). Self-efficacy and disability beliefs in behavioral treatment of pain. *Behaviour Research and Therapy, 25,* 289–299.

Dolce, J. J., Crocker, M. F., Moletteire, C., & Doleys, D. M. (1986). Exercise quotas, anticipatory concern and self-efficacy expectancies in chronic pain: A preliminary report. *Pain, 24,* 365–372.

Fernandez, E., & Turk, D. C. (1989). The utility of cognitive coping strategies for altering pain perception: A meta-analysis. *Pain, 38,* 123–135.

Fishman, B. (1992). The cognitive-behavioral perspective on pain management in terminal illness. In D. C. Turk & C. S. Feldman (Eds.), *Noninvasive approaches to pain management in the terminally ill* (pp. 73–88). New York: Haworth Press.

Flor, H., & Turk, D. C. (1989). The psychophysiology of chronic pain: Do chronic pain patients exhibit symptom-specific psychophysiological responses? *Psychological Bulletin, 105,* 215–259.

Flor, H., Turk, D. C., & Birbaumer, N. (1985). Assessment of stress-related psychophysiological reactions in chronic back pain patients. *Journal of Consulting and Clinical Psychology, 53,* 354–364.

Fordyce, W. E. (1976). *Behavioral methods for chronic pain and illness.* St. Louis, MO: C.V. Mosby.

Fry, P. S., & Wong, P. T. P. (1991). Pain management training in the elderly: Matching interventions with subjects' coping styles. *Stress Medicine, 7,* 93–98.

Gatchel, R. J., & Turk, D. C. (1996). *Psychological approaches to pain management.* New York: Guilford Press.

Geisser, M. E., Robinson, M. E., & Henson, C. D. (1994). The Coping Strategies Questionnaire and chronic pain adjustment: A conceptual and empirical reanalysis. *Clinical Journal of Pain, 10,* 98–106.

Geisser, M. E., Robinson, M. E., Keefe, F. J., & Weiner, M. L. (1994). Catastrophizing, depression and the sensory, affective and evaluative aspects of chronic pain. *Pain, 59,* 79–83.

Grembowski, D., Patric, D., Diehr, P., Durham, M., Beresford, S., Kay, E., & Hecht, J. (1993). Self-efficacy and health behavior among older adults. *Journal of Health and Social Behavior, 34,* 89–104.

Haldeman, S., Shouka, M., & Robboy, S. (1988). Computed tomography, electrodiagnostic and clinical findings in chronic workers' compensation patients with back and leg pain. *Spine, 13,* 345–350.

Hazard, R. G., Benedix, A., & Genwich, J. W. (1991). Disability exaggeration as a predictor of functional restoration outcomes for patients with chronic low-back pain. *Spine, 16,* 1062–1067.

Hill, A., Niven, C. A., & Knussen, C. (1995). The role of coping in adjustment to phantom limb pain. *Pain, 62,* 79–86.

Holroyd, K. A., Nash, J. M., Pingel, J. D., Cordingley, G. E., & Jerome, A. (1991). A comparison of pharmacological (amitriptyline HCl) and nonpharmacological (cognitive-behavioral) therapies for chronic tension headaches. *Journal of Consulting and Clinical Psychology, 59,* 387–393.

Holzman, A. D., & Turk, D. C. (1986). *Pain management: A handbook of psychological treatment approaches.* Elmsford, NY: Pergamon Press.

Jacobsen, P. B., & Butler, R. W. (1996). Relation of cognitive coping and catastrophizing to acute pain and analgesic use following breast cancer surgery. *Journal of Behavioral Medicine, 19,* 17–29.

Jaffe, A., Froom, J., & Galambos, N. (1994). Minor depression and functional impairment. *Archives of Family Medicine, 3,* 1081–1086.

Jensen, M. A., Turner, J. A., & Romano, J. M. (1991). Self-efficacy and outcome expectancies: Relationship to chronic pain coping strategies and adjustment. *Pain, 44,* 263–269.

Jensen, M. P., Turner, J. A., Romano, J. M., & Karoly, P. (1991). Coping with chronic pain: A critical review of the literature. *Pain, 47,* 249–283.

Keefe, F. J., Caldwell, D. S., Williams, D. A., Gil, K. M., Mitchell, D., Robertson, C., Martinez, S., Nunley, J., Beckham, J. C., & Helms, M. (1990). Pain coping skills training in the management of osteoarthritic knee pain—II: Follow-up results. *Behavior Therapy, 21,* 435–447.

Keefe, F., & Williams, D. (1990). A comparison of coping strategies in chronic pain patients in different age groups. *Journal of Gerontology, 45,* 161–165.

Keen, S., Dowell, A. C., Hurst, K., Klaber Moffett, J. A., Tovey, P., & Williams, R. (1999). Individuals with low back pain: How do they view physical activity. *Family Practice, 16,* 39–45.

Kempen, G. I. J. M., & Ormel, J. (1998). The impact of physical performance and cognitive status on subsequent ADL disability in low-functioning older adults. *International Journal of Geriatric Psychiatry, 13,* 480–483.

Kerns, R. D., Turk, D. C., & Rudy, T. E. (1985). The West Haven-Yale Multidimensional Pain Inventory (WHYMPI). *Pain, 23,* 345–356.

Kivinen, P., Sulkava, R., Halonen, P., & Nissinen, A. (1998). Self-reported and performance-based functional status and associated factors among elderly men: The Finnish cohorts of seven countries study. *Journal of Clinical Epidemiology, 51,* 1243–1252.

Klenerman, L., Slade, P. D., Stanley, I. M., Pennie, B., Reilly, J. P., Atchison, L. E., Troup, J. D., & Rose, M. J. (1995). The prediction of chronicity in patients with an acute attack of low back pain in a general practice setting. *Spine, 20,* 478–84.

Kores, R. C., Murphy, W. D., Rosenthal, T. L., Elias, D. B., & North, W. C. (1990). Predicting outcome of chronic pain treatment via a modified self-efficacy scale. *Behavior Research and Therapy, 28,* 165–169.

Lascelles, M. A., Cunningham, S. J., McGrath, P., & Sullivan, M. J. L. (1989).

Teaching coping strategies to adolescents with migraine. *Journal of Pain and Symptom Management, 4,* 135–144.

Melzack, R., & Casey, K. L. (1968). Sensory, motivational and central control determinants of pain: A new conceptual model. In D. Kenshalo (Ed.), *The skin senses* (pp. 137–153). Springfield, IL: Charles C Thomas.

Melzack, R., & Wall, P. D. (1965). Pain mechanisms: A new theory. *Science, 150,* 971–980.

Middaugh, S. J., Kee, W. G., Peters, J., & Herman, K. (1992). Physiological response of older and younger pain patients to biofeedback-assisted relaxation training. *Biofeedback and Self-Regulation, 17,* 304–305.

Middaugh, S. J., Levin, R. B., Kee, W. G., Barchiese, F. D., & Roberts, J. M. (1988). Chronic pain: Its treatment in geriatric and younger patients. *Archives of Physical Medicine and Rehabilitation, 69,* 1021–1025.

Middaugh, S. J., Woods, S. E., Kee, W. G., Harden, R. N., & Peters, J. R. (1991). Biofeedback-assisted relaxation training for the aging chronic pain patient. *Biofeedback and Self-Regulation, 16,* 361–377.

Murphy, J., & Isaacs, B. (1982). The post-fall syndrome: A study of 36 elderly patients. *Gerontology, 28,* 265–270.

Nathan, P. W. (1976). The gate control theory of pain: A critical review. *Brain, 99,* 123–158.

Nicholas, M. K. (1992). Relapse rates following treatment in pain management programs. In P. H. Wilson (Ed.), *Principles and practice of relapse prevention* (pp. 259–271). New York: Guilford Press.

O'Leary, A., Shoor, S., Lorig, K., & Holman, H. R. (1988). A cognitive-behavioral treatment for rheumatoid arthritis. *Health Psychology, 7,* 527–544.

Osterweis, M., Kleinman, A., & Mechanic, D. (1987). *Institute of Medicine's Committee on Pain, Disability, and Chronic Illness Behavior, Pain and Disability: Clinical, behavioral, and public policy perspectives.* Washington, DC: National Academy Press.

Parker, J., & Wright, G. (1995). The implications of depression for pain and disability in rheumatoid arthritis. *Arthritis Care and Research, 8,* 279–283.

Pennix, B. W. J. H., Guralnik, J. M., Ferrucci, L., Simonsick, E. M., Deeg, D. J. H., & Wallace, R. B. (1998). Depressive symptoms and physical decline in community-dwelling older persons. *Journal of the American Medical Association, 279,* 1720–1726.

Phillips, H. (1987). Avoidance behavior and its role in sustaining chronic pain. *Behavior Research and Therapy, 25,* 273–279.

Puder, R. S. (1988). Age analysis of cognitive-behavioral group therapy for chronic pain outpatients. *Psychology and Aging, 3,* 204–207.

Radloff, L. S. (1977). The CES-D scale: A self-report depression scale for research in the general population. *Applied Psychological Measurement, 1,* 385–401.

Ressor, K. A., & Craig, K. D. (1988). Medically incongruent chronic back pain: Physical limitations, suffering, and ineffective coping. *Pain, 32,* 35–45.

Richter, I. L., McGrath, P. J., Humphreys, P. J., Goodman, J. T., Firestone, P., & Keens, D. (1986). Cognitive and relaxation treatment of paediatric migraine. *Pain, 25,* 195–203.

Robinson, M. E., Riley, J. L., Myers, C. D., Sadler, I. J., Kvaal, S. A., Geisser, M. E.,

& Keefe, F. J. (1997). The Coping Strategies Questionnaire: A large sample, item level factor analysis. *Clinical Journal of Pain, 13*, 43–49.

Rosenstiel, A. K., & Keefe, F. J. (1983). The use of coping strategies in chronic low back pain patients: Relationship to patient characteristics and current adjustment. *Pain, 17*, 33–44.

Rozzini, R., Frisoni, G. B., Ferrucci, L., Barbisoni, P., Bertozzi, B., & Trabucchi, M. (1997). The effect of chronic diseases on physical function. Comparison between activities of daily living scales and the physical performance test. *Age Ageing, 26,* 281–287.

Rudy, T. E., & Turk, D. C. (1991). Psychological aspects of pain. *International Anesthesiology Clinics, 29*, 9–22.

Slade, P. D., Troup, J. D. G., Lethem, J., & Bentley, G. (1983). The fear-avoidance model of exaggerated pain perception—II: Preliminary studies of coping strategies for pain. *Behaviour Research and Therapy, 21*, 409–416.

Sorkin, B. A., Rudy, T. E., Hanlon, R. B., Turk, D. C., & Stieg, R. L. (1990). Chronic pain in old and young patients: Differences appear less important than similarities. *Journal of Gerontology, 45*, 64–68.

Turk, D. C., & Flor, H. (1987). Pain > pain behavior: Utility and limitations of the pain behavior construct. *Pain, 31*, 277–295.

Turk, D. C., Meichenbaum, D., & Genest, M. (1983). *Pain and behavioral medicine: A cognitive-behavioral perspective.* New York: Guilford.

Turk, D. C., & Rudy, T. E. (1985, October). Pain experience: *Assessing the cognitive component.* Paper presented at the Annual Meeting of the American Pain Society, Dallas, TX.

Turk, D. C., & Rudy, T. E. (1989). An integrated approach to the treatment of chronic pain: Beyond the scalpel and syringe. In C. D. Tollison (Ed.), *Handbook of chronic pain management* (pp. 222–236). Baltimore: Williams & Wilkins.

Turk, D. C., & Rudy, T. E. (1991). Neglected topics in the treatment of chronic pain patients—relapse, noncompliance, and adherence enhancement. *Pain, 44*, 5–28.

Turk, D. C., & Rudy, T. E. (1992). Cognitive factors and persistent pain: A glimpse into Pandora's box. *Cognitive Therapy and Research, 16*, 99–122.

Turk, D. C., & Rudy, T. E. (1994). A cognitive-behavioral perspective on chronic pain: Beyond the scalpel and syringe. In C. D. Tollison (Ed.), *Handbook of pain management* (pp. 136–151). Baltimore: Williams & Wilkins.

Turk, D. C., Rudy, T. E., Kubinski, J. A., Zaki, H. H., & Greco, C. M. (1996). Dysfunctional patients with temporomandibular disorders: Evaluating the efficacy of a tailored treatment protocol. *Journal of Consulting and Clinical Psychology, 64*, 139–146.

Vlaeyen, J. W. S., Kole-Snijders, A. M. J., Boeren, R. G. B., & van Eek, H. (1995). Fear of movement/(re)injury in chronic low back pain and its relation to behavioral performance. *Pain, 62*, 363–372.

White, A. A., & Gordon, S. L. (1982). Synopsis: Workshop on idiopathic low-back pain. *Pain, 7*, 141–149.

Woodard, N. J., & Wallston, B. S. (1987). Age and health care beliefs: Self-efficacy as a medicator of low desire for control. *Psychology and Aging, 2*, 3–8.

An Approach to Musculoskeletal Disorders

4

Marie Feletar, Stephen Hall,
Paula Breuer, and Ann K. Williams

Rheumatological disease is prevalent in older adults and presents a different spectrum of complaints compared with that of younger patients (Laiho, Tuohimehto, & Tilvis, 2001). Debility related to musculoskeletal conditions is a major variable determining independence and, therefore, the need for institutionalization. Appropriate diagnosis and therapy of some of the more treatable conditions can be very rewarding, facilitating improved quality of life and self-sufficient living. The health and living status of our aging population also has significant economic implications and should provide a complementary reflection of society as a whole.

Rheumatological diagnoses in older adults are based more on clinical acumen than on serologic or radiographic data. Radiographs, computed tomograms (CT), magnetic resonance imaging (MRI) studies, and serological tests show high rates of abnormality with age (Boden, Davis, Dina, Patronas, & Wiesel, 1990). Therefore, they must not be considered diagnostic in the absence of clinical symptoms. These principles arise frequently in this chapter and will be explored in more detail in the discussion of regional problems.

An approach to the older adult with musculoskeletal symptoms is to categorize pathology into that which is degenerative versus that which is inflammatory. Common musculoskeletal problems in older adults related to degenerative pathology include osteoarthritis of the knees, hips, hands, and cervical and lumbar spine. Tendinopathies or tendinoses, usually resulting from chronic microtrauma, are a widespread problem affecting the upper and lower limbs, in particular the rotator cuff mechanism of the shoulder and the Achilles and posterior tibial tendons. Lateral and medial epicondylitis and de Quervain's tenosynovitis also arise from this mechanism. Other regional problems are carpal tunnel syndrome and the syndrome of lateral hip pain. Such processes produce symptoms, which are modified by biomechanical factors. Inflammatory problems such as polymyalgia rheumatica (PMR), giant cell arteritis, and rheumatoid arthritis tend not to be so affected by biomechanical considerations, although of course they are worthy of considerable attention due to their impact, their amenability to drug therapy, and the potential toxicity of such therapy in older adults. This chapter is organized according to regional musculoskeletal syndromes; common systemic musculoskeletal disorders are also discussed. For each disorder, we discuss an approach to diagnosis and treatment, as well as underlying pathophysiology.

EVIDENCE AND PRINCIPLES FOR PRACTICE

Upper Limb

Shoulder

Shoulder pain is a common problem, afflicting up to 21% in one community survey of an older adult population (Chard, Hazleman, Hazleman, King, & Reiss, 1991). Pain of shoulder origin is nearly always associated with significant nocturnal pain and is aggravated by activities of arm elevation, such as combing or brushing hair. Not all pain in the region of the shoulder, however, stems from this joint. A useful rule is that pain proximal to the shoulder generally does not arise from the shoulder and is likely to stem from the cervical spine. Similarly, pain extending distal to the elbow is unlikely to stem from the shoulder and may reflect elbow disorders or cervical radiculopathy. Rarely does shoulder pain stem from more distant pathology, such as diaphragmatic irritation caused by acute cholecystitis.

Physical examination findings are broadly in two groups—those with and without capsular involvement (see Table 4.1). The examiner should be facing the patient, who is in the seated position, and the patient's arm should be cradled in the examiner's opposite arm to elicit maximum relaxation. If pain is equally reproduced in passive as well as active movement, then the pathology is usually capsular. This includes synovitis, adhesive capsulitis, or other conditions involving capsular irritation, such as crystalline or septic arthritis. If pain is found throughout the range of movement, then the pathology may lie within the glenohumeral joint or may be capsular in origin. Rotator cuff disease, however, leads to pain mainly with active rather than passive motion, if adequate relaxation can be achieved.

TABLE 4.1 Differentiating Physical Findings in Common Shoulder Disorders

Physical finding	Acute rotator cuff tear	Chronic rotator cuff disease	Glenohumeral osteoarthritis	Adhesive capsulitis
Age	Any	> 40 yo	> 40 yo	> 40 yo
Pain— passive motion	–	–	+	+
Pain— active motion	+	+	+	+
Impingement	+	+	–	–
Restricted range of motion*	–	–	+	+
Weakness	+	+/–	–	–

* If full relaxation is achieved.

Rotator Cuff Disease   The most pertinent issues of the shoulder in older adults are rotator cuff disease and adhesive capsulitis, or frozen shoulder. Glenohumeral joint osteoarthritis may be secondary to a degenerated rotator cuff, leading to lack of stability stemming from a large rotator cuff tear or other pathology such as basic calcium phosphate (BCP) arthropathy. The glenohumeral joint, however, is not a site of primary (i.e., idiopathic) osteoarthritis. Rotator cuff tears occur with increasing frequency as people age. In one study, 61% of cadaveric specimens were found to have evidence of degenerative changes in the supraspinatus tendon (Hijoka, Suzuki, Makamura, & Hojo, 1993). The number of tendons with degeneration and tear increased from the fifth to the sixth decades and remained at 60% per decade between the ages of 60 and 90. The size of the tear also has been shown to increase with age (Lehman, Cuomo, Kummer, & Zuckerman, 1995). Another cadaveric study suggested that the morphology of the acromion (curved or beaked) correlates with the incidence and severity of the rotator cuff tear (Panni, Milano, Lucania, Fabbriciani, & Logroscino, 1996).

As radiologically evident rotator cuff disruption is not always symptomatic, imaging must be appropriately correlated with clinical findings in the evaluation of the individual patient with a painful shoulder. An x-ray may reveal a subacromial spur. Ultrasound or MRI evidence of rotator cuff disease in an older patient is very common and may represent an incidental finding. A rotator cuff tear (most commonly in the supraspinatus tendon) and subacromial bursitis lead to similar clinical findings. These include a painful arc of abduction, usually between 60 and 120 degrees, and signs of impingement, for example, pain or catching on forced elevation and external rotation.

Initial treatment should usually be conservative, particularly in the older adult population, in whom surgery is a major undertaking with a long (3–9 month) recovery time. Subacromial corticosteroid injection is a simple and effective means of alleviating pain and may need to be repeated once or twice in the setting of an acute tear. Physical therapy is a useful adjunct aiming to strengthen the rotator cuff mechanism. Symptoms, particularly in older adults, frequently recur within 6–24 months; thus periodic injections remain a useful treatment.

Adhesive Capsulitis   Capsulitis causes shoulder pain and stiffness, with findings on physical examination of diffuse tenderness about the glenohumeral joint and restricted active and passive motion in all planes. It is more common in women and in diabetics. Precipitating factors cannot always be identified, but it appears more common following shoulder surgery and after periods of prolonged immobility such as after a cerebrovascular accident.

The natural history is one of progression through three phases over an average period of 30 months (Reeves, 1975). The first stage is increasingly severe pain, with significant nocturnal symptoms, followed by the second phase of progressive stiffness, or "freezing," during which the pain characteristically eases. The duration of this second phase may determine the recovery time. Last, the shoulder "thaws," that is, it starts to regain range of motion. Frequently, range of motion does not return completely to normal, but resulting disability is minimal. Disability is more related to the degree of pain rather than restriction of movement. Eight to fifteen percent develop this condition in the other shoulder. It is said to rarely recur on a previously affected side. A plain x-ray of the shoulder joint will elucidate whether significant glenohumeral disease is present and a major contributor to the restriction of movement. Neither ultrasound nor MRI adds useful information in this clinical scenario.

Treatment regimens vary. Prednisone alleviates nocturnal pain that can appreciably improve the patient's level of comfort but alone may not alter outcome (Binder, Hazleman, Parr, & Roberts, 1986). Intra-articular steroids also may benefit pain and range of movement in the early phase without long-term advantage (Bulgen, Binder, Hazleman, & Roberts, 1984). Hydrodilatation or distension arthrography by injection of 20–100 ml of saline or other media combined with local anesthetic and corticosteroid appear the more definitive treatment, which has been shown to be therapeutic in 80–90% of cases (Gavant, Rizk, Gold, & Flick, 1994; Wybier et al., 1997). Most achieve improvement immediately, but the benefit may be delayed in some by 2–4 weeks. The therapeutic mechanism may lie in achieving disruption of the surrounding bursae (subscapular or subacromial), which may act as a sort of flap valve release mechanism (Gavant et al., 1994). Physical therapy focusing on stretching exercises to improve range of motion and strengthening exercises to prevent reoccurrence is an effective adjunct to these high-volume injection therapies. Oral or intra-articular corticosteroids can be effective in alleviating pain in order to allow the patient to tolerate this quite painful distension procedure. If this fails, surgical capsulotomy, either arthroscopically or open, can be effective (Watson, Dalziel, & Story, 2000).

While rotator cuff disease commonly occurs concurrently in both shoulders, adhesive capsulitis does not. Thus, bilaterally restricted shoulders should raise suspicion of an inflammatory synovitis such as rheumatoid arthritis. A history of marked diffuse shoulder girdle stiffness associated with irritable shoulders on examination and a raised erythrocyte sedimentation rate (ESR), is more consistent with polymyalgia rheumatica (PMR; see discussion below).

Myofascial Pain   Myofascial pain (MP) may exist in the majority of patients who present to pain clinics, although the prevalence of this disorder in the general population is not known. If the practitioner is unfamiliar with its typical signs and symptoms, the older adult patient is likely to suffer from being subjected to unnecessary diagnostic tests, inappropriate treatment, unrelieved pain, and persistent suffering. Thus, it is important that the primary practitioner gain familiarity with this disorder. Typical signs and symptoms of MP include pain referred from trigger points in specific patterns; activation of trigger points by overload, trauma, or chilling; and autonomic responses including sweating or vasoconstriction. Physical findings include tight bands of tissue that restrict motion and are painful upon stretch and palpation. Trigger points occur in the belly of muscles, not in their tendinous insertions. Patients may complain of burning, aching, and/or stabbing that is deep, and referred pain patterns may be poorly localized. A common site for MP is the trapezius, which may cause pain about the shoulder and upper back. Trigger points are commonly located in the attachment of the upper trapezius along the medial border of the scapula, and above the upper medial border of the scapula.

Treatment includes spray and stretch with vapocoolant spray followed by moist heat, digital pressure with ischemic compression to the trigger point in relaxed muscle, friction massage, ice massage, and stretch using hold/relax techniques. Hold/relax stretching involves gentle contraction of the affected muscle followed by passive stretching. Following treatment, the muscle may remain sore for several days but then pain will improve. Long-term treatment of this chronic condition involves teaching patients to learn to manage their pain through self-application of digital pressure, use of heat and cold modalities (see below), use of proper body biomechanics, avoidance of aggravating activities, stretching, relaxation, and a carefully designed fitness program. The appropriate fitness exercises are highly individualized, but activities such as swimming in a warm pool or using a recumbent bicycle are frequently effective in improving strength and endurance without aggravating the condition. The reader is referred to chapter 7 of this book for discussion of the utility of trigger-point injections. For those interested in a comprehensive discussion of MP, J. Travell and D. Simons' book, *Myofascial Pain and Dysfunction,* is an excellent reference for specific trigger-point patterns and treatment regimes.

Calcific Arthritis and Periarthritis   Basic calcium phosphate (BCP) crystals may be associated with several articular and periarticular conditions about the shoulder, including tendonitis, bursitis, periarthritis, intra-articular arthropathies, and tumoral calcinosis. Calcific deposits at the margins of the rotator cuff tendons, frequently the supraspinatus tendon, suggest the presence of degenerative disease. These deposits may be asymptomatic; when symptomatic, they are most typically associated with a single episode of acute periarthritis. A unique form of BCP arthritis that occurs most commonly in older females is Milwaukee shoulder syndrome (McCarty et al., 1981). The disease may be unilateral or bilateral and may be asymptomatic, or may be associated with pain and significant shoulder dysfunction. Effusions are usually noninflammatory and may be large volume, with associated severe glenohumeral joint destruction. X-rays may reveal soft tissue calcifications and upward subluxation of the humeral head. Treatment is often unsuccessful, but analgesics and therapeutic shoulder aspiration should be attempted.

   Chondrocalcinosis (deposition of calcium pyrophosphate dihydrate [CPPD]) of the hyaline cartilage of the shoulder joint, common also in the wrist, knee, and hip with advancing years, may predispose to an acute calcific arthritis (pseudogout) with a joint effusion palpable at the anterior aspect of the joint. Diagnostic aspiration can be performed at the bedside and will help with differentiation of acute pseudogout from a septic joint; the distinction of these two conditions based upon history and physical examination may be impossible.

Elbow

Lateral Epicondylitis   Lateral epicondylitis falls into the category of a tendinosis, which refers more correctly to the degenerative rather than inflammatory pathology underlying this disorder. The pathology discussed here provides insight into other tendinous regions affected by chronic microtrauma. Pain is felt from the extensor origin, in the region of the lateral epicondyle and down the forearm; it is usually aggravated by activity, such as carrying and lifting with a pronated hand. Examination findings confirm this localized tenderness, frequently 2–3 cm distal to the epicondyle. Provocation testing with resisted wrist extension typically enhances the pain.

Ultrasonography has revealed focal areas of degeneration and discrete cleavage tears in the deep part of the tendon. The most common abnormality in a series of 72 patients was a focal hypoechoic area in the deep part of the tendon corresponding to fibers contiguous with the extensor carpi radialis brevis (Connell et al., 2001). Histological examination of these hypoechoic zones revealed collagen degeneration and fibroblastic proliferation. Associated pathological changes in the lateral collateral ligament were found in 8 of 72 elbows (11%). The pathogenesis of this problem is likely to be one of accumulated microtrauma to the tendon causing disruption and tendinosis. Histological changes in a series of nine patients revealed mesenchymal differentiation and vascular hyperplasia, but no inflammation (Nirschl, 1995).

No treatment in isolation appears to provide satisfactory long-term results, that is, more than 6 months. Local corticosteroid injection into the region that is most tender, typically 2–3 cm distal to the epicondyle, does not alter the pathological process but often relieves pain. It appears effective at least in the short term (3 months or so), although there have been no rigorous trials that definitively support the efficacy of this intervention. Hay, Paterson, Lewis, and Croft (1999) performed a randomized controlled trial comparing corticosteroid injection versus naproxen and placebo, without a sham injection included in the naproxen and placebo arms. At four weeks, pain had resolved or improved in 92% of the injection group versus 57% in the naproxen group. At one year, pain scores were low and comparable in all three groups, suggesting the natural history is one of resolution with time.

Extracorporeal shock wave lithotripsy (ECSWL) is a relatively new therapeutic modality for various tendinopathies. Again, clinical trials tend to be methodologically limited. Improvement has been demonstrated in 42% of patients with chronic tennis elbow at 6 months, compared to a placebo group receiving lower intensity and lower frequency impulses (Rompe, Hope, Kullmer, Heine, & Burger, 1996). Sixty-three percent of patients showed good or excellent relief of pain in a trial, however, without a comparison-control group (Hammer, Rupp, Ensslin, Kohn, & Seil, 2000). Resistance-based exercises may help to strengthen the extensor musculature once acute pain has been controlled with anti-inflammatory drugs (NSAIDs), heat treatments, injection, or ECSWL and rest (Solveborn, 1997). Surgery also may be successful in 40–70% of patients.

Hand

Osteoarthritis   Osteoarthritis (OA) of the hand is a major source of disability, deformity, and pain in older adults. Symptoms described by those afflicted include pain, stiffness, and loss of function. Simple tasks such as faucet turning and holding a knife become difficult. Fine motor manipulation becomes impaired so that recreational activities such as knitting, cutting, and holding a bowling ball or golf club also become limited. Hand OA is more prevalent with age and tends to afflict females more often than males. The ability to perform manual tasks using the hands has been shown to correlate with state of dependency (Williams, Hadler, & Earp, 1982); thus hand OA is a potential threat to independence. Genetics is now better understood to play a significant role. There is a greater concordance for hand OA in monozygotic twins than in dizygotic twins and an increased risk of hand OA in first-degree relatives of patients with hand OA (Doherty, 2000).

Pattern recognition helps the clinician to distinguish primary OA in the hands from other disorders. It characteristically affects most severely the distal interphalangeal (DIP) joints of the index and middle fingers as well as the first carpo-metacarpal (CMC) joint of the thumb (Caspi et al., 2001). The remaining DIP, proximal interphalangeal (PIP), and scapho-trapezium joints also are frequently affected. Development of osteophytes leads to the clinical impression of bony enlargement in these zones. Classical radiographic features of OA include osteophytes, joint space narrowing, subchondral sclerosis, and cyst formation. Uptake in osteoarthritic joints on technetium bone scanning correlates with progression of OA in the hands as well as in the knees (Buckland-Wright, Macfarlane, Fogelman, Emery, & Lynch, 1991; Dieppe, Cushnaghan, Young, & Kirwan, 1993).

Simple analgesics such as acetominophen and NSAIDs can be effective. Physical therapy to maintain intrinsic muscle strength and flexibility may be important to improve functional capacity, as intrinsic muscle wasting through disuse is a common accompaniment of hand OA. Oral glucosamine and chondroitin sulphate shows promise as an analgesic agent, either equivalent or superior to NSAIDs (Towheed et al., 2001). Its mode of action is unclear but it may have some cartilage modifying impact. Long-term efficacy and safety, especially with the number of different preparations available, has yet to be determined. A CMC brace for support of the first CMC joint may provide symptomatic relief; this brace immobilizes the joint while allowing the remainder of the hand to be functional. Arthroplasty for the small joints of the hands is a surgical option but is technically more difficult than for large joints. For basal thumb OA, partial or complete trapeziectomy with tendon interposition and ligament reconstruction is used for advanced disease (Barron, Glickel, & Eaton, 2000).

Metacarpophalangeal OA with hook osteophytes most commonly at the second and third joints should raise the suspicion of OA as a secondary rather than a primary phenomenon. Culprit pathologies include calcium pyrophosphate dihydrate (CPPD) crystal deposition disease, hemochromatosis, hyperparathyroidism, and hypothyroidism. Iron studies, serum, calcium, and thyroid function are appropriate screening tests. OA in nonweight-bearing joints such as the wrists, shoulders, and elbows is not considered primary in origin but rather secondary to other pathology, such as trauma, infection, or other diseases. In the wrists, the most common cause is CPPD. It most commonly presents as an incidental radiographic finding. Alternate presentations include acute inflammatory arthritis (pseudogout) or a chronic arthropathy. Radiographic evidence of this condition increases with age (Sanmarti et al., 1993). The classic sites of chondrocalcinosis are the triangular cartilage of the wrist, medial meniscus of the knee, and symphysis pubis. It also may be found in the glenohumeral joint and hip.

Carpal Tunnel Syndrome   Carpal tunnel syndrome (CTS) is a clinical syndrome that gives rise to pain and paresthesias in the palmar surface of the hand corresponding to the distribution of the median nerve. Some patients localize these rather nonspecific symptoms poorly. Discomfort is characteristically worst at night, often awakening patients. CTS is more common in patients with diabetes and rheumatoid arthritis. The pathology is median nerve compression in the carpal tunnel. Clinical examination may yield signs of intrinsic muscle wasting, more marked in the thenar than hypothenar eminence. Phalen's maneuver (appearance or worsening of paresthesia with maximal passive wrist flexion for 1 minute) and Tinel's sign (paresthesia in the median territory elicited by gentle tapping over the carpal tunnel) are not very sensitive though commonly described screening procedures. Sensory loss can be present in the lateral three-and-a-half digits.

Difficulty arises in diagnosing this quite common condition as the presumed gold standard test, nerve conduction studies (NCS), offers poor sensitivity and specificity for analyzing these rather nonspecific symptoms. NCS evidence of CTS has been shown to be prevalent in asymptomatic individuals. Atroshi et al. (1999) found that 354 of 2,466 people responding to a community survey reported symptoms of pain, numbness, and/or tingling in the hand. Ninety-four of these were felt on clinical grounds to have CTS. NCS revealed median neuropathy in 120 symptomatic subjects (prevalence 4.9%). Only 66 symptomatic subjects had clinically and electrophysiologically confirmed CTS (2.7%). Of 125 control subjects clinically examined, NCS evidence of neuropathy of the median nerve was found in 23 (18.4%). It is for this reason that classic symptoms of CTS may lead the clinician to treat based on diagnostic suspicion, as NCS results may not alter management.

Local corticosteroid injection was found by a Cochrane review to be superior to placebo at one month, but results beyond one month are not available (Marshall, Tardif, & Ashworth, 2000). Local injection of methylprednisolone is superior, however, to oral corticosteroids (Wong et al., 2001). A paucity of RCTs does not allow an evidence-based comparison between injection and surgical intervention (i.e., carpal tunnel release).

Inflammatory hand arthritis   Faced with a patient complaining of joint pain and swelling confined to the hand, the clinician's main diagnostic possibilities are OA and inflammatory arthritis. The combination of a classic anatomical pattern and tenderness in the affected joints and the absence of clinically apparent synovitis should leave no doubt about OA accounting for the patient's symptoms. Synovitis from another disorder (e.g., gout, rheumatoid arthritis) may be found in hands already afflicted by OA. Morning stiffness beyond 30 minutes or so should arouse suspicion of a primary inflammatory phenomenon. The presence of synovial thickening ascertained by careful palpation of the joint margins, tenderness, and stress pain in the MCPs, PIPs, and/or the wrists adds to the weight of evidence for joint inflammation.

A common constellation of test results in the older adult with or without a rheumatological disorder includes an accelerated ESR, a rheumatoid factor (RF) that is slightly elevated, and an antinuclear antibody (ANA) that is low titer positive. The prevalence of a positive serum RF increases with age, as does a positive ANA and other autoantibodies (Manoussakis et al., 1987). The prevalence of RF can be as high as 14.1% in apparently healthy people aged 67–95. Thus the diagnosis of rheumatological disorders in older adults must rely primarily on clinical findings; these findings must be prioritized over laboratory data. Thirty percent of rheumatoid arthritis (RA) patients, for example, may be seronegative.

RA that starts when patients are >60 years of age displays some differing features as compared with younger onset disease. The female to male ratio is not as high—1.6:1 vs. 4.4:1, respectively. Constitutional symptoms (fever, weight loss, fatigue) are more common at initial presentation in older onset patients as are polymyalgic features, occurring four times more frequently than in younger onset RA (Bajocchi, La Corte, Locaputo, Govoni, & Trotta, 2000). The presentation may be more acute in older adults and shoulder involvement is more common (Deal et al., 1985). The prognosis has been suggested as worse for older seropositive patients but perhaps better in older seronegative patients compared with younger onset seronegative disease. Allelic differences between the groups may partly account for this (van Schaardenburg & Breedveld, 1994). HLA-DRB1*04 linked alleles, immunogenetic markers associated with disease severity, are not as closely associated with RA in older adults as they are in younger patients. When present, however, these alleles are associated with more severe arthritis in older onset disease (Hellier, Eliaou, Daures, Sany, & Combe, 2001).

RSSSPE Remitting seronegative symmetrical synovitis with pitting edema (RSSSPE or RS3PE) is a syndrome presenting with dramatic acute swelling on the dorsum of the hands. It also may involve the feet. The underlying pathology may include extensor tenosynovitis and acute joint involvement. It is a condition of the older adult responding dramatically to low- to medium-dose corticosteroids. There is frequently some clinical overlap with other inflammatory conditions.

An Italian group prospectively followed 23 patients with RS3PE and 177 PMR patients with MRI (Cantini et al., 1999). Patients with pure RS3PE had a shorter treatment duration, lower cumulative corticosteroid dose, lower frequency of systemic signs/symptoms, and lower rate of relapse than did patients with PMR. Among the seronegative group, there may be some overlapping clinical features between PMR and RS3PE. Gonzalez-Gay et al. (2001) found a similar HLA-DRB1 association between seronegative late-onset RA and PMR. MRI of the hands and feet showed evidence of tenosynovitis in five patients and synovitis in three of the RS3PE group. Two additional groups of patients, each 13 in number, had a benign prognosis (Berthier, Toussirot, & Wendling, 1998; Russell, Hunter, Pearson, & McCarty, 1990). Others have found that some patients with RS3PE ultimately develop other rheumatic diseases such as RA and spondyloarthropathy (Schaeverbeke et al., 1995). Olive, del Blanco, Pons, Vaquero, and Tena, (1997) found 3 of 27 patients developed hematological disease, 2 lymphoma, and 1 myelodysplasia. Classification criteria may have confounded these analyses as some patients presenting with significant peripheral edema and a marked polyarthritis may have been categorized as either RS3PE or RA.

Lower Limb

Hip/Leg

Trochanteric Bursitis   Symptoms of trochanteric bursitis include pain
localized around the lateral hip and buttock with radiation down the lateral aspect of the leg. Pain may be constant or intermittent, occurring particularly at night when lying on the affected side and applying direct
pressure to the bursa. Patients also may complain of pain when descending stairs, a factor that relates to pathology within the gluteus medius and
minimus. Examination reveals tenderness that may be diffuse around the
buttock and lateral thigh but frequently most acute at the posterosuperior aspect of the greater trochanter, which is the point of insertion of the
gluteus medius. Weakness in lateral hip flexion and exacerbation of pain
(provocation testing) is a frequent finding.

There have not been any studies of incidence in the general population, although Howell, Biggs, and Bourne (2001) found that of 176 patients
undergoing total hip arthroplasty, 20% were found to have tears of the
abductor mechanism. Surgically, tears of these muscles are found at their
attachment to the greater trochanter (Bunker, Esler, & Leach, 1997; Kagan,
1999). MRI of 250 patients with buttock and lateral hip pain or groin pain
revealed evidence of gluteus medius tendinopathy in 35 and gluteus minimus involvement in 10; distention of the adjacent bursa also was observed
(Kingzett-Taylor et al., 1999). Surgical proof of tendinosis was found in
six patients who underwent operations. While this study does not provide
direct evidence for the clinical correlation between radiological findings
of tendinopathy and the clinical syndrome of lateral hip pain, there is
growing appreciation that the lateral hip pain syndrome is likely secondary to gluteus medius tendinopathy with or without associated bursitis.
This is analogous to the rotator cuff syndrome involving the shoulder, thus
sometimes the lateral hip syndrome is labeled "rotator cuff of the hip."

Treatment is largely conservative, with corticosteroid/anesthetic injection at the posterosuperior aspect of the greater trochanter, that is, the
site of insertion of the gluteus medius. An unblinded cohort study of 75
patients found up to 61% reporting continued improvement 26 weeks
postinjection, with better responses to higher doses of betamethasone
(24 mg vs. 12 mg or 6 mg; Shbeeb & Matteson, 1996). Low back pain is a
frequent associate of trochanteric bursitis, and physical therapy to effect
spinal stabilization and/or McKenzie passive extension can be helpful.
Furthermore, exercises designed to strengthen hip abduction are of value
(Shbeeb & Matteson). The problem tends to be a recurrent one, similar
to the rotator cuff syndrome. Two or three injections may be required,

due to the poor healing potential of the pathological tendon. Surgery can be used, but there is no sound evidence that it is more effective than conservative treatment. Good surgical results were reported in seven patients by Kagan (1999).

Tensor Fascia Lata Syndrome   Tensor fascia lata (TFL) syndrome is on the list of differential diagnoses for lateral hip pain. Discomfort may occur at the iliac crest or distally around the lateral hip, typically worse with activity such as walking. Stretching the fascia by adducting the affected leg with the patient lying supine may reproduce the symptoms, as will resisted hip abduction. Treatment includes gradual stretching and ultrasound for reduction of inflammation. Injection of the region of greatest tenderness also may alleviate symptoms.

Foot

Persistent foot pain commonly occurs in association with plantar fasciitis, calcaneal bursitis, and metatarsalgia. Plantar fasciitis presents with pain of the plantar surface of the foot that is sharp and particularly severe with the first few steps in the morning. Point tenderness occurs over the medial calcaneal plantar tuberosity. Patients often report a recent increase in activity level prior to the onset of symptoms. Pain relief may be achieved through wearing a heel lift, temporarily reducing aggravating activities, and then gradually increasing them. Ultrasound and roller foot massage also may be helpful. Metatarsalgia presents with pain on the plantar surface of the metatarsal heads that is most pronounced with weight bearing. Patients often will have a hypermobile or pronated foot. Treatment involves modalities for pain relief and orthotics to relieve pressure. Posterior calcaneal bursitis results in posterior heel pain and swelling around the Achilles tendon insertion. Modalities to reduce inflammation and swelling as well as shoe modification can be helpful.

Many older persons exhibit chronic deformities and resultant pain in their feet. Examples include hammer toes and hallux valgus (bunion deformities). While surgical intervention may be the only long-term solution, symptomatic relief may be achieved through foot massage using rollers on the plantar surface of the foot, footwear that provides added room in the toe box, night splints, and pads or orthotics to reduce pressure on the affected areas.

Spine

Low Back Pain

Back pain in the older person presents a different spectrum of diagnostic possibilities as compared with the same complaint in a younger person. The diagnosis is necessarily based largely on clinical features rather than radiological abnormalities, as the latter become increasingly common with advancing years and, therefore, may be incidental. Boden et al. (1990) illustrated this well in a prospective study of abnormal MRI of the lumbar spine in 67 asymptomatic subjects who had never had low back pain, sciatica, or neurogenic claudication. Evaluated independently by three neuroradiologists, one third of scans were found to show substantial abnormality. Of those under the age of 60, 20% revealed herniated nucleus pulposus, and one revealed lumbar canal stenosis. Among those 60 years or older, 57% had abnormal scans, 36% showed herniated nucleus pulposus, and 21% showed lumbar canal stenosis. In 20- to 39-year-olds, 35% of scans revealed a degenerated or bulging disc in at least one lumbar level, in contrast with 60- to 80-year-olds, in whom a degenerated or bulging disc was found in all but one of the subjects. MRI appears more sensitive (91.7% vs. 83.3%) and specific (100% vs. 71.4%) than CT when compared with operative findings (Forristall, Marsh, & Pay, 1988).

The structures in the spine giving rise to mechanical back pain, that is, pain amplified in the erect position and frequently by sitting or bending, are numerous and not biomechanically separable. Discs are composed of an outer layer, termed the annulus fibrosis, and an inner layer, called the nucleus pulposus. Tears of the annulus are a frequent major cause of acute back pain that typically abates in 1–6 weeks. With successive tears over time, increasing amounts of the inner nucleus leak and become permanently lost. Facet joints and surrounding musculo-ligamentous structures also may contribute to back pain.

For straightforward mechanical back pain, a plain x-ray likely revealing degenerative changes, and a CT scan that has been ordered to exclude more sinister pathology are unlikely to change management. Conservative (nonoperative) therapy is appropriate, as the natural history is usually favorable. Disc protrusions have been shown to radiologically regress over a period of 4–12 months, although radiological resolution tends to lag behind clinical improvement (Komori et al., 1996).

Simple analgesia and mobilization as soon as pain permits is appropriate treatment. Physical therapy should focus on retraining of posture and modes of lifting and bending. Lumbar stabilization exercises, as directed by a physical therapist, may help to protect against future episodes of pain (Dettori, Bullock, Sutlive, Franklin, & Patience, 1995; Hides, Jull,

& Richardson, 2001). Warning signs and symptoms for more serious causes of back pain, for example, fractures, tumor, and infection, include severe nocturnal pain, the presence of neurological compromise, and systemic systems such as fevers, sweats, and weight loss. These signs and symptoms demand more detailed imaging using MRI to better define anatomy. A bone scan is useful to highlight the presence of a fracture within the last 12 months, or to suggest widespread bony malignancy, but does not offer information about the state of neural structures.

Sciatica

Sciatica is defined as radicular type of pain in one or both lower extremities that results from inflammation or pressure on one or more nerve roots of the lumbosacral plexus. In the older adult, sciatica is more likely to result from spinal canal stenosis than disc prolapse, and occasionally may be due to uncommon causes such as intraspinal tumor or metastatic malignancy. The key features distinguishing sciatica caused by disc prolapse compared with lumbar spinal stenosis are listed in Table 4.2. Leg pain from a herniated nucleus pulposus typically subsides within 2–12 weeks, representing alleviation of nerve root encroachment by the disc; the patient is then left with mechanical back pain that may persist and fluctuate for a longer period. The natural history of sciatica caused by spinal stenosis is less well characterized, although it is likely that most cases resolve spontaneously (Johnsson, Rosen, & Uden, 1992). CT will most often provide adequate imaging of the lumbar spine when the history and physical findings are straightforward. In this situation, radiographic findings typically correlate with clinical signs and symptoms. When inadequate resolution is achieved, an MRI is appropriate.

If simple analgesics and rest have failed to manage pain or the pain is very severe, lumbar epidural injection of corticosteroid and local anesthetic is a therapeutic option for symptom relief, as discussed in chapter 7 of this book. It is not effective, however, for the treatment of the more mechanical causes of low back pain. While it is commonly used in community practice, studies to date do not allow us to scientifically evaluate the efficacy of this mode of treatment. Most of our information comes from series of patients and limited clinical trials (Spaccarelli, 1996). The best trial to date is that by Carette et al. (1997), which concluded that epidural corticosteroids lead to short-term improvement in leg pain and sensory deficits but not in functional status. The numbers of patients that proceeded to surgery over the 12-month follow-up period was not significantly different between groups. Two meta-analyses have yielded conflicting conclusions as to the effectiveness of this treatment modality (Koes, Scholten, Mens, & Bouter, 1995; Watts & Silagy, 1995). It is likely that the

TABLE 4.2 Differentiating Physical Examination Findings in Sciatica: Disc Herniation Versus Lumbar Spinal Stenosis

Signs & Symptoms	Disc Herniation	Spinal Canal Stenosis
Back Pain	+/−	+/−
Leg pain uni/bilateral	Unilateral	Uni- or bilateral
Postural variation standing/walking	+/−	++
sitting	+	−
recumbent	−	−
Neurological deficit	Often	+/−
Straight leg raising*	+	−

* With patient supine and knee fully extended, the examiner passively raises the leg. The normal angle (without pain) achieved between the leg and the table is about 80°. If straight leg raising is painful, stop and lower the leg slightly. Then, dorsiflex the foot to put stretch on the sciatic nerve; precipitation of pain makes sciatic nerve pathology more likely. The absence of pain suggests that the positive straight leg raise may be related to hamstring tightness.

longer the duration of sciatica, the less likely epidural steroid injection will be effective. Surgery is generally reserved for those whose symptoms fail to settle with conservative treatment. Indications for surgery are (1) progressive motor neurological deficit, (2) sphincter loss, and (3) pain unrelieved by other treatments (the usual indication for surgery). Sciatica in the setting of fixed neural exit foraminal stenosis due to facet joint enlargement and spondylolisthesis does not have as favorable a natural history and is, therefore, more likely to warrant surgical intervention.

Epidural Lipomatosis

A less common etiology of lumbar spinal stenosis is epidural lipomatosis, a condition thought to be most commonly related to a history of oral or epidural corticosteroid therapy (McCullen, Spurling, & Webster, 1999; Robertson, Tratnelis, Follett, & Menezes, 1997). So-called idiopathic cases occur most commonly in obese individuals, perhaps related to endogenous hypercortisolism (Koch, Doppman, Patronas, & Chrousos, 2000). CT imaging reveals not just preservation of the fat plane around the epidural space, but also an excess of adipose tissue. This is in stark contrast to the usual loss of the fat plane seen in lumbar canal stenosis secondary to bony, ligamentous, and discogenic encroachment upon the spinal canal. A patient with symptoms of canal stenosis and CT evidence of excessive adipose tissue around the epidural space, therefore, may have epidural lipomatosis. Both the thoracic and lumbar regions may be affected. Only case reports of this condition are found in the literature.

Piriformis Syndrome

Some have proposed piriformis syndrome (PS) as a differential diagnosis for sciatica-like pain. The sciatic nerve lies below the piriformis and may course through its fibers. Patients complain of deep gluteal pain that may radiate down the posterior thigh. PS is a clinical diagnosis with a wide range of proposed etiologies, such as spasm, nerve entrapment, or displacement of the sciatic nerve by an enlarged piriformis muscle. The pain of PS may be aggravated by sitting, squatting, and/or forceful external rotation of the hip. The patient will exhibit deep pain in the buttock lateral and inferior to the posterior iliac spine. Physical examination should occur with the patient in the supine position. The knee and hip of the affected leg are flexed to right angles; the examiner then internally rotates and passively adducts the thigh. Precipitation or worsening of sciatica symptoms with this maneuver is supportive of PS. Palpation of the piriformis also will typically elicit tenderness. Treatment includes deep friction massage and gradual stretching of the piriformis using hold/relax techniques (see under Myofascial Pain above). Direct injection of the muscle, best performed under fluoroscopic guidance, also may provide symptomatic relief.

Ischiogluteal Bursitis

Ischiogluteal bursitis, traditionally termed "Weaver's Bottom," also leads to deep buttock pain, characteristically with sitting, when direct pressure is placed over this bursa. Point tenderness at the ischial tuberosity is a clue. Injection is made difficult by proximity to the sciatic nerve.

Kyphosis

Kyphosis is most commonly the result of either spondylotic change in the thoracic spine or multiple vertebral fractures stemming from osteoporosis. This may be painful or painless but the deformity does compromise balance mechanisms. This is not a reversible condition and functional improvement requires attention to paraspinal strengthening through rehabilitative exercises. At times formal bracing is needed such as a full-length thoracolumbar brace with shoulder straps and semirigid stays. In addition, any component of osteoporosis mandates the use of an increasingly wide range of effective therapies.

Lifelong habits of flexed posture, vertebral body fractures associated with osteoporosis, and reduced flexibility in proximal joints can be associated with increased muscular activity in postural muscles leading to pain complaints in the cervical and scapular regions as well as the parathoracic and paralumbar regions. For example, an increased thoracic kyphosis following osteoporotic fractures results in increased extension of the cervical spine and forward position of the scapulas. Postural muscles in the cervical spine and shoulder girdle then must become increasingly active, resulting in chronic muscular strain. Treatment includes medications for pain relief and exercise to improve spinal flexibility and increased posterior muscle strength. Activities should emphasize spinal extension to reduce postural muscle hyperactivity. Short-term treatments for paravertebral spasm include heat modalities, electrotherapy, and soft tissue mobilization through friction, digital pressure, and general massage. Long-term management includes patient education and development of an exercise routine to strengthen postural muscles and improve body mechanics.

Camptocormia

Camptocormia is a condition of reversible thoracic kyphosis that is distinguished from rigid kyphosis by asking the patient to stand, upon which the kyphosis is quite apparent, and then lie down, when the patient "unrolls" to become supine. A secondary flexion contraction of the hip may develop in long-standing cases. This condition was initially described in young soldiers in World War I, and was felt to be psychogenic. Subsequently, it has come to be recognized as a distinct organic condition that usually occurs in the older adult and is caused by abnormal paraspinal muscles (Legaye & Dimbolu, 1995; Perez-Sales, 1990).

MRI of the paraspinal muscles in a series of 27 patients (5M, 22F, mean age 69) revealed a heterogeneous appearance of the spinal muscles, with areas of low density similar to those found in primary muscular dystrophies (Laroche, Delisle, Aziza, Lagarrigue, & Mazieres, 1995). Histology of the musculature shows an increase in fibrous tissue with a lobulated pattern and nonspecific findings of type 2 atrophy and some ragged red fibers. Response to corticosteroids has been quoted by some authors in case series, but no randomized control trial has been performed, an issue made more difficult by the perceived rarity of this condition (Karbowski, 1999). While most cases appear idiopathic, camptocormia may be associated with motor neuron disease (Van Gerpen, 2001) or Parkinson's disease (Djaldetti, Mosberg-Galili, Sroka, Merims, & Melamed, 1999).

Role of the Physical Therapist in Evaluation and Treatment

The physical therapist plays a key role in the evaluation and treatment of the vast majority of older adults with persistent pain caused by musculoskeletal disorders. The therapist serves three vital functions: (1) evaluation, (2) education regarding philosophy/techniques that will promote adherence to prescribed treatments, and (3) administration of passive treatment modalities. An overview of these roles is summarized in Table 4.3. In this age of managed care, assessment and treatment are often too narrowly focused. Because of the older adult's duration of symptoms, comorbid medical conditions, cognitive and sensory changes, and change in physical activity, the musculoskeletal screening process needs to be both careful and comprehensive. Persistent pain is frequently accompanied by decreased activity and disuse, which, in and of itself, requires treatment. Thus, we favor a general functional and musculoskeletal screening examination, followed by an in-depth evaluation of the area of pain. The older adult with back pain, for example, will require evaluation of the back, but also of endurance, balance, gait, postural abnormalities, and leg-length discrepancy, all of which may serve to perpetuate pain, decrease mobility, and promote disability.

One of the principal roles of the physical therapist who treats the older adult with persistent pain is to educate the patient adequately about a variety of issues. These include (1) why it is important to comply with treatment recommendations, (2) how to incorporate self-management techniques into daily routines, and (3) other techniques to promote treatment adherence and decrease pain flares. A key teaching point for the older adult with persistent pain is the need to be an active participant in the treatment process (see chapter 3). Patients seeking only passive modalities (e.g., medication, massage) typically are poor pain rehabilitation candidates.

Physical Therapy Modalities for the Treatment of Regional Musculoskeletal Disorders

This section discusses physical therapy (PT) modalities for the treatment of regional musculoskeletal pain syndromes. These modalities include heat and cold, massage, and various forms of electrical stimulation. There is a paucity of rigorous investigation examining the efficacy of these ther-

TABLE 4.3 Role of the Physical Therapist in Evaluation and Treatment of Older Adults With Painful Musculoskeletal Disorders

Role	Ultimate Beneficial Effect

Assessment
 Comprehensive biomechanical and
   functional assessment, including
     musculoskeletal examination
     balance, gait, & mobility
     endurance
     posture
     leg length discrepancy
     proper use of assistive device
     shoes, braces, inserts
	Identifies all factors that contribute
	   to continued pain and impaired
	   function, so that an optimal
	   treatment program can be
	   devised to (1) diminish pain
	   (2) ameliorate disability, &
	   (3) maintain independence
	
	Avoids an overly focused assessment
	   that runs the risk of applying a
	   "band-aid" but not preventing
	   future problems

Treatment
 Education
 Teach patient the difference
   between "exercise" and "work"
   and the importance of exercise
 	
Remove barriers to exercise
   performance (e.g., fear,
   environmental barriers)
 	
Teach patients about exercise/
   flexibility techniques that can
   be incorporated into daily
   routines (e.g., activity pacing,
   movement strategies to avoid
   pain flares)
 	
Teach patients techniques (e.g.,
   heat, ice, massage) to help with
   management of pain flares
 	
Teach proper stretching
   techniques
 	
Administration of Modalities
 Deliver massage, heat, cold,
   ultrasound, TENS
	Patient will perform exercise
	   that will improve functional
	   capacity and sense of well-being
	
	Enhances adherence to treatment
	
	Maintains optimal function;
	   enhance adherence to treatment
	
	Gives patient sense of control over
	   pain; decrease health care
	   utilization
	
	Avoids overstretching that will
	   cause pain and diminish
	   adherence to prescribed
	   treatment
	
	Views modalities as analgesics
	   whose purpose is to decrease pain
	   in order to enhance adherence to
	   exercise and maintain function

apies, but they have withstood the test of time and remain valuable clinical tools. Their purpose is not simply to provide pain relief but, as with systemic medications, to promote adherence to other treatments such as exercise. An excellent reference to which the reader is referred for more information on these modalities as well as other PT techniques is *Geriatric Physical Therapy* (Guccione, 2000).

Thermal modalities such as hot and cold packs should always be used with caution, especially when the patient has compromised circulation, reduced sensation, or altered mental status. Thermal injuries can occur quickly and take many weeks to heal. Generally, heat is advised for chronic conditions or when increased flexibility is desired. Heat acts by increasing tissue perfusion and aids in the removal of metabolites from muscles in chronic spasm. Increased extensibility of tissues as well as reduction in pain perception also may result. Gentle exercise also improves blood flow to musculotendinous tissue and is an excellent adjunct to heat. Cold or cool treatments may be helpful for acute problems or for flares of persistent pain conditions. Cold will reduce the production of pain producing chemicals and may interfere with pain transmission. It may be applied with cold packs or ice massage.

Massage and soft tissue manipulation of tendon and ligamentous structures can improve extensibility and tolerance to biomechanical stresses. Relaxation routines, including deep breathing, visual imagery, and progressive relaxation, can reduce pain and associated muscle tension. These techniques are discussed in greater detail in chapter 3. Exercise can promote feelings of well-being and reduce pain through stimulation of circulation, improved flexibility, and improved muscle balance. Daytime activity can also serve to promote nighttime sleep.

Ultrasound uses the production of high-frequency sound waves to increase circulation, improve extensibility of soft tissue, and reduce pain. The pain reduction associated with ultrasound may be due to increased circulation or modification of neural tissue. Physical therapists choose between various frequencies and intensities of ultrasound, depending upon the acuity of the problem and desired outcomes. Phonophoresis combines anti-inflammatory medications (typically hydrocortisone, lidocaine, or salicylate) with ultrasound to help reduce localized inflammation.

Transcutaneous electrical nerve stimulation (TENS) delivers electrical nerve stimulation through electrodes placed on the skin's surface. This modality is used for a wide variety of neuropathic and musculoskeletal conditions associated with persistent pain. Portable battery units usually provide a balanced asymmetric biphasic wave. In conventional TENS, high-frequency low-amplitude current provides a cutaneous stimulation without muscle contraction. Other modes of TENS also are used, including high-amplitude, low-frequency, or brief-intense mode. Electrode placement varies, but patterns frequently used include electrodes placed proximal to the painful area, bracketing the painful area, or one electrode over the site of the pain and the other paraspinally over the related nerve root. Acupuncture sites also may be used. Generally, a trial period of 14 days to one month is recommended for TENS with persons who have persistent pain.

The demonstrated efficacy of TENS for both acute and persistent pain is theoretically based on several mechanisms. It may modify the sensitivity of peripheral receptors or free nerve endings responsible for the transmission of nociceptive stimuli, or block transmission of impulses from afferent A-delta and C fibers. Autonomic effects and increased production of endogenous opioids also have been demonstrated. The original gate control theory of Melzack and Wall hypothesized that TENS stimulation of large diameter A-beta afferents inhibited nociceptive input in the dorsal horn of the spinal cord. This theory has undergone many revisions and exact mechanisms of action remain unclear.

Contraindications to TENS include placement near demand-type pacemakers and use when operating automobiles or power machinery. Precaution should be exercised in patients with fixed-rate pacemakers, a history of cardiac problems, and when use is anticipated over the carotid sinus. Caution is important when the cause of the pain is undiagnosed or when intense stimulation is being considered in the vicinity of fragile tissues. Skin irritation under the electrodes may require modification of the mode of stimulation.

Pulsed and alternating currents also are used to promote cellular stimulation and beneficial tissue changes. When used at muscle contraction levels, the muscle-pumping action may improve lymphatic drainage and blood flow and promote relaxation after stimulation. *Interferential current* is popular in Europe and the United States and is purported to reach deeper tissues; however, studies indicate that any benefit over TENS is questionable. *Iontophoresis* uses direct current to drive analgesic and anti-inflammatory medications into specific tissue areas. Ions commonly used are similar to those used in phonophoresis and include hydrocortisone, mecholyl, lidocaine, and salicylate.

Fibromyalgia Syndrome

Fibromyalgia Syndrome (FMS) is a condition characterized by chronic widespread musculoskeletal pain, marked fatigue, and disturbed sleep. The American College of Rheumatology (ACR) in 1990 published criteria to render uniformity to the classification of this problem (Wolfe et al., 1990). While it is clear that examination of a patient suffering from FMS often elicits widespread muscular tenderness, nine pairs of tender point locations are described by the ACR in their definition, as these have been shown to be sensitive and reproducible sites of pain elicitation. They are examined by applying firm pressure of 4 kg/m² with the thumb or forefinger. Skin fold tenderness (i.e., light skin-fold pinching eliciting a painful response) is also a frequent examination finding.

In the setting of persistent pain such as in FMS, severity of symptoms is usually disproportionate to the degree of objective pathology found by the clinician. FMS affects women much more commonly than men, and has a prevalence in the general population of 2% (Wolfe, Ross, Anderson, Russell, & Hebert, 1995). Prevalence increases with age, with rates of 7% in women aged 60 to 79. FMS may be associated with other diseases. For example, it has an incidence of 12% in rheumatoid arthritis patients and up to 22% in systemic lupus erythematosus (SLE) (Morand, Miller, Whittingham, & Littlejohn, 1994). FMS symptoms overlap somewhat with those of chronic fatigue syndrome (CFS). Irritable bowel syndrome (IBS), migraines, and CFS are conditions commonly associated with FMS (Hudson, Goldenberg, Pope, Keck, & Schlesinger, 1992). There are likely to be shared physiological and psychological factors that account for this. Depression, affective disorders, and anxiety are more prevalent in FMS than in the general population (Moldofsky & Scarisbrick, 1976). Psychological disturbance that contributes to pain amplification and sleep difficulty is identified more often among FMS patients than in patients with other rheumatological disorders (Ahles, Yunus, Riley, Bradley, & Masi, 1984; Payne et al., 1982).

The clinical presentation of FMS is one of long-standing diffuse musculoskeletal pain, affecting the upper limbs, lower limbs, and trunk. Patients describe their discomfort as "pain all over." They may complain that physical contact such as a hug is very uncomfortable, that massages are intolerable, and that simple knocks against furniture amplify pain significantly. The pattern of pain is fairly constant in nature, though it typically increases on exertion, and is present nocturnally. Fatigue, as well as pain, limits physical activity. Patients also may describe stiffness. Nonrestorative sleep is reported in up to 70–80% of FMS patients. Sleep is described as light and restless and patients awaken easily. Abnormal electroencephalographic (EEG) activity has been found during sleep in FMS sufferers (Branco, Atalaia, & Paiva, 1994; Harding, 1998). While FMS patients with mild symptoms are aware of background pain but maintain normal working hours and social lives, others are so greatly incapacitated that they can participate in few or no daytime activities. Physical immobility, functional losses, and psychological factors then come into play and sometimes promote long-term disability.

Muscle biopsy has not demonstrated consistent pathological abnormality (Kalyan-Raman, Kalyan-Raman, Yunus, & Masi, 1984). As integrated mechanisms of the stress response, the sympathetic and hypothalamic-pituitary-adrenal axes have been studied, looking for physiological aberrations to account for FMS. Aberrations in autonomic nervous system regulation have been found. These include diminished heart rate variability (Martinez-Lavin, Hermosillo, Rosas, & Soto, 1998), impaired baroreflex response (Kelemen, Lang, Balint, Trocsanyi, & Muller, 1998), reduced peripheral cutaneous adrenergic activity and increased cholinergic activity in response to stressors (Qiao, Vaeroy, & Morkrid, 1991; Vaeroy, Qiao, Morkrid, & Forre, 1989).

Research into the role of the hypothalamic-pituitary-adrenal (HPA) axis in FMS supports the notion of a hypoadrenal state. The usual diurnal pattern of cortisol secretion in FMS is disturbed (Bengtsson & Bengtsson, 1988). Following HPA axis stimulation, a high ACTH response is achieved without a parallel increase in the cortisol response (Crofford et al., 1994; Griep, Boersma, & deKloet, 1994; Griep et al., 1998). In response to insulin-induced hypoglycemia, a reduced ACTH and adrenaline response has been demonstrated, in further support of an attenuated stress reaction (Adler, Kinsley, Hurwitz, Mossey, & Goldenberg, 1999). As yet, these abnormalities do not provide us with a cohesive explanation for the phenomenon of FMS.

While sympathetic blockade has been shown to significantly reduce rest pain and the number of tender points in FMS for the duration of the block (Bengtsson & Bengtsson, 1988), this mode of therapy does not provide a helpful avenue for long-term management. Treatment importantly includes reassurance and education about the nature of the diagnosis. There is often a high level of anxiety about more sinister causes of persistent pain. Patients frequently are reassured simply that there is an explanation for their symptoms. Pharmacological intervention has a limited role and is not the mainstay of treatment. Depression, if present, should be treated. Low-dose tricyclic antidepressants such as nortriptyline improve sleep quality and symptoms on the global assessment scale and lead to improvement in tender point score, pain, and fatigue (Carette, McCain, Bell, & Fam, 1986). Fluoxetine alone or in combination with amitriptyline also has beneficial effects (Goldenberg, Mayskiy, Mossey, Ruthazer, & Schmid, 1996), although both of these medications have substantial potential for adverse reactions in older adults. Attention to physical fitness is a key element in management. Aerobic exercise reduces tender point pain, increases work capacity, and improves global status (Melworm, Jakob, Walker, Peter, & Keul, 2000; Jentoft, Kvaivik, & Mengshoel, 2001). Management of psychosocial factors perpetuating pain, apart from treating depression, is the other focus of therapy. Interdisciplinary treatment programs may therefore be quite beneficial.

Systemic Inflammatory Disorders

PMR and Giant Cell Arteritis

Polymyalgia rheumatica (PMR) and giant cell arteritis share the same demographic pattern. They occur almost exclusively in those over the age of 50, with 90% of patients over 60 years of age (Hunder, 1997). The mean age of onset is 70 and the female-to-male ratio is in the order of 2:1. PMR is a syndrome of marked early morning stiffness, often hours in duration, with pain in the neck, shoulder girdle, hip girdle, and buttocks. It may be confined to either the upper or lower limbs, and symptom onset may be quite abrupt. An elevated ESR is typical. Examination reveals irritable shoulders and hips, representing the underlying pathology of synovitis in these joints.

PMR is usually exquisitely sensitive to oral corticosteroids in a dose of 15 mg of prednisone or less. A common mistake is using excessive doses in an older adult population more susceptible to the significant morbidity of this treatment. Robb-Nicholson et al. (1988) found that over a 5-year follow-up of 62 patients treated for PMR, 25% developed cataracts, a 4-fold increase when compared to untreated patients, and 19% developed vertebral fractures, 6-fold more than in untreated patients. The usual treatment duration is 12–24 months. It is our practice to start dose reduction once symptoms have stabilized after 3–4 weeks of treatment. Too rapid reduction will inevitably bring about a recurrence of symptoms. When the dose has been tapered to 10 mg, additional tapering by 1 mg every 3–4 weeks, guided by clinical symptoms and ESR monitoring, may help minimize relapse.

PMR in the older adult may present as an isolated syndrome or occur as the presenting feature of RA, in which case peripheral arthritis will develop. The association of PMR and giant cell arteritis in the older adult is well established. Symptoms of GCA, often referred to as temporal arteritis, should be explored in all patients ≥ age 50 with PMR. Other vasculitides such as Wegener's, Churg-Strauss, and polyarteritis nodosa, also may have polymyalgic symptoms as a clinical feature. These conditions must be borne in mind by the clinician treating a patient with PMR who is either unable to come off prednisone, has a persistently raised ESR despite low- to medium-dose corticosteroids, or develops a peripheral arthritis.

Giant cell arteritis (GCA) is the most common form of vasculitis in the older adult, with incidence rates varying between 0.26 per 100,000 in Japan, to 27/100,000 in Finland (the highest rates in northern Europe). Comparable rates of up to 24.0/100,000 exist in Olmsted County, Minnesota (Emmerich & Fiessinger, 1998; Franzen, Sutinen, & von Knorring, 1992). The label "temporal arteritis" is a misnomer, discounting the possibility of systemic vascular involvement; thus the name giant cell arteritis (GCA) is more appropriate.

GCA affects large and medium-sized arteries with well-developed internal and external elastic laminae. It preferentially affects the upper extremity branches of the aorta, in particular the extracranial vessels of the head. In deceased patients with active GCA, the highest incidence of severe artery involvement, in descending order, is: superficial temporal, vertebral, ophthalmic, and posterior ciliary. Almost any vascular bed, however, can be affected and rare cases of histologically proven gynecological, breast, prostate, coronary, and respiratory involvement have been reported (Bretal-Laranga et al., 1995; Cook, Bensen, Carroll, & Joshi, 1988; Ormsby & Haskell, 1997; Sendino et al., 1992; Stephenson & Underwood, 1986).

Ten to fifteen percent of GCA patients will have large-vessel involvement that may be the sole feature (Klein, Hunder, Stanson, & Sheps, 1975). Symptoms of upper limb claudication predominate, with pallor and pain involving the whole upper limb, not to be confused with the proximal muscle pain of PMR. Absent upper limb pulses and blood pressure in the affected arm provide strong clues to large-vessel disease, as do prominent vascular bruits. This group of patients is predominantly female, tends to be younger than the mean for GCA, has a longer duration of symptoms before the diagnosis is made, and has less frequent symptoms pertaining to cranial involvement (Brack, Martinez-Taboada, Stanson, Goronzy, & Weyand, 1999). Up to 50% will, therefore, have negative temporal artery biopsies. They also may have lower ESRs. Aortic rupture is a major risk. It is likely that the incidence is somewhat underestimated. Ostberg (1973) found that among 889 postmortem cases, 1.6% showed histological evidence of arteritis. His analysis included just two sections of the aorta and the temporal artery.

The clinical presentation of GCA depends on the vascular bed involved. New onset temporal headaches, scalp tenderness, and jaw claudication relate to temporal artery inflammation. Jaw claudication is defined as a clear history of jaw pain after commencement of chewing, but not at rest. It is caused by masseter and temporalis ischemia. This is not to be confused with temporomandibular OA, also more common in the older adult, which leads to more constant jaw pain and may be supported by the presence of radiographic changes and localized tenderness over the joint.

Ten percent of patients with GCA will present with purely constitutional symptoms. A raised ESR should raise suspicion of vasculitis. Visual loss is the most feared complication and is most frequently due to posterior ciliary artery inflammation leading to anterior ischemic optic neuropathy (Hayreh, Podharsky, & Zimmerman, 1998). Warning symptoms include transient visual loss or amaurosis fugax (a "curtain" coming down over the patient's field of vision); these should lead to prompt administration of corticosteroids. Other visual phenomena such as blurred vision, diplopia, and eye pain are less common. Respiratory tract symptoms such as cough, sore throat, and hoarse voice may occur in approximately 10% of patients (Larson, Hall, Hepper, & Hunder, 1984). Ischemia secondary to bronchial artery involvement that accounts for these symptoms has been found at autopsy in patients with GCA.

We now better understand that one requires only a low index of suspicion to proceed with temporal artery biopsy. Buchbinder and Dietsky (1992) confirmed this in a decision analysis. The gold standard of treatment is corticosteroids. Though effective, they are associated with significant potential side effects in the older adult population. The diagnosis, therefore, must be made with certainty if therapy is to be continued for the usual 12–18 months. Bilateral 4 cm biopsies are advised to maximize the chance of identifying GCA, as histologically it is characterized by skip lesions. Unilateral biopsy will miss 15% of cases. A biopsy is most helpful in its high negative predictive value for the condition. Visual loss almost never occurs in the setting of a negative temporal artery biopsy in untreated patients and is very unlikely to occur after treatment is initiated. The Mayo Clinic series from 1965–1980 supports this, demonstrating 134 biopsies (46 positive, 88 negative) in which no patient with a negative temporal artery biopsy who was not treated for GCA developed visual loss (Hall et al., 1983). Other vasculitides such as Wegener's granulomatosis and polyarteritis nodosa also may be found in the temporal arteries (Brack et al., 1999; Ostberg, 1973).

SETTING-SPECIFIC CONSIDERATIONS

Care of older adults with persistent pain from musculoskeletal disorders should be guided by functional status and comorbidities, rather than setting of care per se. For example, the older athlete who is otherwise healthy may present with injuries similar to younger active persons, while the frail older adult who lives in a long-term-care facility may have multiple medical, cognitive, and psychiatric comorbidities accompanying musculoskeletal disorder. These individuals on opposite ends of the older adult physiologic/functional spectrum require different therapeutic approaches. With the older athlete, one should remember the importance of earlier mobilization, longer healing times, and a higher incidence of previous contributing injuries and overuse syndromes. The treatment, however, may be similar to that prescribed for a younger individual. Frail older adults, on the other hand, may require more education and involvement of their caregivers and support network. Cognitive deficits, depending on their severity, mandate intimate involvement of the caregiver in the plan of care.

Mild deficits may simply require very explicit and simplified written and pictorial instructions.

Because of the many potential toxicities associated with pharmacological treatments in older adults, it behooves the practitioner, when appropriate, to first consider nondrug management such as those discussed in this chapter. While nursing home residents are in many ways viewed as a disadvantaged population, they are advantaged in their ready access to physical therapists trained to deliver these safe nonpharmacologic modalities. For older adults who reside in the community, physical therapy services may be limited by Medicare restrictions, depending on the nature of the underlying condition; private reimbursement or education of caregivers to provide services may be necessary. Issues of transportation also may be restrictive. In-home physical therapy services to frail older persons may be limited by the amount of equipment that is practical to carry into the home. Generally, the breadth of services available to older adults with musculoskeletal disorders reflects the specialized knowledge of the primary practitioner and/or rheumatologist and physical therapist. The ultimate goal of all providers of care must be optimizing the patient's function and quality of life.

SUMMARY/RECOMMENDATIONS

1. Musculoskeletal disorders associated with a wide variety of underlying physical pathology are the most common cause of pain-associated disability in older adults. In order to provide optimal care for the older adult persistent pain sufferer, primary practitioners should know how to evaluate and manage these disorders, and refer for consultative care when necessary.
2. Because of the prevalence of minor serologic abnormalities in healthy older adults, the evaluation and treatment of patients with musculoskeletal pain should focus on clinical signs and symptoms.
3. Radiographic imaging studies (e.g., plain films, MRI, CT) commonly reveal pathology in asymptomatic older adults (e.g., osteoarthritis, CPPD deposition); thus they should be obtained only after thorough clinical evaluation and only if their results will alter management.
4. Myofascial pain is very common in persistent pain sufferers; the primary practitioner should be familiar with the historical features and physical examination findings that support this diagnosis.
5. Although systemic medications often are prescribed to treat persistent pain in older adults with musculoskeletal disorders, noninvasive physical therapy modalities may serve as useful primary or adjunctive treatment. It is important, therefore, to involve a physi-

cal therapist in both the evaluation and the treatment of the majority of older adults with persistent musculoskeletal pain.

6. In addition to underlying dense tissue pathology, biomechanical abnormalities (e.g., poor posture, leg length discrepancy), and generalized weakness may contribute to and complicate pain in older adults. A physical therapist skilled in the evaluation and treatment of persistent pain conditions should be an integral part of the treatment team.

7. Inflammatory arthritides are less common than noninflammatory causes of musculoskeletal pain in older adults. Familiarity with their presentation, however, is essential because of the frequent need to manage them using toxic medications. Referral to a rheumatologist should be considered early.

8. Some musculoskeletal disorders, such as myofascial pain and fibromyalgia, may be difficult to manage with medications and physical therapy alone. Involvement of a psychologist for the treatment of psychosocial contributors may be a key component of treatment.

CASE STUDIES

Case 1

A 91-year-old woman was referred to the pain clinic for evaluation and treatment of a 2–3-year history of right-sided headaches, neck pain, and facial pain. She also reported difficulty turning her head, but no weakness or radiation of pain into the upper extremities. She started to wear a soft collar a year ago and to sleep with three pillows to support her head. The patient stated, "I can control the pain by not doing anything." She had significantly curtailed her involvement in social activities, and her ADLs had become increasingly difficult to complete independently. She was reluctant to come to the clinic, stating, "I've tried physical therapy before; it didn't help." Plain x-rays showed osteoarthritis of the cervical spine. Prior treatment included chiropractic manipulation, physical therapy, and electrical stimulation, without improvement in her symptoms. Physical examination revealed marked anterior positioning of the head, kypho-scoliosis, and markedly restricted cervical range of motion in axial extension (chin tuck), axial rotation, and lateral flexion accompanied by pain. All cervical musculature was hypertonic and tender to palpation. There were multiple taut bands and trigger points. The patient also had an unsteady gait and decreased standing balance.

Physical therapy diagnoses were (1) myofascial and mechanical head and neck pain, (2) deconditioning, (3) postural abnormalities, and (4) abnormal/unsteady gait. Treatment goals were to (1) decrease pain, (2) increase cervical motion, (3) correct posture and gait, and (4) enhance ADL and AADL performance. The patient received eight treatments consisting of heat; soft tissue massage, including trigger point treatment and gentle passive stretches; and a home exercise program (HEP) with instruction in correct stretching techniques, posture and gait exercises, flare management techniques, and proper head and neck positioning. She was extensively educated to improve her HEP adherence, particularly with regard to her need to take an active approach to the pain problem. Over the course of treatment, the patient's pain decreased, cervical range of motion increased, muscle tone normalized, and she began to engage in more social activities, including planning a family dinner party at her home.

Discussion

This case is instructive in several ways. Often patients are quite discouraged if previous physical therapy treatment has not been successful. If improper techniques have been used in the past, therapeutic inefficacy or exacerbation of pain may result. In the case of myofascial pain as experienced by this patient, specific passive techniques including skin mobilization, deep tissue massage, and trigger point techniques must be used before progressing to active stretching and strengthening exercises. If an active approach is used early on, worsening of pain and nonadherence to treatment recommendations are likely to result. Use of myofascial techniques (at least 15–20 minutes are recommended) and gentle stretches can be quite effective in reducing muscular discomfort, resulting in encouraging the patient. This encouragement will help to institute and maintain the patient's active involvement in treatment, which will in turn produce a lasting therapeutic effect with regard to reduced pain and improved functional status. This case also teaches us the importance of educating older adults with persistent pain regarding the pain cycle (i.e., the spiraling detrimental effect of pain, rest, and inactivity) in order to promote HEP adherence. Finally, we are taught the importance of a careful and comprehensive assessment of the older adult with regional musculoskeletal pain. This patient's primary complaint was neck pain and headaches, but she also had significant impairment of her balance and gait that impaired her ADL independence. The treatment program was necessarily broadly focused and resulted in significant improvement in the patient's quality of life.

Case 2

An 82-year-old woman with fibromyalgia and generalized pain complaints for 24 years was referred to the pain clinic's fibromyalgia interdisciplinary treatment program. Her other diagnoses included cervical spine osteoarthritis, tension-type headaches, mechanical shoulder pain, fatigue, and depression. She had been treated over the years with nerve blocks, physical therapy, chiropractic manipulation, and multiple medication trials, none of which provided significant or lasting relief. The patient was in the midst of a pain flare lasting several months that caused her to reduce participation in social activities. She was independent in all ADLs, but she found them difficult because of pain. She used heat, rest, and over-the-counter analgesics for pain relief. Physical examination revealed postural changes, a guarded gait pattern with sufficient standing balance, and 18/18 fibromyalgia tender points. Strength was 3+ – 4–/5 throughout, indicative of general deconditioning.

The patient was enrolled in a 3-week (9 separate days, 6 hours/day) interdisciplinary treatment program. Physical therapy consisted of instruction in proper exercise techniques (patients are asked to stretch to a point of a "feel good" stretch without increasing their baseline pain), whole-body stretching, and a strengthening and conditioning program including aerobic exercises. A key component of the program is education regarding pain self-management techniques and development of a progressive HEP that patients are to perform twice a day for one hour.

The patient was initially very skeptical about her ability to tolerate the program, so it was modified in order to allow her to take a nap at lunchtime. With this minor adaptation the patient was able to complete the program. She initially needed frequent encouragement to exercise because she was fearful about increasing her pain and injuring herself, stating, "I am much older than the other patients [in the group]." She quickly realized, however, that her fears and worries were similar to the other fibromyalgia patients in the program. Over the course of the program she was able to actively decrease her pain with exercises and manage it with flare management techniques. She developed high self-efficacy, improved mobility, and ease of ADL performance. The patient thought that the program was very beneficial and she felt a sense of accomplishment in her ability to follow it through to completion.

Discussion

This patient had a long-standing pain problem that had never been addressed in a comprehensive way. Treatment had been focused on regional pain, but her fibromyalgia per se was never dealt with. With only minor modifications to the treatment program the patient was able to benefit substantially. She ultimately learned that her pain and functional compromise were related to her fibromyalgia rather than to her age. She benefited from sharing her experiences with the other fibromyalgia patients in the group even though most were younger. Group therapy can be a very powerful tool in pain rehabilitation of the older adult and certainly should be considered for the older pain patient who is not limited by significant medical comorbidities. This case also demonstrates the effectiveness of interdisciplinary treatment programs for older adults with refractory pain syndromes.

REFERENCES

Adler, G. K., Kinsley, B. T., Hurwitz, S., Mossey, C. J., & Goldenberg, D. L. (1999). Reduced hypothalamic-pituitary and sympathoadrenal responses to hypoglycemia in women with fibromyalgia syndrome. *Am J Med, 106,* 534–543.

Ahles, T. A., Yunus, M. B., Riley, S. D., Bradley, J. M., & Masi, A. T. (1984). Psychological factors associated with primary fibromyalgia syndrome. *Arthritis Rheum, 27*(10), 1101–1106.

Atroshi, I., Gummeson, C., Johnsson, R., Ornstein, E., Ranstam, J., & Rosen, I. (1999). Prevalence of carpal tunnel syndrome in a general population. *JAMA, 14*(282), 153–158.

Bajocchi, G., La Corte, R., Locaputo, A., Govoni, M., & Trotta, F. (2000). Elderly onset rheumatoid arthritis: Clinical aspects. *Clin Exp Rheumatol, 18*(4 Suppl. 20), S49–S50.

Barron, O. A., Glickel, S. Z., & Eaton, R. G. (2000). Basal joint arthritis of the thumb. *J Am Acad Orthop Surg, 8*(5), 314–323.

Bengtsson, A., & Bengtsson, M. (1988). Regional sympathetic blockade in primary fibromyalgia. *Pain, 33,* 161–167.

Berthier, S., Toussirot, E., & Wendling, D. (1998). Acute benign edematous polyarthritis in the elderly (or RS3PE syndrome): Clinical course apropos of 13 cases. [Article in French]. *Presse Med, 27*(34), 1718–1722.

Binder, A., Hazleman, B. L., Parr, G., & Roberts, S. (1986). A controlled study of oral prednisolone in frozen shoulder. *Br J Rheumatol, 25*(3), 288–292.

Boden, S. D., Davis, D. O., Dina, T. S., Patronas, N. J., & Wiesel, S. W. (1990). Abnormal magnetic-resonance scans of the lumbar spine in asymptomatic subjects: A prospective investigation. *J Bone Joint Surg Am, 72*(3), 403–408.

Brack, A., Martinez-Taboada, A., Stanson, A., Goronzy, J. J., & Weyand, C. M. (1999). Disease pattern in cranial and large-vessel giant cell arteritis. *Arthritis Rheum, 42,* 311–317.

Branco, J., Atalaia, A., & Paiva, T. (1994). Sleep cycles and alpha delta sleep in fibromyalgia syndrome. *J Rheumatol, 21*, 1113–1117.

Bretal-Laranga, M., Insua-Vilarino, S., Blanco-Rodriguez, J., Caamano-Freire, M., Mera-Varela, A., & Lamas-Cedron, P. (1995). Giant cell arteritis limited to the prostate. *J Rheum, 22*(3), 566–568.

Buchbinder, R., & Dietsky, A. S. (1992). Management of suspected giant cell arteritis: A decision analysis. *J Rheumatol, 19*(8), 1220–1228.

Buckland-Wright, J. C., Macfarlane, D. G., Fogelman, I., Emery, P., & Lynch, J. A. (1991). Technetium 99m methylene diphosphonate bone scanning in osteoarthritic hands. *Eur J Nucl Med, 18*, 12–16.

Bulgen, D. Y., Binder, A. I., Hazleman, B. L., & Roberts, S. (1984). Frozen shoulder: Prospective clinical study with an evaluation of three treatment regimens. *Ann Rheum Dis, 43*(3), 353–360.

Bunker, T. D., Esler, C. N., & Leach, W. J. (1997). Rotator cuff tear of the hip. *J Bone Joint Surg Br, 79*(4), 618–620.

Cantini, F., Salvarini, C., Olivieri, I., Barozzi, L., Macchioni, L., Niccoli, L., Padula, A., Pavlica, P., & Boiardi, L. (1999). Remitting seronegative symmetrical synovitis with pitting oedema (RS3PE) syndrome: A prospective follow up and magnetic resonance imaging study. *Ann Rheum Dis, 58*(4), 230–236.

Carette, S., Leclaire, R., Marcoux, S., Morin, F., Blaise, G. A., St-Pierre, A., Truchon, R., Parent, F., Levesque, J., Bergeron, V., Montminy, P., & Blanchette, C. (2997). Epidural corticosteroid injections for sciatica due to herniated nucleus pulposus. *NEJM, 336*(23), 1634–1640.

Carette, S., McCain, G. A., Bell, D. A., & Fam, A. G. (1986). Evaluation of amitiyptyline in primary fibrositis: A double blinded placebo controlled study. *Arthritis Rheum, 29*(5), 655–659.

Caspi, D., Flusser, G., Farber, I., Ribak, J., Leibovitz, A., Habot, B., Yaron, M., & Segal, R. (2001). Clinical, radiologic, demographic, and occupational aspects of hand osteoarthritis in the elderly. *Semin Arthritis Rheum, 30*(5), 321–331.

Chard, M. D., Hazleman, R., Hazleman, B. L., King, R. H., & Reiss, B. B. (1991). Shoulder disorders in the elderly: A community survey. *Arthritis Rheum, 34*(6), 766–769.

Connell, D., Burke, F., Coombes, P., McNealy, S., Freeman, D., Pryde, D., & Hoy, G. (2001). Sonographic examination of lateral epicondylitis. *Am J Roentgenol, 176*(3), 777–782.

Cook, D. J., Bensen, W. G., Carroll, J. J., & Joshi, S. (1988). Giant cell arteritis of the breast. *CMAJ, 139*, 513–515.

Crofford, L. J., Pillemer, S. R., Kalogeras, K. T., Cash, J. M., Michelson, D., Kling, M. A., Sternberg, E. M., Gold, P. W., Chrousos, G. P., & Wilder, R. L. (1994). Hypothalamic-pituitary-adrenal axis perturbations in patients with fibromyalgia. *Arthritis Rheum, 37*(11), 1583–1592.

Deal, C. L., Meenan, R. F., Goldenberg, D. L., Anderson, J. J., Sack, B., Pastan, R. S., & Cohen, A. S. (1985). The clinical features of elderly-onset rheumatoid arthritis: A comparison with younger-onset disease of similar duration. *Arthritis Rheum, 28*(9), 987–994.

Dettori, J. R., Bullock, S. H., Sutlive, T. G., Franklin, R. J., & Patience, T. (1995). The effects of spinal flexion and extension exercises and their associated postures in patients with acute low back pain. *Spine, 20*(21), 2303–2312.

Dieppe, P., Cushnaghan, J., Young, P., & Kirwan, J. (1993). Prediction of the progression of joint space narrowing in osteoarthritis of the knee by bone scintigraphy. *Ann Rheum Dis, 52*(8), 557–563.

Djaldetti, R., Mosberg-Galili, R., Sroka, H., Merims, D., & Melamed, E. (1999). Camptocormia (bent spine) in patients with Parkinson's disease—characterisation and possible pathogenesis of an unusual phenomenon. *Mov Disord, 14*(3), 443–447.

Doherty, M. (2000). Genetics of hand osteoarthritis. *Osteoarthritis Cartilage, 8*(Suppl. A), S8–S10.

Emmerich, J., & Fiessinger, J. N. (1998). Epidemiology and etiological factors in giant cell arteritis (Hortons disease and Takayasu's disease). *Ann Med Interne, 149*(7), 425–432.

Forristall, R. M., Marsh, H. O., & Pay, N. T. (1988). Magnetic resonance imaging and contrast CT of the lumbar spine: Comparison of diagnostic methods and correlation with surgical findings. *Spine, 13*(9), 1049–1054.

Franzen, P., Sutinen, S., & von Knorring, J. (1992). Giant cell arteritis and polymyalgia rheumatica in a region of Finland: An epidemiologic, clinical and pathologic study, 1984–1988. *J Rheumatol, 19,* 273–276.

Gavant, M. L., Rizk, T. E., Gold, R. E., & Flick, P. A. (1994). Distention arthrography in the treatment of adhesive capsulitis of the shoulder. *J Vasc Interv Radiol, 5,* 305–309.

Goldenberg, D., Mayskiy, M., Mossey, C., Ruthazer, R., & Schmid, C. (1996). A randomised double-blind crossover trial of fluoxetine and amitiyptyline in the treatment of fibromyalgia. *Arthritis Rheum, 39*(11), 1852–1859.

Gonzalez-Gay, M. A., Hajeer, A. H., Dababneh, A., Makki, R., Garcia-Porrua, C., Thomson, W., & Ollier, W. (2001). Seronegative rheumatoid arthritis in elderly and polymyalgia rheumatica have similar patterns of HLA association. *J Rheumatol, 28,* 122–125.

Griep, E. N., Boersma, J. W., & deKloet, R. (1994). Pituitary release of growth hormone and prolactin in the primary fibromyalgia syndrome. *J Rheum, 21,* 2125–2130.

Griep, E. N., Boersma, J. W., Lentjes, E. G. W. M., Prins, P. A., Van der Korst, J. K., & de Kloet, R. (1998). Function of the hypothalamic-pituitary-adrenal axis in patients with fibromyalgia and low back pain. *J Rheumatol, 25,* 1374–1381.

Guccione, A. A. (2000). *Geriatric physical therapy* (2nd Ed.). St. Louis, MO: Mosby.

Hall, S., Persellin, S., Lie, J. T., O'Brien, P. C., Kurland, L. T., & Hunder, G. G. (1983). The therapeutic impact of temporal artery biopsy. *Lancet, 2*(8361), 1217–1220.

Hammer, D. S., Rupp, S., Ensslin, S., Kohn, D., & Seil, R. (2000). Extracorporeal shock wave therapy in patients with tennis elbow and painful heel. *Arch Orthop Trauma Surg, 120*(5–6), 304–307.

Harding, S. M. (1998). Sleep in fibromyalgia patients: Subjective and objective findings. *Am J Med Sci, 315*(6), 367–376.

Hay, E. M., Paterson, S. M., Lewis, M., & Croft, P. (1999). Pragmatic randomised controlled trial of local corticosteroid injection and naproxen for treatment of lateral epicondylitis of elbow in primary care. *BMJ, 319*(7215), 964–968.

Hayreh, S. S., Podharsky, P. A., & Zimmerman, B. (1998). Ocular manifestations of giant cell arteritis. *Am J Opthalmol, 125*(4), 509–520.

Hellier, J. P., Eliaou, J. F., Daures, J. P., Sany, J., & Combe, B. (2001). HLA-DRB1 genes and patients with late onset rheumatoid arthritis. *Ann Rheum Dis, 60*(5), 531–535.

Hides, J. A., Jull, G. A., & Richardson, C. A. (2001). Long-term effects of specific stabilizing exercises for first-episode low back pain. *Spine, 26,* e243–e248.

Hijoka, A., Suzuki, K., Makamura, T., & Hojo, T. (1993). Degenerative change and rotator cuff tears. An anatomical study in 160 shoulders of 80 cadavers. *Arch Orthop Trauma Surg, 112,* 61–64.

Howell, G. E. D., Biggs, R. E., & Bourne, R. B. (2001). Prevalence of abductor mechanism tears of the hips in patients with osteoarthritis. *J Arthroplasty, 16,* 121–123.

Hudson, J. I., Goldenberg, D. L., Pope, H. G., Keck, P. E., & Schlesinger, L. (1992). Comorbidity of fibromyalgia with medical and psychiatric disorders. *American Journal of Medicine, 92,* 363–367.

Hunder, G. G. (1997). Giant cell arteritis and polymyalgia rheumatica. *Med Clin North Am, 81,* 195–219.

Jentoft, E. S., Kvaivik, A. G., & Mengshoel, A. M. (2001). Effects of pool-based and land-based aerobic exercise on women with fibromyalgia/chronic widespread muscular pain. *Arthritis Rheum, 45,* 42–47.

Johnsson, K-E, Rosen, I., & Uden, A. (1992). The natural course of lumbar spinal stenosis. *Clin Orthop, 279,* 82–86.

Kagan, A., II. (1999, November). Rotator cuff tears of the hip. *Clin Orthop, 368* 135–140.

Kalyan-Raman, U. P., Kalyan-Raman, K., Yunus, M. B., & Masi, A. T. (1984). Muscle pathology in primary fibromyalgia syndrome: A light microscopic, histochemical and ultrastructural study. *J Rheumatol, 11*(6), 808–813.

Karbowski, K. (1999). The old and the new camptocormia. *Spine, 24*(14), 1494–1498.

Kelemen, J., Lang, E., Balint, G., Trocsanyi, M., & Muller, W. (1998). Orthostatic sympathetic derangement of baroflex in patients with fibromyalgia. *J Rheumatol, 25*(4), 823–824.

Kingzett-Taylor, A., Tirman, P. F., Feller, J., McGann, W., Prieto, V., Wischer, T., Cameron, J. A., Cvitanic, O., & Genant, H. K. (1999). Tendinosis and tears of gluteus medius and minimus muscles as a cause of hip pain: MR imaging findings. *Am J Roentgenol, 173*(4), 1123–1126.

Klein, R. G., Hunder, G. G., Stanson, A. W., & Sheps, S. G. (1975). Large artery involvement in giant cell (temporal) arteritis. *Ann Int Med, 83*(6), 806–812.

Koch, C. A., Doppman, J. L., Patronas, N. J., & Chrousos, G. P. (2000). Do glucocorticoids cause spinal epidural lipomatosis? When endocrinology and spinal surgery meet. *Trends Endocrinol Metab, 11*(3), 86–90.

Koes, B. W., Scholten, R. J. P. M., Mens, J. M. A., & Bouter, L. M. (1995). Efficacy of epidural steroid injections for low back pain and sciatica: A systematic review of randomised clinical trials. *Pain, 63,* 279–288.

Komori, H., Shinomiya, K., Nakai, O., Yamaura, I., Takda, S., Furuya, K. (1996). The natural history of herniated nucleus pulposis with radiculopathy. *Spine, 15*(21), 225–229.

Laiho, K., Tuohimehto, J., & Tilvis, R. (2001). Prevalence of rheumatoid arthritis and musculoskeletal disease in the elderly population. *Rheumatol Int, 20*(3), 85–87.

Laroche, M., Delisle, M. B., Aziza, R., Lagarrigue, J., & Mazieres, B. (1995). Is camptocormia a primary muscle disease? *Spine, 20*(9), 1011–1016.

Larson, T. S., Hall, S., Hepper, N. G., & Hunder, G. G. (1984). Respiratory tract symptoms as a clue to giant cell arteritis. *Ann Intern Med, 101*(5), 594–597.

Legaye, J., & Dimbolu, D. (1995). Camptocormia or reducible lumbar kyphosis in elderly subjects. Apropos of 2 cases of lipoid degeneration of the paravertebral muscles. [Article in French]. *Acta Orthop Belg, 61,* 278–281.

Lehman, C., Cuomo, F., Kummer, F. J., & Zuckerman, J. D. (1995). The incidence of full thickness rotator cuff tears in a large cadaveric population. *Bull Hosp Jt Dis, 54,* 30–31.

Manoussakis, M. N., Tzioufas, A. G., Silis, M. P., Pange, P. J., Goudevenos, J., & Moutsopoulos, H. M. (1987). High prevalence of anti-cardiolipin and other autoantibodies in a healthy elderly population. *Clin Exp Immunol, 69,* 557–565.

Marshall, S., Tardif, G., & Ashworth, N. (2000). Local corticosteroid injection for carpal tunnel syndrome (Cochrane Review). *Cochrane Database Syst Rev, 4,* CD001554.

Martinez-Lavin, M., Hermosillo, A. G., Rosas, M., & Soto, M. E. (1998). Circadian studies of autonomic nervous balance in patients with fibromyalgia. A heart rate variability analysis. *Arthritis and Rheumatism, 41*(11), 1966–1971.

McCarty, D. J., et al. (1981). Milwaukee shoulder: Association of microspheroids containing hydroxyapatite crystals, active collagenase and neutral protease with rotator cuff defects—I. Clinical aspects. *Arthritis & Rheumatism, 24,* 464–473.

McCullen, G. M., Spurling, G. R., & Webster, J. S. (1999). Epidural lipomatosis complicating lumbar steroid injections. *J Spinal Disord, 12*(6), 526–529.

Melworm, L., Jakob, E., Walker, U. A., Peter, H. H., & Keul, J. (2000). Patients with fibromyalgia benefit from aerobic endurance exercise. *Clin Rheumatol, 19*(4), 253–257.

Moldofsky, H., & Scarisbrick, P. (1976). Induction of neurasthenic musculoskeletal pain syndrome by selective sleep stage deprivation. *Psychosomat Med, 38,* 35–44.

Morand, E. F., Miller, M. H., Whittingham, B., & Littlejohn, G. O. (1994). Fibromyalgia syndrome and disease activity in systemic lupus erythematosis. *Lupus, 3*(3), 187–191.

Nirschl, R. P. (1995). Tennis elbow tendinosis: Pathoanatomy, nonsurgical and surgical management. In S. L. Gordon, S. J. Blair, & L. J. Fine (Eds.), *Repetitive motion disorders of the upper extremity* (pp. 467–479). Rosemont, IL: American Academy of Orthopaedic Surgeons.

Olive, A., del Blanco, J., Pons, M., Vaquero, M., & Tena, X. (1997). The clinical spectrum of remitting seronegative symmetrical synovitis with pitting edema. The Catalan Group for the study of RS3PE. *J Rheumatol, 24,* 333–336.

Ormsby, A. H., & Haskell, R. (1997). Giant cell arteritis of the uterus: Case report and review. *Pathology, 29,* 227–230.

Ostberg, G. (1973). On arteritis with special reference to polymyalgia arteritica. *Acta Pathol Microbiol Scand, 237*(Suppl.), 1–59.

Panni, A. S., Milano, G., Lucania, L., Fabbriciani, C., & Logroscino, C. A. (1996). Histological analysis of the coracoacromial arch: Correlation between age-related changes and rotator cuff tears. *Arthroscopy, 12*(5), 53, 1040.

Payne, T. C., Leavitt, F., Garron, D. C., Katz, R. S., Golden, H. E., Glickman, P. B., & Vanderplate, C. (1982). Fibrositis and psychological disturbance. *Arthritis Rheum, 25*(2), 213–217.

Perez-Sales, P. (1990). Camptocormia. *Br J Psychiatry, 157*, 765–767.

Qiao, Z., Vaeroy, H., & Morkrid, L. (1991). Electrodermal and microcirculatory activity in patients with fibromyalgia during baseline, acoustic stimulation and cold pressor tests. *J Rheum, 18*(9), 1383–1389.

Reeves, B. (1975). The natural history of the frozen shoulder syndrome. *Scand J Rheumatol, 4*(4), 193–196.

Robb-Nicholson, C., Chang, R. W., Anderson, S., Roberts, W. W., Longthe, J., Carson, J., Larson, M., George, D., Green, J., & Bryant, G., et al. (1988). Diagnostic value of the history and examination in giant cell arteritis: A clinical pathological study of 81 temporal artery biopsies. *J Rheumatol, 15*(12), 1793–1796.

Robertson, S. C., Tratnelis, V. C., Follett, K. A., & Menezes, A. H. (1997). Idiopathic spinal epidural lipomatosis. *Neurosurgery, 41*, 68–74.

Rompe, J. D., Hope, C., Kullmer, K., Heine, J., & Burger, R. (1996). Analgesic effect of extracorporeal shock-wave therapy on chronic tennis elbow. *J Bone Joint Surg Br, 78*, 233–237.

Russell, E. B., Hunter, J. B., Pearson, L., & McCarty, D. J. (1990). Remitting seronegative symmetrical synovitis with pitting edema—13 additional cases. *J Rheumatol, 17*(5), 633–639.

Sanmarti, R., Panella, D., Brancos, M. A., Canela, J., Collado, A., & Brugues, J. (1993). Prevalence of articular chondrocalcinosis in elderly subjects in a rural area of Catalonia. *Ann Rheum Dis, 52*(6), 418–422.

Schaeverbeke, T., Fatout, E., Marce, S., Vernhes, J. P., Halle, O., Antoine, J. F., Lequen, L., Bannwarth, B., & Dehais, J. (1995). Remitting seronegative symmetrical synovitis with pitting edema: Disease or syndrome? *Ann Rheum Dis, 54*(8), 681–684.

Sendino, A., Barbado, F. J., Gonzalez-Anglada, I., Aton, E., Lopez-Barea, F., & Vazquez, J. J. (1992). Temporal arteritis: A form of systemic panarteritis. *Ann Rheum Dis, 51*(9), 1082–1084.

Shbeeb, M. I., & Matteson, E. L. (1996). Trochanteric bursitis (greater trochanter pain syndrome). *Mayo Clin Proc, 71*(6), 565–569.

Solveborn, S. A. (1997). Radial epicondylalgia ("tennis elbow") treatment with stretching or forearm band: A prospective study with long term follow-up including range of motion measurements. *Scand J Med Sci Sports, 7*(4), 229–237.

Spaccarelli, K. C. (1996). Lumbar and caudal epidural corticosteroid injections. *Mayo Clin Proc, 71*, 169–178.

Stephenson, T. J., & Underwood, J. C. E. (1986). Giant cell arteritis: An unusual cause of palpable masses in the breast. *Br J Surg, 73*, 105.

Towheed, T. E., Anastassiades, T. P., Shea, B., Houpt, J., Welch, V., & Hochberg, M. C. (2001). Glucosamine therapy for treating osteoarthritis (Cochrane Review). *Cochrane Database Syst Rev* 1, CD002946.

Vaeroy, H., Qiao, Z., Morkrid, L., & Forre, O. (1989). Altered sympathetic nervous system response in patients with fibromyalgia (fibrositis syndrome). *J Rheum, 16*(11), 1460–1465.

Van Gerpen, J. A. (2001). Camptocormia secondary to early amyotrophic lateral sclerosis. *Mov Disord, 16*, 358–360.

van Schaardenburg, D., & Breedveld, F. C. (1994). Elderly-onset rheumatoid arthritis. *Semin Arthritis Rheum, 23*(6), 367–378.

Watson, L., Dalziel, R., & Story, I. (2000). Frozen shoulder: A 12-month clinical outcome trial. *J Shoulder Elbow Surg, 9*, 16–22.

Watts, R. W., & Silagy, C. A. (1995). A meta-analysis on the efficacy of epidural corticosteroids in the treatment of sciatica. *Anaesth Intens Care, 23*, 564–569.

Williams, M. E., Hadler, N. M., & Earp, J. A. (1982). Manual ability as a marker of dependency in geriatric women. *J Chronic Dis, 35*, 115–122.

Wolfe, F., et al. (1990). The American College of Rheumatology 1990 criteria for the classification of fibromyalgia. Report of the Multicentre Committee. *Arthritis Rheum, 33*(2), 160–172.

Wolfe, F., Ross, K., Anderson, J., Russell, I. J., & Hebert, L. (1995). The prevalence and characteristics of fibromyalgia in the general population. *Arthritis Rheum, 38*, 19–28.

Wong, S. M., Hui, A. C., Tang, A., Ho, P. C., Hung, L. K., Wong, K. S., Kay, R., & Li, E. (2001). Local vs systemic corticosteroids in the treatment of carpal tunnel syndrome. *Neurology, 56*(11), 1565–1567.

Wybier, M., Parlier-Cuau, C., Baque, M. C., Champsaur, P., Haddad, A., & Laredo, J. D. (1997). Distension arthrography in frozen shoulder syndrome. *Semin Musculoskeletal Radiol, 1*, 251–256.

Functional Assessment and Outcomes

5

Joan C. Rogers and Sharon M. G. Gwinn

The term *function* as used in reference to functional assessment, functional outcomes, functional status, or functional abilities, applies to multiple and diverse concepts. Rehabilitation professionals refer to limited muscle or arm function, restricted function in walking, or the inability to function as a mother or a carpenter. In these examples, function refers to a body organ or part, an activity of daily living, and participation in societal roles. Because of these different applications of the term, the meaning of functional assessment in relation to pain is unclear. Will the assessment focus on an organ, organ system, or body part with the intent of clarifying the origins and nature of pain? Or will it focus on pain-related restrictions in daily living activities or age-appropriate social roles? A similar confusion arises in regard to functional outcomes, functional status, and functional abilities. To clarify these ambiguities in terminology, the model of disablement proposed by the World Health Organization labeled dysfunctions at the level of body structures or functions as *impairments,* those at the level of activities of daily living as *activity limitations* or *disability,* and those at the level of social roles as *participation restrictions* or *handicap* (World Health Organization, 1980, 2001).

A comprehensive assessment of pain-related impairment takes into account the nature of the pain itself: pain location (where the pain occurs); pain duration (how long the pain has been ongoing, when the pain started, what caused it); pain timing (when the pain occurs and its constancy); pain intensity (how strong the pain is); and pain perception (what the pain feels like—tingling, aching, etc.). The assessment of pain-related impairment is dealt with elsewhere in this book (see chapter 2) and will not be expanded on here. The emphasis of this chapter on functional assessment and outcomes is on the effects of pain in daily life. The World Health Organization disablement model portrays these effects at two levels: activities and participation. When pain intensity is low, older adult patients may be able to carry out their usual activities of daily living. When it is intensified, however, they may no longer be able to perform their usual activities or may perform them with considerable difficulty. Hence, activity limitations emerge. When only a few activities are limited, role performance, which spans spousal, parental, familial, self-care, occupational, leisure, and health responsibilities, may be largely unaffected. For example, if pain occurs only when the arm is raised above 100°, it may be possible to rearrange task materials so that movements requiring more than 100° arm flexion are avoided. When adaptation does not occur, however, and when a substantial number of one's usual activities are negatively influenced by pain, role dysfunction appears. Thus, in the model of disablement, pain-related impairment may lead to restrictions in activities and participation. Adaptations in task performance designed to alleviate or eliminate the effects of pain may improve overall activity and role participation. Hence, a major goal of rehabilitative interventions is to enhance adaptive capacity.

Functional assessment instruments may concentrate on pain-related impairment, activity limitations, or participation restrictions, or they may span one, two, or all of these dimensions of disablement. Although a positive association is generally found between pain-related impairment and restrictions in activity and societal participation, the association is very complex. Despite severe pain, older adult patients may adapt the way they engage in activities to enable them to continue to pursue valued tasks (Arnoff, Feldman, & Campion, 2000). Thus, measures of pain-related impairment, activity limitations, or participation restrictions may yield differential and/or conflicting results. The intensity of pain experienced by patients may remain the same following rehabilitative interventions but their disability may lessen. Support for this observation comes from studies demonstrating modest or complex relationships between the severity of pain and disability (Fordyce et al., 1984; Grönblad et al., 1993; Hopman-Rock, Odding, Hofman, Kraaimaat, & Bijlsma, 1996; Leveille et al., 1999). A primary implication of the disparity between impairment and restrictions in activity and participation is that each of these dimensions of disablement contributes something unique to pain assessment. Hence, if information about patients' daily functioning despite pain is needed, it should be measured directly, and disability prognoses should not be projected from pain-related impairment measures.

EVIDENCE AND PRINCIPLES FOR PRACTICE

Pain, Activity Limitations, and Participation Restrictions

Studies of both community-based and institutionalized older adults suggest that persistent pain is highly prevalent in older adults. In one study (Brochet, Michel, Barberger-Gateau, & Dartigues, 1998), 33% of the community-based older adults experienced persistent pain, with the joints of the extremities (19%) and the back (12%) the most common sites. Other epidemiologic studies have yielded estimates between 25% and 75% for any type of pain and between 10% and 71% for musculoskeletal pain alone (Scudds & Robertson, 1998). Estimates of pain prevalence in long-term-care facilities are even higher, ranging from 49% to 83% (Fox, Raina, & Jadad, 1999).

Not only is pain highly prevalent in the older adult, it is also highly disabling. In a recent study, community-dwelling older adults with musculoskeletal pain indicated that they had the most difficulty performing household chores, such as vacuuming or yard work. In descending order of difficulty, the following daily living tasks also were named: rising from an armless chair, reaching above the head to retrieve a 5-pound object, climbing 5 stairs, bathing in the tub, bending to pick up an object from the floor, walking outdoors on level ground, shopping, and dressing. Less problematic, but still causing difficulty for at least 10% of the sample, were bed, car, and toilet transfers; washing and drying the body and hair; opening jars (previously opened), milk cartons and car doors; and turning faucets (Scudds & Robertson, 1998). The negative influence of low back pain is exhibited most often in bending over, but also has a prevalence in excess of 10% in walking, sitting, lying down, performing household chores, and sleeping (Lavsky-Shulan et al., 1985). Among institutionalized older adults, complaints of pain-related disability were expressed by 71% to 83% of the residents (Ferrell, Ferrell, & Osterweil, 1990). In addition to activity limitations, persistent pain is known to decrease quality of life (Hopman-Rock, Kraaimaat, & Bijlsma, 1997).

Categories of Activities

The effects of pain on activity are generally exhibited as difficulty performing an activity rather than inability to perform it (Leveille et al., 1999). Symptoms of increased difficulty in performing activities are awkward body mechanics, which are often instituted in attempts to avoid pain; slowed or retarded movement, resulting in activities taking longer to perform; modifications of the way activities are usually performed; and less frequent performance. In the case of persistent pain, these symptoms of task difficulty are generally present before patients actually stop performing activities.

Pain influences activities differentially depending on the location of pain and the movements involved in the activity. If pain is located in the joints of the dominant hand, pain will likely influence all upper-extremity activities, for example, buttoning buttons on the front of a shirt, obtaining a cup from an overhead cupboard, and stirring a pot of stew. If, however, the pain only occurs when the arm is moved above 45° flexion and abduction, buttoning buttons may not be problematic, while reaching overhead to obtain the cup and static holding of the arm over the pot are likely to be difficult. Thus, the primary questions to be answered in assessing pain-related activity limitations are: (1) Because of your pain, which of your usual daily living activities are difficult for you to perform? and (2) Which activities are you doing less often or have you stopped doing due to pain?

For the purposes of functional assessment, activities of daily living are generally grouped into four major categories: basic activities of daily living, instrumental activities of daily living, advanced activities of daily living, and work.

Basic activities of daily living

The term *basic activities of daily living* (BADL) refers to activities involving functional mobility and personal care (Rogers & Holm, 1997). Functional mobility includes ambulation or wheelchair mobility on different types of surfaces (e.g., pavement, gravel) and transfers from one surface to another (e.g., from standing to sitting on a kitchen chair or commode). Personal care includes feeding, hygiene, toileting, bathing, and dressing. BADL are viewed as essential to life. Patients typically perform BADL themselves independently, unless they have sufficient financial resources to hire a valet or personal maid. Exceptions may occur in regard to hair and nail care, where the services of beauticians or barbers, manicurists, and podiatrists may be substituted for self-performance.

Instrumental activities of daily living

Grouped under instrumental activities of daily living (IADL) are activities associated with independent living in the community (Lawton & Brody, 1969; Rogers & Holm, 1997). Although there is less agreement among clinicians about the specific activities included under IADL than under BADL, the listing generally includes using the telephone, getting to places beyond walking distance, shopping for groceries and other necessities, preparing meals, doing housework, taking medications, and managing money. At times, clothing care, handyman chores, and leisure activities are also listed as IADL. Whereas BADL are essential for human survival, IADL are essential for independent living in the community. Unlike BADL, older adults have more options for fulfilling IADL responsibilities. In regard to cooking for example, if older adults do not care to prepare meals or are unable to prepare them, they may have someone else in the household cook, go out to eat at a restaurant, or have meals delivered to their homes. Because of the various options available for fulfilling IADL, the assessment process must distinguish between activity limitations that are pain related and those that are due to personal preference. In other words, the baseline assessment covers patients' premorbid activity level or usual daily living activities.

Advanced activities of daily living

The category *advanced activities of daily living* (AADL) was devised by Reuben, Laliberte, Hiris, and Mor (1990) to capture activities that are more physically and socially challenging than IADL. AADL include participating in active sports that may cause one to become winded or work up a sweat, walking a mile or more without resting, walking a quarter mile or more without resting, entertaining in one's home, visiting the homes of others, going out to eat with others, working at a hobby, and traveling out of town.

Work

Because of the perception that housework is the only work that older adults engage in, work has been neglected in geriatric functional assessment. However, several societal trends suggest that work needs to be brought into the mainstream of geriatric practice. These trends include the escalating costs of consumer goods resulting in the financial need to work, the shrinking labor force that encourages older workers to remain at their jobs or to return to work, and the numbers of older adults serving as caregivers for their grandchildren, disabled spouse, family members, or friends. In addition, older adults may be committed to volunteer positions, such as delivering meals-on-wheels. Because of the diversity of work activities, disability assessment typically focuses on components of activities associated with work rather than on work tasks themselves. Examples of these components are walk one quarter mile; walk up 10 steps; stand for 2 hours; sit for 2 hours; reach overhead; reach forward to shake hands; grasp, lift, or carry 10 or 25 pounds; and stoop, crouch, or kneel (National Center for Health Statistics, 1987).

Hierarchy of activity categories

The four activity categories create a hierarchy, with each higher category encompassing activities that are more complex and physically demanding than the one below it. Thus, BADL are easier to perform than IADL, IADL are easier than AADL, and AADL are easier than work. Theoretically, the effects of pain-related impairment will be manifested first in work, followed by AADL, IADL, and last by BADL. Indeed, research suggests that when back pain interferes with the performance of BADL, activity limitation is predictive of relapse (Infante-Rivard & Lortie, 1997) and delayed return to usual activities (Coste, Delecoeuillerie, Cohen, Le Parc, & Paolaggi, 1994). The hierarchy is beneficial for directing clinicians' attention to the full range of daily living activities, including those beyond the bare essentials that lead toward an improved quality of life.

Assessment of Activity Limitations (Disability) and Participation Restrictions (Handicap)

Pain-related activity limitations may be assessed either through a patient's self-report or a clinician's ratings. The patient report includes interviews, questionnaires, diaries, and subjective summary indices. Clinician ratings incorporate performance testing and objective summary indices. Assessment of participation restrictions is generally restricted to self-reports because of the breadth, diversity, and personalized nature of the activities that comprise any role.

Patient report: Interview

The clinical interview is perhaps the most common method of assessment used in patient care. Interviewing may be restricted to patients or may include family members and friends. Patients are generally motivated to tell the "story" of their pain experience. Inquiry about the influence of pain on lifestyle should focus on (1) activities that patients perform that do not elicit pain; (2) activities that patients perform that do elicit pain and the level of pain that accompanies performance; (3) activities that patients refrain from performing or perform less often due to pain; (4) accommodations that patients have made in activity performance or participation due to pain; (5) patients' understanding of pain, especially their perceptions about their ability to control pain; and (6) patients' activity and participation goals. Because the significance of any activity varies from patient to patient, it is important to ascertain the specific activities that patients perceive as problematic. A simple way of obtaining this information is to inquire about a patient's chief activity complaint. Interestingly, however, the severity of patients' primary pain complaint has not been found to be particularly sensitive to change (Beurskens, de Vet, & Koke, 1996). The clinical interview targets patients' priorities for activity and participation, and hence for intervention; furnishes insight into disparities in performance and participation patterns (e.g., why watching television is painful but going out to movies is not); and yields an assessment of patients' problem-solving and coping abilities.

Patient report: Questionnaires

The need to demonstrate the effectiveness and efficacy of pain interventions has spurred the development of standardized self-report functional assessment questionnaires. A comprehensive review of these instruments is beyond the scope of this chapter. Instruments were selected for inclusion that are commonly used in practice and that reflect a variety of instrument types. The Pain Disability Index and Medical Outcome Survey-Pain Index are generic pain instruments. The Oswestry Disability Questionnaire, Roland and Morris Disability Questionnaire, Quebec Back Pain Disability Scale, and Neck Pain and Disability Scale are pain instruments devised for specific body parts. The Functional Status Index is a generic functional assessment instrument for chronic disabling conditions. The presentation of each instrument includes information about content (the activities or roles covered), reliability (the extent to which scores are reproducible), validity (the extent to which the instrument measures what it purports to measure), responsiveness (the ability to detect clinically important change), and practicality (ease of administration and scoring).

Although most of these questionnaires have included older adults in the development process, none has been specifically tested on older adults. Hence, clinicians need to be aware that their content may not include activities that are most relevant to pain elicitation in older adults and that they may not be as valid or as reliable in this population as they are in younger populations. Further, unless the pain-eliciting activities are included on the questionnaire, it cannot document improvement following intervention. Therefore, using a questionnaire in combination with an interview is recommended because this procedure allows information obtained from the questionnaire to be cross-validated with that obtained from the interview and vice versa. There is suggestive evidence that, compared to younger adults, older adults underreport pain-related disability (Tait, Chibnall, & Krause, 1990). A recently devised instrument, the Geriatric Pain Measure (Ferrell, Stein, & Beck, 2000) holds promise because it was specifically developed for use with older adults. Further, it uses a simple dichotomous rating system (no, yes) and summarizes the experience of activity-related pain into clinically useful categories: disengagement from activities due to pain and pain with ambulation, strenuous activities, and other activities.

Pain Disability Index (PDI) (Tait, Chibnall, & Krause, 1990)

The PDI is a 7-item self-report questionnaire that measures pain interference with the performance of 7 social roles: family and home responsibilities, recreation, social activity, occupation, sexual behavior, self-care, and life-support (e.g., eating, breathing). Sample activities are provided for each role. Each role is rated on an ordinal scale ranging from 0 (no disability) to 10 (total disability). The total PDI score can range from 0 to 70. The PDI has high internal consistency (Cronbach's alpha = 0.86) (Tait et al., 1990). Test-retest reliability, using prehospital and hospital admission scores, was modest ($r = 0.44$). Compared to patients with low PDI scores, patients with high PDI scores reported more psychological distress, severe pain characteristics, and activity limitations, thus providing evidence of construct validity. They also exhibited higher levels of objectively assessed pain behaviors (Tait et al., 1990). Former inpatients scored higher than former outpatients (Tait, Pollard, Margolis, Duckro, & Krause, 1987) and working patients scored higher than patients on sick leave (Grönblad, Järvinen, Hurri, Hupli, & Karaharju, 1994).

Medical Outcomes Survey Pain Index (MOS-PI) (Sherbourne, 1992)

Of the 12 items on the MOS-PI, 6 comprise the Pain Effects subscale and inquire about the effects of pain on mood, mobility, sleep, work inside and outside the house, recreation, and enjoyment. Pain effects are rated on a 5-point scale (1 = low pain interference, 5 = extreme pain interference). Higher scores indicate greater activity limitations. An additional item, Days Pain Interfered, records the number of days over the past 4 weeks that pain interfered with usual activities. The remainder of the survey involves pain severity. The MOS-PI requires about 5 minutes to complete. A total score can be calculated for all items (MOS-PI) or three subscale scores can be derived (Pain Effects, Days Pain Interfered, Pain Severity). The MOS-PI and Pain Effects subscale have high internal consistency ($r = 0.93$ and 0.91 respectively). The Pain Effects subscale correlated $r = 0.95$ with the MOS-PI and $r = 0.71$ with the Days Pain Interfered subscale. Higher validity coefficients were obtained between the Pain Effects subscale and a physical role limitation measure ($r = 0.66$) than with an emotional role limitation measure ($r = 0.39$).

Oswestry Disability Questionnaire (ODQ) (Fairbank, Davies, Couper, & O'Brien, 1980)

The ODQ, a self-administered questionnaire, includes 10 performance sections selected from other disability questionnaires for their relevance to the daily living problems experienced by people with low back pain. The sections inquire about pain intensity, personal care, lifting, walking, sitting, standing, sleeping, sex life, social life, and traveling. Each section is rated on a 6-point ordinal scale, consisting of statements indicative of progressively greater difficulty. The ratings range from 0 to 5, with 5 representing the greatest disability. For example, on the walking section, a rating of 0 indicates that pain does not interfere with walking, while a score of 5 indicates that patients spend most of their time in bed and have to crawl to the toilet. Patients select the statement that most accurately describes their performance. A total score (maximum = 50) is derived by summing the section scores and doubling this figure to obtain a total score expressed as a percentage. The ODQ can be completed in 3.5 to 5 minutes and scored in 1 minute. Test-retest reliability of the ODQ using scores obtained on 2 consecutive days yielded a coefficient of $r = 0.99$ (Fairbank et al., 1980). An intraclass correlation coefficient of 0.83 was obtained for test-retest reliability (Grönblad et al., 1993). Validity is based on the weekly improvement observed over 3 weeks in patients with a first occurrence of low back pain (Fairbank et al.). Further evidence of validity comes from significant associations (Kendall's tau) of performance-based assessments of lifting, sitting, and walking tasks with relevant ODQ items (Fisher & Johnston, 1997). Research suggests that ODQ is more responsive to change in low back patients than the SF-36 (Taylor, Taylor, Foy, & Fogg, 1999) and comparable to the Roland-Morris Disability Questionnaire (Stratford, Binkley, Solomon, Gill, & Finch, 1994).

Disability Questionnaire (DQ) (Roland & Morris, 1983)

The DQ is a 24-item self-report questionnaire that measures self-rated disability due to low back pain. Statements from the Sickness Impact Profile that seemed most applicable to back pain were selected for inclusion on the DQ. The phrase "because of my back or back pain" was added to each statement so that only disability due to back pain would be rated. A dichotomous response format is used, with yes indicating that patients have difficulty with that particular activity and no indicating that they do not have difficulty. One point is given for every item answered yes. The total score may range from 0 (no disability) to 24 (severe disability). The DQ can be completed in 5 minutes and scored in 1 minute. Test–retest reliability, with both tests done on the same day, was established as $r = 0.91$. Validity was established by comparing DQ ratings to a 6-point pain severity scale. All results fell within the 95% confidence interval, indicating good agreement between the disability and impairment instruments. Agreement between physical signs (e.g., physician rating of spine flexion) and DQ scores was not as clear. Evidence of scale responsiveness comes from correlations of change scores on the DQ with improvements in spine flexion, straight-leg raising, and self-rated pain severity (Deyo & Centor, 1986). The ROC curve of the score change for the DQ was greater than that of the ODQ, indicating its greater sensitivity (Beurskens, de Vet, & Koke, 1996). For making decisions in regard to individual patients, the DQ performs best when patients' baseline scores are between 4 and 20 (Stratford et al., 1996).

The Quebec Back Pain Disability Scale (QBPD) (Kopec et al., 1995)

The QBPD is a 20-item self-report instrument designed to assess the level of functional disability in individuals with back pain. The items include actions (e.g., stand up for 20–30 minutes), BADL (e.g., put on socks), and IADL (e.g., carry two bags of groceries). Items are rated on a 0 (not difficult at all) to 5 (unable to do) scale. A disability score is expressed as a mean score calculated as the total divided by the number of items answered. The QBPD can be completed in less than 5 minutes. Cronbach's alpha coefficient was 0.96 and test-retest reliability, with retesting done within 2 to 4 days, was high (intraclass correlation coefficient = 0.92). Evidence of validity is gleaned from the strong correlations between the OBPD and other disability scales: $r = 0.77$ with the DQ, $r = 0.80$ with the ODQ, and, $r = 0.72$ with the physical function scale of the SF-36. Correlations between the QBPD and a 7-point pain impairment scale were lower, ranging from $r = 0.51$ to 0.54. Patients having prior back surgery, previous hospitalizations, or using injections and drugs for pain had higher QBPD scores than patients not having these characteristics. Mean QBPD scores improved significantly over 6 months.

Functional Status Index (FSI) (Jette, 1987)

The FSI, a self-report instrument, includes 18 items in 5 categories: mobility, personal care, hand activities, home chores, and social role activities. Each item is rated for (1) difficulty experienced while doing the task (1 = no, 4 = severe), (2) pain experienced while doing the task (1 = no pain; 4 = severe); and (3) the assistance needed to complete the task (0 = independent, 4 = unable or unsafe). Patients rate their experience over the past 7 days. Internal consistency estimates for the FSI pain indices, calculated with Cronbach's alpha, ranged from 0.66 (hand activities) to 0.90

(social role). Intraclass correlation coefficients ranging from 0.69 (personal care) to 0.88 (gross mobility) were obtained for test-retest reliability and from 0.71 (gross mobility) to 0.82 (social role) for interrater reliability. The FSI pain index yielded a correlation coefficient of $r = 0.40$ with a functional classification scheme and of $r = 0.43$ with professional judgment.

Neck Pain and Disability Scale (NPAD) (Wheeler, Goolkasian, Baird, & Darden, 1999)

The NPAD is a 20-item, self-report instrument designed to assess the intensity of neck pain and its interference with vocational, recreational, social, and self-care activities as well as to identify pain-related emotional factors. Items are rated on a 10-cm visual analog scale with scale points ranging from 0 (no pain or interference) to 5 (severe pain or complete interference). The maximum score is 100 and higher scores indicate greater neck pain and disability. The NPAD is usually completed in 5 minutes. It demonstrates high internal consistency (coefficient alpha = 0.93) and compares favorably to other pain-disability instruments with correlations of $r = 0.80$ with the PDI and $r = 0.78$ with the ODQ. Patients with neck pain scored higher than pain-free controls and patients with lower back and leg pain.

Patient report: Daily activity diaries

The daily diary provides a feasible mechanism for obtaining behavioral data about the effects of pain on daily functioning. Diary content consists of postures (e.g., sitting), activity (e.g., cooking), pain relief measures (e.g., use of heating pads), use of analgesic medications, and pain intensity. Time spent alone and with others and setting (e.g., restaurant) may also be recorded to take into account environmental considerations. Diaries are completed for every quarter-, half-, or full hour, with patients recording the behavior that predominated over the designated interval. Diaries may be kept for varying durations (e.g., 2 weeks). Scoring takes into account the amount and distribution of time spent in the various activities and postures. Using 112 hours (16 hours of uptime per day) as the norm for weekly uptime, an uptime of less than 80 hours per week due to pain would be viewed as a significant reduction of overall activity level (Fordyce, Brena, Holcomb, de Lateur, & Loeser, 1978).

Follick, Ahern, and Laser-Wolston (1984) concluded that daily activity diaries were valid activity measures when compared with spousal diaries and objective measurement of uptime and downtime with an electronic monitor. Reliability data indicated that activity patterns were relatively consistent from day to day. Fordyce et al. (1984) found significant relationships between persistent pain patients' reports of pain severity and amount of activity limitation but few relationships with other common measures of pain behavior, such as medication use and health care utilization.

Patient report: Subjective summary indices

As a summary indicator of activity and participation restrictions, patients may be asked the number of days or half days over the past month that they have not been able to carry out their usual activities due to pain, or the number of hours or days over the past week that they have spent in bed or resting due to pain.

Clinician ratings

In addition to being easy to administer, self-reports of activity limitations and participation restrictions have the advantage of being able to obtain information about a wide range of behaviors cost effectively. Their disadvantage lies in the disparities or mismatches that commonly occur between how people say they perform and how they actually perform. Objective assessment, including performance testing and objective summary indices, provides objective evidence about performance.

Performance testing

Ideally, behavioral assessment involves observation of pain-associated behaviors in the activity context (e.g., home, car) where the behaviors occur. Naturalistic or ecological observation, with or without the use of videotaping of behavior, is labor intensive, costly, and largely impractical, although at times it is used by insurance companies investigating disability claims. Performance testing provides a feasible alternative. It involves observation of behavioral samples under controlled, usually standardized conditions. The activities to be observed may be selected from the perspective of their relevance to (a) the daily life of the patient (e.g., client-centered approach) or (b) the pain diagnosis, such as low back pain or shoulder pain (e.g., population-based approach). Unlike the subjective methods, by observing patients' body mechanics during performance testing, clinicians can give patients feedback about their movement skills. Hence, it is often the method of choice in clinical settings.

Keefe and Block (1982) devised a 10-minute standardized protocol for chronic low back pain involving walking (1 minute, repeated twice), sitting (1, 2 minutes), reclining (1 minute, repeated twice), and standing (1, 2 minutes). Performance is videotaped and rated for the occurrence of five pain behaviors: guarding, rubbing, grimacing, bracing, and sighing. Interrater reliability for this protocol is excellent, with percent agreement ranging from 93% to 99% (Keefe & Block). The system has been adapted for patients with osteoarthritis (Keefe & Williams, 1992) and rheumatoid arthritis (McDaniel et al., 1986). In a sample of community-dwelling older adults with chronic low back pain, stronger correlations with self-reported pain and disability were found with an ADL simulation protocol than with the Keefe and Block protocol (Weiner, Pieper, McConnell, Martinez, & Keefe, 1996). In the ADL simulation, task components were performed to elicit pain behaviors. The simulations were long-leg sit, as in bending to don socks and shoes; bridging, as in lower-body dressing in bed; moving supine to prone, as in turning over in bed; and moving supine to sit, as in getting out of bed. An intraclass correlation coefficient of 0.60 was obtained for the protocol.

Another performance-based protocol specific for low back pain devised by Simmonds et al. (1998) includes measures of reach and upper body endurance not covered in the other protocols reviewed. In the low back pain group, excellent interobserver (intraclass correlation ≥ 0.98) and within session test-retest coefficients (r = > 0.91) were obtained, except for sit-to-stand and trunk flexion.

Performance assessment for persistent pain was expanded by Harding et al. (1994) to highlight speed and endurance through measures of walking, stair climbing, chair transfers, balance, sit-ups, arm endurance, grip strength, and peak flow. Interobserver reliability results, using intraclass correlation coefficients or kappa coefficients, depending on the data, were excellent (above 0.98). Test-retest reliability coefficients were fair-to-good (0.70 to 0.99) except for balance. All performance measures indicated significant improvement from pretreatment to posttreatment, and the improvement increased or was maintained at the 1-month follow-up.

Clinician ratings: Objective summary indices

Work status, in terms of either being employed or unemployed or number of days of work lost, is a commonly used objective measure of activity and participation restriction. Because many factors other than work capacity determine work status, the utility of summary indices is limited, particularly among older adults where retirement is common.

Instrument Comparison

Table 5.1 compares the content of the instruments presented in this chapter. The seven roles delineated under *Participation* were abstracted from the PDI, which provides the most comprehensive assessment of social roles. Because of its comprehensiveness, the PDI is the preferred instrument for assessing participation. Participation is either the only or the primary dimension of disablement assessed on the PDI and MOS-PI. The four pain-site specific instruments (ODQ, Quebec, DQ, NPAD) and the FSI span participation and activity. Excluding the PDI, participation is most comprehensively covered on the NPAD, followed by the ODQ. No role is included on all instruments reviewed but pain in relation to sleep is found on all instruments except the MOS-PI and FSI (sleep is included under *Life support*).

Functional assessment instruments for pain-related impairment have been studied for their application to older adults, with and without cognitive impairment. Unfortunately, the same attention has not been directed toward functional assessment instruments for either participation or activity, although Weiner et al. (1996) successfully used the DQ with a sample of community-dwelling older adults. The household or home management role is of particular interest for geriatric assessment because this role often stands at the interface between independent and dependent living. On the PDI, household tasks appear to be assessed in two categories (family and home responsibilities, occupation) without a clear delineation of the distinguishing tasks allocated to each category. On the DQ, home management is included under "doing any of the jobs that I usually do around the house" and "avoiding heavy jobs around the house," while on the MOS-PI, NPAD, and FSI, it is embedded in the interpretation of work. On the PDI, driving is incorporated into both the self-care and family and home roles, creating ambiguity similar to that noted above for household tasks. This problem is avoided on the Quebec, NPAD, and FSI because driving is treated as a separate item (driving is not represented on Table 5.1).

To provide a geriatric framework for activity assessment, the activities identified by Scudds and Robertson (1998) as most problematic for older adults with musculoskeletal pain were matched to the activities assessed on the instruments. On Table 5.1, under *Activity*, the activities are listed from most to least difficult to perform. Using this listing as a guide, the FSI provides the most comprehensive activity assessment, specifically evaluating about half of the 20 activities. It is the only instrument that includes the most difficult activities (vacuuming and yard work, which are considered in separate items) as well as bathing and opening containers. Many of the most problematic activities are covered on the Quebec and DQ; however, some problematic activities are not included on any measure reviewed, namely, bathing in the tub, running errands or shopping, transferring into cars and onto the commode, washing hair, opening car doors, turning faucets, cutting meat, and lifting full cups or glasses. Walking is the most commonly assessed activity. Because the Quebec and DQ were

TABLE 5.1 Comparison of Self-Report and Performance Instruments

	Self-report instruments							Performance instruments			
	PDI	MOS-PI	ODQ	DQ	Quebec	NPAD	FSI	Keefe	Weiner	Simmonds	Harding
Participation											
Life support	X		X	X	X	X					
Self-care	X		X			X					
Family, home	X			X							
Occupation	X	X				X	X				
Recreation	X	X				X					
Social	X		X			X	X				
Sexual	X		X			X					
Activity											
Chores							X				
Transfer: chair				X			X			X	X
Reach overhead					X						
Climb 5 steps				X	X		X			X	
Bathe in tub											
Bend down				X	X		X		X	X	
Walk outdoors		X	X	X	X	X	X	X		X	X
Run errands, shop											
Dress				X	X		X		X		
Transfer: bed				X	X				X		
Transfer: car											
Wash, dry body							X				
Open jars							X			X	
Shampoo hair											
Transfer: commode											
Open milk carton							X			X	
Open car doors										X	
Turn faucets										X	
Cut meat										X	
Lift full cup/glass											
Activity Components											
Stand			X	X	X	X		X			
Sit			X	X	X			X			
Lie								X	X		
Lift			X							X	
Push, pull					X						

devised specifically for disability related to back pain, only lower extremity tasks are included on these instruments. The utility of activity assessments based on pain sites, such as the back, warrants study in older adults because their pain may be more generalized. For example, older adults with low back pain secondary to osteoarthritis may also have hand involvement.

The final segment of Table 5.1, *Activity Components*, takes into account the actions that enable activity performance. Standing is included on the four pain-site specific instruments, while sitting is restricted to the back pain disability scales. Interestingly, lifting is singled out only on the ODQ. As static body positions, standing and sitting are contrasted with the dynamic movement involved in the activities.

Moving to the four performance instruments, it is apparent from Table 5.1 that their content is distributed between activity and activity components. Activities tend to be measured in terms of simulations, such as the lumbar flexion and long-leg sitting tasks on the protocols by Simmonds and Weiner, respectively, which approximate "bending down to pick up clothing." Walking is included on the persistent pain protocol (Harding) and two of the three protocols devised for low back pain (Keefe, Simmonds). Other than walking, there are few commonalities among these instruments. The Keefe, Simmonds, and Harding protocols try to capture the endurance aspect of activity performance through repeated testing (e.g., repeated sit-to-stand) and graded performance (walk, speed walk). These protocols involve tasks that are similar to those typically assessed in relation to capacity for work and the AADL.

SETTING-SPECIFIC CONSIDERATIONS

Postacute Care: Skilled Nursing Facilities and Home Health Care

Over the past decade, several standardized assessments have been devised for use in postacute care settings. The Minimum Data Set for Long Term Care (MDS) and the Outcome and Assessment Information Set (OASIS) were developed for use in skilled nursing facilities and home health care, respectively. The Minimum Data Set for Post-Acute Care (MDS-PAC) is proposed for use in rehabilitation. Each assessment has its own unique approach to pain assessment.

On the MDS, Version 2.0 (Health Care Financing Administration, 1998), pain is assessed in three items in Section J, Health Conditions. Data are sought on pain frequency, intensity, and location over the past 7 days. The MDS-PAC, Version 1.0 (Health Care Financing Administration, 2000) also contains three pain items (Section I, Pain Status) but inquiry is made for the past 3 days. In addition to data about pain frequency and intensity, patients are asked to compare pain at the assessment point to pain at the time of the precipitating event. On the OASIS (Center for Health Services and Policy Research, 1998), pain is considered under Sensory Status (M0420, M0430). The first pain item assesses the frequency with which pain interferes with activity or movement. The second assesses the intractability or constancy of pain and whether or not pain interferes with behaviors such as sleep, appetite, energy, concentration, social relationships, emotions, and the performance of physical activity. Thus, the MDS and MDS-PAC assess pain only in terms of impairment, while the OASIS considers disability attributable to pain. Although all three instruments use a self-report format, each allows for observational input from caregivers, such as nurses, nursing assistants, spouses, or relatives. In addition to the MDS items, the MDS incorporates an automatic system for triggering more in-depth assessment of problem areas identified through its screening process. The intent of the Resident Assessment Protocols (RAPS) is to link assessment data concerning 18 problem conditions (e.g., falls, pressure ulcers) to care plans. Given the prevalence and incidence of pain in nursing home residents, pain is significantly absent from the problem list.

Persons With Cognitive Impairment

For cognitively impaired clinical populations secondary to mental retardation, dementia, or delirium, the validity of self-report assessment methods has been questioned because of the limited ability or the actual inability that these patients have to express pain verbally. The need for valid pain assessments is particularly apparent in nursing homes where the prevalence of dementia and musculoskeletal impairments secondary to arthritis and old fractures is high. Ferrell, Ferrell, and Rivera (1995) found that 17% of their nursing home sample was unable to complete any pain scale, prompting them to conclude that cognitive impairment was a substantial barrier to pain assessment and management. Although some cognitively impaired nursing home residents are unable to respond to pain instruments, research by Parmelee, Smith, and Katz (1993) supports the validity of pain reporting in those who are able to respond.

Observing behavior has been proposed as a viable alternative to self-reports of disability for patients who are cognitively impaired, nonverbal, or confused. Ferrell et al. (1995) noted that nursing home residents who were unable to complete any pain scales were able to communicate their needs qualitatively. Marzinski (1991), Parke (1992), and Simons and Malabar (1995) suggested that changes in typical behavior be analyzed for their potential for being pain induced. A sudden increase or decrease in overall activity level or the replacement of usual moaning and rocking with quiet and withdrawn behaviors may be indicative of pain. From the perspective of disability assessment, the question that is being raised is, How do patients with extremely limited verbal communication abilities express their basic needs related to pain perception and control? Behaviorally, pain is typically evidenced in facial expressions (e.g., grimacing), body postures (e.g., guarding an extremity, rubbing a painful body part), vocalizations (e.g., moaning, sighing) and avoidance of activities (e.g., refusal to get out of bed).

Hurley, Volicer, Hanrahan, Houde, and Volicer (1992) identified nine behaviors indicative of discomfort, including but not limited to pain, from their observations of noncommunicative patients with advanced Alzheimer's disease: "noisy breathing, negative vocalization, absence of a look of contentment, looking sad, looking frightened, having a frown, absence of a relaxed body posture, looking tense, and fidgeting" (p. 372). The magnitude of each item is scored on a visual analogue scale, with the anchors absent (0) and extreme (100). Overall discomfort observed is scored on a visual analogue scale, extending from completely comfortable to extremely uncomfortable. Reliability estimates for the scale are acceptable, including internal consistency (coefficient alpha = 0.77), test-retest reliability (r = 0.60), and interrater reliability (r = 0.90). Evidence of construct validity was obtained from the scales' ability to detect differences in discomfort precipitated by fever.

SUMMARY/RECOMMENDATIONS

1. A pain-related functional assessment should consider impairment, activity limitations, and participation restrictions.
2. Pain-related activity restrictions are highly prevalent in older adults, with activity limitations in vacuuming and yard work being most problematic and restricting performance of the home management role.
3. Assessment of activity restrictions should include BADL, IADL, AADL, and work, with specific attention directed toward a patient's most valued tasks.
4. Pain-related activity limitations may be assessed subjectively and objectively, while participation restrictions are assessed only subjectively. Subjective methods include interviews, questionnaires, diaries, and subjective summary indices. Objective methods include performance testing and objective summary indices.
5. Self-reports of function are easier to administer and score, can cover a broader range of behaviors, and are more cost-effective than performance tests. However, patients may under- or overre-

port their pain-related disability. Performance testing is particularly useful for clinical assessment because it enables clinicians to assess the body mechanics patients use to perform tasks and their potential for eliciting pain.

6.   Although instruments and protocols for assessing activity limitations and participation restrictions have included older adults in their development, except for the Weiner at al. protocol, none has been specifically devised for or evaluated in older adults. The PDI and FSI provide the most comprehensive assessment of participation and activity, respectively.

7.   Because pain may be more generalized in older adults than in younger adults, a generic instrument, such as the FSI, may be preferable to pain-site specific instruments.

8.   None of the standardized instruments used or proposed for use in postacute care provide an adequate assessment of pain-related restrictions in activity and participation.

9.   For older adults who are cognitively impaired, confused, or nonverbal, changes in their usual behavior should be evaluated for their potential for being pain induced.

10.   Functional outcomes following rehabilitative interventions are manifested by reductions in impairment and disability.

CASE STUDIES

Ms. Nettie: Pain Measures—PDI and ODQ

Case

Nettie, an 83-year-old woman who lives alone in a senior citizens' high-rise apartment building, has diagnoses of osteoporosis, spinal compression fractures, and osteoarthritis coexisting with slight weakness secondary to an old cerebral vascular accident. Her chief complaint is constant low back pain that interferes with her daily functioning. She scored 49 on the PDI and 70% on the ODQ, which indicates very severe disability. She complained most about pain during tasks requiring bending, twisting, and lifting. The specific tasks that she asked for help with were removing wet clothes from the washer and placing them into the dryer, lifting grocery bags from her cart into her car trunk, changing bed linens, and running the vacuum.

In occupational therapy, oral and written instruction was given about body mechanics to eliminate twisting during activities and to minimize lifting heavy objects. Proper techniques were practiced in the clinic until four simulation tasks (e.g., lifting sugar from a low shelf, moving a heavy sofa, moving items from the refrigerator to the sink, sweeping) were performed correctly three times in sequence. A home program was established to increase awareness of correct and incorrect body mechanics. During the three subsequent outpatient visits, task simulations became increasingly more complex and training was done to remediate incorrect techniques. At discharge, Ms. Nettie's scores on the PDI decreased to 40 and on the ODQ to 46%, indicating a change from very severe to severe disability. She reported feeling happier, sleeping better, and having more energy.

Discussion

Ms. Nettie lives alone at home. If she became more disabled, she would need to move to a more restricted environment. The desired outcome was reduction in disability to allow her to maintain her current residence. The PDI and ODQ were chosen because they provide summary disability levels and help to identify specific tasks that are problematic and contribute to disability. Any decrease in summary disability scores indicates improvement in the ability to live independently in the community.

Mr. Carl: Pain Measure—Pain Diary

Case

Mr. Carl, a 65-year-old, retired tool and die maker, lives with his wife in a three-story home. He was referred to occupational therapy for home health care due to a progressive decrease in self-care abilities. Because his wife is unable to care for him, his ability to complete his BADL independently and to prepare light meals was essential in order for him to remain at home. During the intake interview, Mr. Carl reported feeling "unwell," but he could not identify any specific reason for his decrease in functioning. During performance testing, he frequently winced and groaned. When specifically asked about pain, he stated, "Yes, I have pain, but that is normal, I'm old." On a pain diagram (see chapter 2), he indicated severe pain in three sites (hands, shoulders, low back), and mild pain in two sites (feet, neck). However, he also reported that these sites and intensities varied daily, depending on his activities. To clarify the influence of pain on Mr. Carl's daily activities, he kept a pain diary for the next week. Analysis of his pain diary revealed that he experienced severe pain in activities requiring a strong grasp or pushing or pulling objects of about 10 pounds in weight. Further, he was spending about 10 hours out of 24 sleeping and an additional 3 hours resting.

Initially in occupational therapy, Mr. Carl was educated about the activities and the specific movements associated with these activities that were prone to elicit pain. After the therapist observed Mr. Carl push, pull, and lift heavy objects, his use of good body mechanics for "sliding" objects was reinforced while his poor leverage in bending at the back to lift objects was pointed out and the appropriate procedures were taught (e.g., bending at the knees). He was encouraged to use a cart on wheels to move objects in his home. The size of the handles on his ADL tools, including his toothbrush and kitchen cutlery, were made larger with thermopellets or foam pipe insulation in order to alleviate his problems in grip.

Discussion

Mr. Carl is able to maintain residence in the community. The primary focus of intervention is to increase ease of task performance. Of the available instruments, only a pain diary allows description of the nature, frequency, and duration of task-associated pain. Using a pain diary focuses attention on task performance difficulties and provides a starting point for intervention. After four visits, the number of pain sites remained the same but pain intensity was reduced to mild in the three sites previously reported as severe and remained mild in the other two sites. He was now completing BADL and meal preparation with less difficulty and pain, had expanded his home responsibilities to include dusting and shopping, and had reduced his sleep to 9 hours and daytime rest to 1 hour. He also reported that he resumed "meeting with the boys for morning coffee and donuts." Because pain, in part, is subjective in nature, an important outcome is perceived reduction in pain. Mr. Carl reported substantively reduced pain, indicating that intervention had a positive outcome.

Ms. Carol: Pain Measure—Observation of Behavior

Case

Ms. Carol is 78-year-old nursing home resident with arthritis and dementia of the Alzheimer's type. During her quarterly assessment on the MDS (Minimum Data Set for Long Term Care), the treatment team noted declining function in basic activities of daily living (BADL) and requested an occupational therapy assessment from her physician. When approached Ms. Carol was alert and pleasant and essentially nonverbal. She responded correctly to one- and two-step commands involving simple movements, but was unable to answer questions about her self-care abilities reliably. The certified nursing assistants (CNAs) assigned to her reported that she was actively resistive when being showered and dressed and that by the time morning care was completed she was moaning and crying. The observational assessment was done the following day during routine morning care. While being bathed and dressed, Ms. Carol winced, cried out, and became combative when her arms were raised for application of spray deodorant and to don an over-the-head shirt. She also had difficulty reaching food items on the far side of her breakfast tray. These observations led the occupational therapist to suspect that Ms. Carol had compromised shoulder movement. An upper extremity assessment of range of motion revealed crepitus in the shoulder joints and resistance to movement above shoulder height (90° of flexion) as evidenced by combativeness accompanied by wincing and crying.

Occupational therapy interventions included educating Ms. Carol's assigned CNAs about joint stiffness and pain and the potential role of passive movement of the shoulder joint during bathing and dressing in eliciting pain behaviors, including resistance and combativeness. Training in how to bathe Ms. Carol without raising her arms above shoulder height was given. The family caregiver, the resident's son, was asked to replace the spray deodorant with a roll-on deodorant because Ms. Carol could operate this herself and its application did not require her to raise her arms as high. The CNAs were encouraged to use front-opening rather than pullover garments because they could be donned more readily with minimal shoulder movement; they were also shown how to don overhead garments while protecting the shoulder joint. Similarly, training was given in how to avoid shoulder pressure when assisting Ms. Carol with transfers and walking. For dining, her bedside table was lowered to lap level to facilitate access to food and eliminate shoulder hiking. To supplement these adaptations, recommendations were made to provide analgesics half an hour before beginning morning care; a warm compress to her shoulders before morning care, as needed; and a bed bath rather than a shower, which could potentially increase fear and agitation. These recommendations were all accepted. The occupational therapist observed the CNA implementing these procedures during morning care the following day. Ms. Carol was calm throughout the session and made no attempt to strike out at the CNA.

Follow-up observational assessment conducted 2 weeks after the initial assessment indicated that the CNAs continued to provide morning care as directed. Two incidents of disruptive behaviors were documented in the nursing record. One incident was attributed to a CNA providing care who was unfamiliar with Ms. Carol and the other when analgesics were not provided before beginning care. Ms. Carol had also gained a pound, which was most likely due to her ability to self-feed more easily.

Discussion

Due to Alzheimer's disease, Ms. Carol is unable to use self-report measures of pain. Hence, the best option for obtaining reliable data is to observe her during task performance and document the type and frequency of pain behaviors and their relationship to performance of BADL. This approach forms the basis for trial clinical interventions to eliminate or decrease pain cause by task performance. As mandated by the Omnibus Budget Reconciliation Act (OBRA, 1987), rehabilitation services must be focused on attaining or maintaining the resident's highest level of functioning. Ms. Carol's renewed ability to self-feed and cooperate with morning care demonstrates the use of pain assessment and intervention to comply with federal regulations.

Following therapy, the activity limitations initially exhibited by Ms. Nettie, Mr. Carl, and Ms. Carol were alleviated to some extent, as evidenced by reduction in disability level, increased activity and decreased inactivity, and increased independence or cooperativeness with ADL, respectively. Cutler, Fishbain, Rosomoff, and Rosomoff (1994) concluded that older adults (> 64 years of age) achieve improved functional status comparable to that of younger adults following intervention. Typically, rehabilitation is a multifaceted intervention conducted by a multidisciplinary team targeted toward reducing impairment (pain intensity, etc.) as well as disability (task performance), with positive functional outcomes at both levels of intervention (Kankaanpää, Taimela, Airaksinen, & Hänninen, 1999).

REFERENCES

Arnoff, G. M., Feldman, J. B., & Campion, T. S. (2000). Management of chronic pain and control of long-term disability. *Occupational Medicine, 15*, 755–770.
Beurskens, A. J. H. M., de Vet, H. C. W., & Koke, A. J. A. (1996). Responsiveness of functional status in low back pain: A comparison of different instruments. *Pain, 65*, 71–76.

Brochet, B., Michel, P., Barberger-Gateau, P., & Dartigues, J. F. (1998). Population-based study of pain in elderly people: A descriptive study. *Age and Aging, 27,* 279–284.

Center for Health Services and Policy Research. (1998). *Outcome and Assessment Information Set (OASIS-B1).* Denver, CO: Author.

Coste, J., Delecoeuillerie, G., Cohen, de L. A., Le Parc, J. M., & Paolaggi, J. B. (1994). Clinical course and prognostic factors in acute low back pain: An inception cohort study in primary care practice. *British Medical Journal, 308,* 577–580.

Cutler, R. B., Fishbain, D. A., Rosomoff, R. S., & Rosomoff, H. L. (1994). Outcomes in treatment of pain in geriatric and younger age groups. *Archives of Physical Medicine and Rehabilitation, 75,* 457–464.

Deyo, R. A., & Centor, R. M. (1986). Assessing responsiveness of functional scales to clinical change: Analogy to diagnostic test performance. *Journal of Chronic Diseases, 39,* 897–906.

Fairbank, J. C. T., Davies, J. B., Couper, J., & O'Brien, J. P. (1980). The Oswestry Low Back Pain Disability Questionnaire. *Physiotherapy, 66,* 271–273.

Ferrell, B. A., Ferrell, B. R., & Osterweil, D. (1990). Pain in the nursing home. *Journal of the American Geriatrics Society, 38,* 409–414.

Ferrell, B. A., Ferrell, B. R., & Rivera, L. (1995). Pain in cognitively impaired nursing home patients. *Journal of Pain and Symptom Management, 10,* 591–598.

Ferrell, B. A., Stein, W. M., & Beck, J. C. (2000). The Geriatric Pain Measure: Validity, reliability and factor analysis. *Journal of the American Geriatrics Society, 48,* 1669–1673.

Fisher, K., & Johnston, M. (1997). Validation of the Oswestry Low Back Pain Disability Questionnaire, its sensitivity as a measure of change following treatment and its relationship with other aspects of chronic pain experience. *Physiotherapy Theory and Practice, 13,* 67–80.

Follick, M. J., Ahern, D. K., & Laser-Wolston, N. (1984). Evaluation of a daily diary for chronic pain patients. *Pain, 19,* 373–382.

Fordyce, W. E., Brena, S. F., Holcomb, R. J., De Lateur, B. J., & Loeser, J. D. (1978). Relationship of patient semantic pain descriptions to physician diagnostic statements, activity level measures and MMPI. *Pain, 5,* 293–303.

Fordyce, W. E., Lansky, D., Calsyn, D. A., Shelton, J. L., Stolov, W. C., & Rock, D. L. (1984). Pain measurement and pain behavior. *Pain, 18,* 53–69.

Fox, P. L., Raina, P., & Jadad, A. (1999). Prevalence and treatment of pain in older adults in nursing homes and other long-term care institutions: A systematic review. *Canadian Medical Association Journal, 160,* 329–333.

Grönblad, M., Hupli, M., Wennerstrand, P., Järvinen, E., Lukinmaa, A., Kouri, J.-P., & Karaharju, E. O. (1993). Intercorrelation and test–retest reliability of the Pain Disability Index (PDI) and the Oswestry Disability Questionnaire (ODQ) and their correlation with pain intensity in low back pain patients. *Clinical Journal of Pain, 9,* 189–195.

Grönblad, M., Järvinen, E., Hurri, H., Hupli, M., & Karaharju, E. O. (1994). Relationship of the Pain Disability Index (PDI) and the Oswestry Disability Questionnaire (ODQ) with three dynamic physical tests in a group of patients with chronic low-back and leg pain. *Clinical Journal of Pain, 10,* 197–203.

Harding, V. R., Williams, A. C. de C., Richardson, P. H., Nicholas, M. K., Jackson, J. L., Richardson, I. H., & Pither, C. E. (1994). The development of a battery of measures for assessing physical function of chronic pain patients. *Pain, 58,* 367–375.

Health Care Financing Administration. (1998). *Minimum Data Set, 2.0.* Washington, DC: U.S. Government Printing Office.

Health Care Financing Administration. (2000, February 23). *Minimum Data Set-Post Acute Care (MDS-PAC)—Version 1.0.* Washington, DC: U.S. Government Printing Office.

Hopman-Rock, M., Kraaimaat, F. W., & Bijlsma, J. W. J. (1997). Quality of life in elderly subjects with pain in hip or knee. *Quality of Life Research, 6,* 67–76.

Hopman-Rock, M., Odding, E., Hofman, A., Kraaimaat, F. W., & Bijlsma, J. W. J. (1996). Physical and psychosocial disability in elderly subjects in relation to pain in the hip and/or knee. *Journal of Rheumatology, 23,* 1037–1044.

Hurley, A. C., Volicer, B. J., Hanrahan, P. A., Houde, S., & Volicer, L. (1992). Assessment of discomfort in advanced Alzheimer patients. *Research in Nursing and Health, 15,* 369–377.

Infante-Rivard, C., & Lortie, M. (1997). Relapse and short sickness absence for back pain in the six months after return to work. *Occupational Environmental Medicine, 54,* 328–334.

Jette, A. M. (1987). The functional status index: Reliability and validity of a self-report functional disability measure. *Journal of Rheumatology, 14*(Suppl. 15), 15–19.

Kankaanpää, M., Taimela, S., Airaksinen, O., & Hänninen, O. (1999). The efficacy of active rehabilitation in chronic low back pain: Effect on pain intensity, self-experienced disability, and lumbar fatigability. *Spine, 24,* 1034–1042.

Keefe, F. J., & Block, A. R. (1982). Development of an observational method for assessing pain behavior in chronic low back pain patients. *Behavior Therapy, 13,* 363–375.

Keefe, F. L., & Williams, D. A. (1992). Pain behavior assessment. In D. C. Turk & R. Melzack (Eds.), *Handbook of pain assessment* (pp. 277–292). New York: Guilford Press.

Kopec, J. A., Esdaile, J. M., Abrahamowicz, M., Abenhaim, L., Wood-Dauphinee, S., Lamping, D. L., & Williams, J. I. (1995). The Quebec Back Pain Disability Scale: Measurement properties. *Spine, 20,* 341–352.

Lavsky-Shulan, M., Wallace, R. B., Kohout, F. J., Lemke, J. H., Morris, M. C., & Smith, I. M. (1985). Prevalence and functional correlates of low back pain in the elderly: The Iowa 65+ rural health study. *Journal of the American Geriatrics Society, 33,* 23–28.

Lawton, M. P., & Brody, E. M. (1969). Assessment of older people: Self-maintaining and instrumental activities of daily living. *Gerontologist, 9,* 179–186.

Leveille, S. G., Guralnik, J. M., Hochberg, M., Hirsh, R., Ferrucci, L., Langlois, J., Rantanen, T., & Ling, S. (1999). Low back pain and disability in older women: Independent association with difficulty but not inability to perform daily activities. *Journal of Gerontology: Medical Sciences, 54A,* M487–M493.

Marzinski, L. R. (1991). The tragedy of dementia: Clinically assessing pain in the confused, nonverbal elderly. *Journal of Gerontological Nursing, 17,* 25–28.

McDaniel, L. K., Anderson, K. O., Bradley, L. A., Young, L. D., Turner, R. A., Agudelo, C. A., & Keefe, F. J. (1986). Development of an observation method for assessing pain behavior in rheumatoid arthritis patients. *Pain, 24*, 165–184.

National Center for Health Statistics: M. G. Kovar & A. Z. LaCroix. (1987). Ability to perform work-related activities: Data from the Supplement on Aging to the National Health Interview Survey, United States, 1984. Advance Data From Vital and Health Statistics. No. 136. DHHS Publication No. (PHS) 87–1250. Hyattsville, MD: Public Health Service.

Omnibus Budget Reconciliation Act (OBRA) of 1987. Public Law 100-203, § 101.

Parke, B. (1992). Pain in the cognitively impaired elderly. *Canadian Nurse, 88*, 17–20.

Parmelee, P. A., Smith, B., & Katz, I. R. (1993). Pain complaints and cognitive status among elderly institution residents. *Journal of the American Geriatrics Society, 41*, 517–522.

Reuben, D. B., Laliberte, L., Hiris, J., & Mor, V. (1990). A hierarchical exercise scale to measure function at the advanced activities of daily living (AADL) level. *Journal of the American Geriatrics Society, 38*, 855–861.

Rogers, J. C., & Holm, M. B. (1997). Evaluation of activities of daily living. In M. E. Neistadt & E. B. Crepeau (Eds.), *Willard and Spackman's occupational therapy*, 9th ed. (pp. 185–208). Philadelphia: Lippincott.

Roland, M., & Morris, R. (1983). A study of the natural history of back pain, part I: Development of a reliable and sensitive measure of disability in low-back pain. *Spine, 8*, 141–144.

Scudds, R., & Robertson, J. M. (1998). Empirical evidence of the association between the presence of musculoskeletal pain and physical disability in community-dwelling senior citizens. *Pain, 75*, 229–235.

Sherbourne, C. D. (1992). Pain measures. In A. L. Steward & J. E. Ware, Jr. (Eds.), *Measuring functioning and well-being: The Medical Outcomes Study approach* (pp. 220–234). Durham, NC: Duke University Press.

Simmonds, M. J., Olson, S. L., Jones, S., Hussein, T., Lee, C. E., Novy, D., & Radwan, H. (1998). Psychometric characteristics and clinical usefulness of physical performance tests in patients with low back pain. *Spine, 23*, 2412–2421.

Simons, W., & Malabar, R. (1995). Assessing pain in elderly patients who cannot respond verbally. *Journal of Advanced Nursing, 22*, 663–669.

Stratford, P. W., Binkley, J., Solomon, P., Finch, E., Gill, C., & Moreland, J. (1996). Defining the minimum level of detectable change for the Roland-Morris Questionnaire. *Physical Therapy, 76*, 359–365.

Stratford, P. W., Binkley, J., Solomon, P., Gill, C., & Finch, E. (1994). Assessing change over time in patients with low back pain. *Physical Therapy, 74*, 528–533.

Tait, R. C., Chibnall, J. T., & Krause, S. (1990). The Pain Disability Index: Psychometric properties. *Pain, 40*, 171–182.

Tait, R. C., Pollard, C. A., Margolis, R. B., Duckro, P. N., & Krause, S. J. (1987). The Pain Disability Index: Psychometric and validity data. *Archives of Physical Medicine and Rehabilitation, 68*, 438–441.

Taylor, S. J., Taylor, A. E., Foy, M. A., & Fogg, A. J. B. (1999). Responsiveness of common outcome measures for patients with low back pain. *Spine, 24*, 1805–1812.

Weiner, D., Pieper, C., McConnell, E., Martinez, S., & Keefe, F. (1996). Pain measurement in elders with chronic low back pain: Traditional and alternative approaches. *Pain, 67*, 461–467.

Wheeler, A. H., Goolkasian, P., Baird, A. C., & Darden, B. V. (1999). Development of the neck pain and disability scale. *Spine, 24*, 1290–1294.

World Health Organization. (1980). *The international classification of impairments, disabilities, and handicaps—A manual relating to the consequences of disease.* Geneva, Switzerland: Author.

World Health Organization. (2001). International classification of functioning, disability, and health. Geneva, Switzerland: Author.

Pharmacologic Management: Noninvasive Modalities

6

David R. P. Guay, Thomas E. Lackner, and Joseph T. Hanlon

Although nonpharmacological pain management modalities should be utilized whenever possible in older individuals with persistent pain, most individuals will require the use of analgesic medications to achieve an optimal response. It is important that health care professionals learn how to use a few agents well rather than attempt to learn how to use the entire cadre of available therapies. Moreover, for persistent pain, regularly scheduled dosing is preferred to "as-needed" dosing of rapid-acting analgesics (Jacox et al., 1994).

Utilizing pain medications for older persons is more complex than for younger ones. Older adults frequently take multiple medications and are prone to adverse drug reactions. To avoid these, one should consider significant age-related changes in the pharmacokinetics and pharmacodynamics of medications (Hanlon, Ruby, Shelton, & Pulliam, 1999). For most drugs, there is no change in oral absorption. However, there is a decreased first-pass effect and increased bioavailability for certain medications (e.g., morphine and certain tricyclic antidepressants). Distribution of drugs may be affected by either decreases or increases in plasma protein binding of drugs. Many medications are primarily metabolized via the liver. It is notable that there may be decreased clearance (CL) and increased terminal disposition half-life (t $^{1}/_{2}$) for some phase I oxidatively metabolized drugs (e.g., piroxicam) and decreased CL and t $^{1}/_{2}$ of drugs with high extraction ratios (e.g., morphine, certain tricyclic antidepressants). Finally, there can be decreased CL and increased t $^{1}/_{2}$ of renally eliminated drugs (e.g., gabapentin).

The purpose of this chapter is to review the noninvasive pharmacotherapy of persistent pain in older adults. Specifically, we will review nonopioids, opioids, and adjunctive agents; their mechanism of action, clinical efficacy, pharmacokinetics, adverse events/drug-drug interactions, contraindications/drug-disease-state interactions/precautions; and dosing and administration as it pertains to older adults.

EVIDENCE AND PRINCIPLES FOR PRACTICE

Nonopioid Analgesics

The nonopioid analgesics (i.e., acetaminophen, salicylates, and other nonsteroidal anti-inflammatory drugs [NSAIDs]) are first-line drug therapy for mild to moderate pain (American Pain Society, 1992). The acetylated (aspirin) and nonacetylated salicylates (magnesium, choline, and sodium salicylate) and other NSAIDs primarily produce analgesia by inhibiting cyclooxygenase (COX), the enzyme that catalyzes the conversion of arachidonic acid to prostaglandin precursors. Prostaglandins are inflammatory mediators that sensitize peripheral nociceptors (Vane, 1971). Two COX isoforms (COX-1 and COX-2) have been identified. Specifically, the inhibition of COX-2 is believed to be responsible for the anti-inflammatory and analgesic effects of NSAIDs. COX-1 is involved in the production of protective prostaglandins (PGD_2, PGE_2, PGF_2) that are responsible for preserving gastrointestinal mucosa, and thromboxane A_2 that promotes platelet aggregation. The conventional NSAIDs and salicylates inhibit both COX-1 and COX-2, whereas the more selective NSAIDs inhibit COX-1 to a lesser extent than COX-2 (Crofford et al., 2000). The principal mechanism by which acetaminophen produces an analgesic effect is most likely by inhibition of cyclooxygenase and related prostaglandin synthesis within the central nervous system. Acetaminophen exhibits little, if any, anti-inflammatory activity (Insel, 1996).

With the exception of pain accompanying substantial inflammation (e.g., rheumatoid arthritis, musculoskeletal trauma, serositis, bone metastasis, soft tissue infiltrates) for which nonacetylated salicylates and other NSAIDs can provide superior pain relief, all of the nonopioid analgesics are similarly effective and have a similar time to onset of effect and time to maximum analgesia. In the setting of inflamation, no NSAID (whether conventional or COX-2 selective) is consistently more effective than any other, and patient response and tolerance to side effects dictate choice of agents (Crofford et al., 2000).

Nonsteroidal Anti-inflammatory Drugs

Pharmacokinetic Considerations   In general, NSAIDs are well absorbed after oral administration, exhibit low non–flow-dependent hepatic clearance and low to nonexistent first-pass metabolism, are highly plasma-protein-bound (principally to albumin), and have small distribution volumes (Guay, 1995). Most NSAIDs are bound extensively ($\geq 95\%$) to albumin, and the drug-free fraction may be increased in patients with hypoalbuminemia. Protein binding is saturable in the usual dose range for some NSAIDs (salicylate, naproxen, ibuprofen), so that increasing daily doses lead to a less-than-proportional increase in steady-state trough concentrations; in contrast, free drug concentrations increase proportionally with dose. Several factors have been assessed for their effect on NSAID plasma protein binding. Female gender has been linked to a decrease in naproxen plasma protein binding. Increasing age has been associated with variable effects on NSAID plasma protein binding: decreased binding for diflunisal, salicylate, ketorolac; no change for etodolac, ibuprofen, oxaprozin; and conflicting data for piroxicam and naproxen. Hepatic and renal disease may be associated with reduced NSAID plasma protein binding as well, in the latter case primarily due to the presence of small-molecular-weight endogenous binding inhibitors. The plasma protein binding of salicylate, diflunisal, naproxen, oxaprozin, and sulindac (+ metabolites) is reduced in patients with renal disease.

All NSAIDs except indomethacin and oxaprozin are virtually entirely dependent on hepatic metabolism for elimination, either through oxidation or glucuronidation. The isozymes of cytochrome P-450 requisite for NSAID metabolism and the possibility of phenotypic differences in NSAID metabolism have not been explored. Limited data are available regarding enterohepatic circulation of NSAIDs, but they suggest that there is a potential for this to occur with indomethacin and sulindac due to their extensive degree of biliary excretion.

The renal elimination of parent compound constitutes only a small proportion of the clearance mechanism of most NSAIDs. The clearance of agents such as ketoprofen, fenoprofen, naproxen, and indomethacin may be decreased to a variable degree in patients with renal impairment or in those taking probenecid concurrently, due to the retention of unstable acylglucuronide metabolites that may hydrolyze to re-form the parent compound. This recycling is one reason for caution in the use of these agents in patients with renal impairment. Urine pH plays a major role in the elimination of salicylate when urine pH exceeds 6.5, as renal clearance increases markedly in this urine pH range.

Adverse Effects/Drug-Drug Interactions   Potentially serious adverse effects of salicylates and other NSAIDs include renal impairment, peripheral edema, precipitation of heart failure, hyperkalemia, gastrointestinal disorders, and central nervous system disturbances (Brater, 1999; Griffin, & Ray, 2000). NSAID-induced renal impairment and fluid retention is secondary to decreased vasodilatory renal prostaglandin production. Adverse gastrointestinal effects, which can often occur without warning symptoms, can range in severity from gastrointestinal distress (e.g., nausea, diarrhea, abdominal discomfort) to life-threatening gastrointestinal perforation, symptomatic gastroduodenal ulcers, and bleeding, as well as esophageal erosion and stricture (Jaspersen, 2000; Walt, Katschinski, Logan, Ashley, & Langman, 1986).

A number of NSAID-related drug-drug interactions are noteworthy. NSAIDs can increase the plasma concentrations and toxicity of lithium and methotrexate and, therefore, concurrent therapy should be avoided. If they are used concurrently, more careful clinical and therapeutic drug monitoring is recommended (Hansten, Horn, Koda-Kimble, & Young, 2000). The concomitant use of NSAIDs with diuretics and other antihypertensives may decrease their effectiveness. The use of NSAIDs with corticosteroids increases the risk of peptic ulcer disease. Finally, the use of drugs that affect platelet function or coagulation can be problematic. In particular, there is an increased risk of hemorrhagic peptic ulcer disease when warfarin and NSAIDs are taken together (Shorr et al., 1993).

Contraindications/Drug-Disease-State Interactions/Precautions   Patients hypersensitive to aspirin or other NSAIDs may experience severe bronchospasm and anaphylactic reactions with any member of the drug class. Nonacetylated salicylates are less likely to precipitate these reactions and acetaminophen infrequently (mild bronchospasm in less than 5%) cross-reacts with NSAIDs (*Drug Facts and Comparisons*, 2000). Celecoxib (Celebrex®), but not rofecoxib (Vioxx®), contains a cross-reactive sulfonamide moiety and can cause reactions in patients allergic to sulfonamides.

There are several disease states (i.e., chronic renal failure, heart failure, hypertension, and peptic ulcer) in which NSAIDs should be used with caution. In particular, the risk of NSAID-induced renal impairment and fluid retention is enhanced in individuals whose renal homeostasis is markedly prostaglandin dependent. Such individuals include those who have volume contraction (e.g., following overly aggressive diuresis or hemorrhage), a functional decrease in circulating blood volume (e.g., congestive heart failure, preexisting renal impairment, cirrhosis), or diabetes mellitus.

Dosing and Administration   Recommended doses for selected NSAIDs are illustrated in Table 6.1. NSAIDs not recommended for use in older patients because of their potential for toxicity include indomethacin (Indocin®), ketorolac (Toradol®), mefenamic acid (Ponstel®), piroxicam (Feldene®), and phenylbutazone (Beers, 1997; McLeod et al., 1997).

TABLE 6.1 Recommended Selected Nonopioid Analgesics

Chemical class and agents	Total daily dose	Dosing interval	Terminal disposition Half-life (hr.)
Nonacetylated salicylate Salsalate (Disalcid® & others)	1.0–3.0 gm	bid–tid	2–20
Propionic acid nsaid Ibuprofen (Motrin®, Advil®, & others)	1.2–3.2 gm	tid–qid	1–3
Cox II inhibitor Rofecoxib (Vioxx®)	12.5–50 mg	qd	17
Acetaminophen[a] (Tylenol® & others)	2.6–4.0 gm	qid	1–3

[a] Drug of choice for noninflammatory disorders

Acetaminophen

Pharmacokinetic Considerations   The t $1/2$ of acetaminophen may be prolonged in older adults, but not enough to warrant routine dosage adjustment (Divoll et al., 1982; Triggs et al., 1975). However, it may be possible to achieve adequate analgesia with a lower total daily dosage by extending the dosing interval to at least 6 hours in individuals with a creatinine clearance of 10–50 mL/minute (Bennett et al., 1994).

Adverse Effects/Drug-Drug and Drug-Disease Interactions/Precautions
Acetaminophen can cause hepatotoxicity following the acute ingestion of greater than 10 grams or chronic use of greater than 4 grams/day. The known risk factors for toxicity from chronic use include alcoholism or regular and heavy use of alcohol, use of hepatic enzyme inducers (e.g., rifampin, phenytoin, carbamazepine, barbiturates) and other hepatotoxic drugs, malnourishment or recent fasting, dehydration, and preexisting liver disease. The risk of hepatotoxicity from chronic use is decreased by using the lowest effective dose or a maximum daily dose of 4 grams including multi-ingredient products (e.g., acetaminophen and opioid combinations), assuring adequate nutrition and hydration, and avoiding

concurrent hepatotoxic drugs. The chronic use of acetaminophen also appears to be an independent, dose-dependent risk factor for nephropathy but it is unknown whether the use of acetaminophen alone increases the extent or rate of progression of renal impairment (Matzke, 1997). Acetaminophen in doses exceeding 2 grams/day for more than 1 week may potentiate the effect of warfarin. Routine prothrombin time (PT/INR) monitoring is recommended in patients receiving both agents.

Topical Agents

Topical capsaicin (Zostrix®) can be effective, after 2–6 weeks, in relieving localized pain due to postherpetic neuralgia, osteoarthritis, and possibly other pain disorders, and works by depleting the pain neurotransmitter substance P in small afferent neurons from the periphery (Bernstein, 1988; Bernstein et al., 1989; Fitzgerald, 1983; Lynn, 1990). The comparative pharmacokinetics and pharmacodynamics of capsaicin in older and younger adults are unknown. Local burning, stinging, and erythema occur frequently, are most prevalent with less than 3 to 4 times daily applications, and usually subside with frequent repeated application but sometimes necessitate discontinuation. Good hand-washing following application is critical. Inadvertent inhalation of the aerosolized dried cream residue can cause coughing, sneezing, and respiratory irritation with a potential for bronchospasm.

A lidocaine 5% skin patch (Lidoderm®) has been shown to be effective in the treatment of postherpetic neuralgia by blocking voltage-regulated neuronal sodium channels without a complete sensory block. The lidocaine patch is well tolerated (i.e., local mild to moderate skin rash, redness, and irritation) without reports of systemic toxicity (Comer & Lamb, 2000).

EMLA 5% cream for topical administration is a eutectic mixture of the anesthetics lidocaine and prilocaine that is a suggested, but not established, treatment for localized peripheral neuropathic pain. However, it is cumbersome to use, requiring thick application and an occlusive dressing (Vaillancourt & Langevin, 1999).

A recent small study suggests that topical ketamine may be effective for the treatment of neuropathic pain (Gammaitoni et al., 2000). Larger studies are required before definitive recommendations can be made.

Nutraceuticals

Glucosamine and chondroitin are nutraceuticals whose analgesic mechanism of action is unclear. Both exhibit anti-inflammatory properties and may favorably affect cartilage metabolism (Delafuente, 2000). While a meta-analysis of 15 controlled studies in osteoarthritis pain found moderate pain relief and improved mobility with glucosamine and a large positive effect for chondroitin, other studies have found no benefit with glucosamine. A recent study provided preliminary evidence that glucosamine sulfate may retard disease progression (Reginster et al., 2001). Additional studies are needed to clearly define efficacy (Leeb et al, 2000; McAlindon, LaValley, Gulin, & Felson, 2000; Rindone, Hiller, Collacott, Nordhaugen, & Arriola, 2000).

There is no evidence that the dosage of glucosamine and/or chondroitin needs to be changed in older adults. However, little is known about their pharmacokinetics or pharmacodynamics in either older or younger adults. The short-term safety of glucosamine and chondroitin appears to be good, while safety with chronic use is not established. The most common adverse effects of glucosamine include gastrointestinal upset (e.g., nausea, epigastric pain), leg pain and edema, and pruritus. The only contraindication to the use of either product is previous hypersensitivity. Glucosamine has been shown to promote insulin resistance in animals but no effect on plasma glucose has been established in humans.

Summary

Nonopioid analgesics can be effective in the management of mild to moderate pain in older adults. It is recommended to maximize the use of acetaminophen for noninflammatory pain prior to exploring further options. Underdosing of this agent is a significant clinical problem. The use of NSAIDs should be restricted to inflammatory pain states, based on their substantial adverse event risk in older adults. Topical agents (e.g., capsaicin) may be helpful in some persistent pain disorders and avoids the systemic side effects seen with oral analgesics.

Opioids and Related Analgesics

Persistent pain conditions (e.g., cancer and neuropathic pain) can be effectively treated with opioids (Abraham, 1999; American Pain Society, 1997; Harati et al., 1998; Watson & Babul, 1998). Most opioid analgesics are equally efficacious when given in equianalgesic doses (Table 6.2). The exception to this is propoxyphene, which has been shown to be no more effective when given alone than placebo (Moertel et al., 1972). The mechanism of action for most opioid analgesics is binding to mu opioid receptors in the central nervous system (Forman, 1996). Although tramadol does not fulfill the classic definition of an opioid, it will be considered here since it too binds to mu opioid receptors. In addition, like tricyclic antidepressants, tramadol also blocks the reuptake of norepinephrine (*Drug Facts and Comparisons*, 2000).

These agents can be used as monotherapy, or a nonopioid can be added. Combination therapy provides additive analgesia to monotherapy and can decrease the opioid dose needed to relieve moderate to severe pain (i.e., be "opioid sparing"). When pain is constant or frequent, these agents should be taken on a scheduled basis with the schedule determined by the pattern of pain and drug-specific pharmacokinetic/pharmacodynamic properties.

Pharmacokinetic Considerations There are few studies of the effect of age on the pharmacokinetics of opioid analgesics. Specifically, data are available for only five commonly used opioid agonists for persistent pain: morphine, meperidine, fentanyl, dihydrocodeine, and propoxyphene. Information about the pharmacokinetics of other opioids must be inferred from data obtained from younger individuals. The following focuses on those agents with specific age-related data.

Morphine given orally is well absorbed but subject to a significant first-pass effect. Morphine primarily undergoes hepatic metabolism via phase II conjugative biotransformation and yields two active metabolites, morphine-6-glucuronide (M-6-G) and morphine-3-glucuronide (M-3-G). These

TABLE 6.2 Recommended Selected Opioid Analgesic Starting Regimens[a]

Drug	*Dosage regimen*	*Terminal disposition Half-life (hr.)*
Codeine 30 mg with acetaminophen 325 mg tablets (Tylenol#3® and others)	1 tablet po q 6h	3–4
Oxycodone 5 mg with acetaminophen 325 mg tablets (Percocet® and others)	1 tablet po q 6h	3–4
Liquid morphine 10 mg/5 ml–500 ml (various) and acetaminophen 325 mg tablets	2.5 mg po q 4h	2–3.5

[a] Dosage regimens approximately equianalgesic—assumes patient is opioid naive

active metabolites are renally cleared and thus can accumulate in patients with renal dysfunction. Morphine is a high hepatic-extraction-ratio drug and is theoretically susceptible to age-related decreases in hepatic blood flow. Several studies have specifically examined the pharmacokinetics of morphine in older adults. After both intravenous and oral administration, older individuals exhibit significantly higher initial and maximum plasma morphine concentrations and reduced total CL compared to younger individuals (Baillie et al., 1989; Owen et al., 1983; Stanski, Greenblatt, & Lowenstein, 1978).

Meperidine has poor potency after oral administration due to a significant first-pass effect and undergoes phase I oxidative hepatic metabolism that yields a renally excreted active metabolite, normeperidine. There are conflicting reports regarding meperidine pharmacokinetics in older adults. One study found a lower meperidine CL with no change in volume of distribution (Vd) in older adult patients (mean age 74 years) when compared to younger ones (mean age 21 years) (Holmberg et al., 1982). In contrast, Herman and colleagues (1985) found no differences in meperidine CL between older adults (mean age 71 years) and younger subjects (mean age 28 years). Odar-Cedarloft and colleagues (1985) documented reduced renal excretion of normeperidine in older versus younger patients. With routine dosing of meperidine, patients may experience central nervous system hyperirritability, including mild nervousness, tremors, myoclonus and seizures due to normeperidine accumulation (Hanlon & O'Brien, 1989).

Despite the popularity of fentany when administered topically, limited information exists regarding the effect of age on its pharmacokinetics. It is not well absorbed orally, explaining its availability in parenteral, transdermal, and transmucosal dosage formulations. In general, the pharmacokinetics of transdermal fentanyl are not altered in older as compared to younger individuals (Scott & Stanski, 1987; Thompson et al., 1998). However, one study did document a significantly enhanced bioavailability of fentanyl after transdermal application in older as compared to younger individuals (Holdsworth et al., 1994).

The pharmacokinetics of two agents, dihydrocodeine and propoxyphene, which are both available in combination with nonopioid analgesics, have been studied in single studies in older adults. Flanagan, Johnston, White, and Crome (1989) studied the single and multiple dose pharmacokinetics of propoxyphene in 12 healthy young (median age 26 years) and 12 healthy older (median age 75 years) adult subjects. The median single- and multiple-dose propoxyphene t $^{1}/_{2}$ were significantly longer in the older adults compared to the younger group. Propoxyphene t $^{1}/_{2}$ was also found to be negatively correlated with creatinine clearance. Moreover, median propoxyphene area under the serum concentration-versus-time curve (AUC) and peak serum concentration (C_{max}) values were higher in older adults compared to the younger group. Davies, Castleden, McBurney, and Jagger (1989) conducted a single- and multiple-dose study of dihydrocodeine pharmacokinetics in 8 young (mean age 24 years) and 8 older (mean age 80 years) adult subjects. After multiple dosing, C_{max} and AUC were significantly higher in the older adults compared to the younger group. Again, there was a significant negative correlation between creatinine clearance and t $1/2$.

Adverse Events/Drug-Drug Interactions There is clear evidence that older adults have an increased pharmacodynamic sensitivity to opioid analgesics (Bellville et al., 1971; Kaiko, 1980; Scott & Stanski, 1987). Therefore, older adults taking opioids may be at greater risk for experiencing sedation, nausea, vomiting, constipation, urinary retention, respiratory depression, falls/fractures, and cognitive impairment. Sedation and mental confusion can be particularly disturbing in older adult patients (Gray, Lai, & Larson, 1999). Sedation is usually transient when initiating opioid use in patients exhausted by severe pain and may continue for several days. Downward dose adjustments should be made in patients when sedation persists beyond this time interval. Occasionally, the use of methylphenidate in low doses may be helpful to reduce opioid sedation (Bruera, Fainsinger, MacEachern, & Hanson, 1992; Walsh, 2000). Cognitive impairment with opioids is common in the older adult and attention should be paid to discontinuing other central nervous system–active drugs associated with cognitive impairment (Gray et al., 1999). Constipation routinely occurs in patients receiving opioid analgesics and should be anticipated by instituting a prophylactic bowel regimen that includes daily doses of stimulant laxatives such as bisacodyl or senna extract. Initial dosing of opioid analgesics can cause nausea and vomiting but these effects are usually transient because continued use of opioid analgesics actually depresses the vomiting center (Hanlon & O'Brien, 1989).

Respiratory depression can be produced by opioids, especially in opioid-naive patients who are receiving high-dose therapy, have cancer involving the lung, have chronic obstructive pulmonary disease, or have recently received nonpharmacologic palliative treatments (e.g., radiation treatment for lytic lesions with multiple myeloma) without subsequent tapering of opioids. Naloxone, an opioid antagonist given parenterally, can reverse respiratory depression as well as analgesic opioid effects. However, with careful oral dose titration, respiratory depression rarely occurs. Tolerance to this effect develops and pain itself is a powerful antagonist to respiratory depression (Hanlon & O'Brien, 1989). Urinary retention is associated with opioid use and thought to be caused by increased smooth muscle and sphincter tone (Hanlon & O'Brien, 1989).

Finally, the use of opioids has been associated with an increased risk of falls and fractures in older adults (Hanlon, Custon, & Ruby, 1996; Shorr, Griffin, Daugherty, & Ray, 1992; Weiner, Hanlon, & Studenski, 1998). The practitioner should exercise caution when prescribing opioids for older adults who already suffer from dysmobility, particularly when they live alone. The prescription of an assistive device should be considered for these individuals.

There are few clinically significant drug-drug interactions involving the use of opioids (*Drug Facts and Comparisons*, 2000). Propoxyphene has been shown to increase the plasma concentrations of carbamazepine. Meperidine given to patients taking a nonselective monoamine oxidase inhibitor (MAOI) such as phenelzine or tranylcypromine, or MAOI-B inhibitor such as selegiline, can cause life-threatening serotonin syndrome. Phenytoin may decrease methadone concentrations. Quinidine and perhaps other cytochrome P450 isozyme 2D6 inhibitors (e.g., paroxetine) can inhibit the analgesic effect of codeine by blocking its metabolism to morphine. This problem can also be seen in older adults who are CY2D6 slow metabolizers (5–10% of Caucasians and 1–3% of Asians and African Americans).

Contraindications/Drug-Disease State Interactions/Precautions There are few absolute contraindications to the use of opioids. Few patients have true allergies to them. In those cases where patients have had an idiosyncratic allergic reaction to a naturally occurring opioid (e.g., morphine), switching to a synthetic opioid (e.g., methadone) can circumvent the problem. There are few clinically significant drug-disease-state interactions to consider with opioids (Beers, 1997; McLeod et al., 1997). They include exacerbation of preexisting constipation and precipitating urinary retention in older adult men with benign prostatic hypertrophy, which may require management with urethral catheterization.

Tolerance and dependence are issues that deserve mention. Physical dependence does occur in patients taking regularly scheduled opioids. However, "addictive drug-seeking behavior" or psychological dependence is not usually exhibited. There is considerable disagreement as to the significance of tolerance and the need to increase the analgesic dose. There is, however, no maximal effective dose for opioids, and pain can be controlled on stable doses for long periods of time. Dosage increases are usually needed because of disease progression.

Dosing and Administration For moderate pain, a combination product containing codeine or oxycodone with acetaminophen is recommended. For patients titrated to a maximum dose of the nonopioid analgesic (4gm/day of acetaminophen), clinicians should consider changing patients to an immediate-release opioid product such as oxycodone or morphine. The reader is referred to Table 6.2 to aid in calculation of the approximate equivalent dose. Because of incomplete cross-tolerance, one half to two thirds of this dose should be prescribed, along with a fast acting as-needed rescue dose (10% of daily dose given every 2 hours; Abraham, 1999). When pain has been stabilized with an immediate-release product, patients may be switched to equivalent doses of available sustained-release oxycodone or morphine products that can be given two or three times daily.

There are several opioids that are not recommended for use in older adults due to their potential for toxicity (meperidine and pentazocine) or lack of efficacy (propoxyphene; Beers, 1997; McLeod et al., 1997). Levorphanol (Levo-Dromoran®) or methadone (Dolophine®) should be used with caution, if at all, in older adults as they are both very lipophilic drugs and thus their long t 1/2 may be further prolonged. Clinicians should also avoid the use of topical fentanyl (Duragesic®) patches in opioid-naive patients, given the lag time to onset of pain relief and the prolonged action even after patch removal. Its use should be reserved for those patients who cannot take oral medications and for whom rectal administration (i.e., hydromorphone, morphine) of other opioids is impractical. Caution should be exercised in the conversion of patients taking low-dose opioids to the fentanyl patch as often the 25 mcg/hour patch may be too large an initial dose for older adults.

Summary

Opioids can be useful in treating persistent pain in older adults. Clinicians should titrate doses to pain relief and anticipate and preemptively treat opioid-induced constipation with a stimulant laxative (see Case 2 below), an adverse effect towards which tolerance will not develop. Moreover, use longer acting opioids, where possible, to allow for more convenient dosing (e.g., extended-release morphine or oxycodone). The use of propoxyphene, meperidine, and pentazocine should be avoided.

Adjunctive Analgesics

Tricyclic Antidepressants

Tricyclic antidepressants (TCAs) have been considered first-line systemic therapy for many neuropathic pain syndromes, including diabetic neuropathy (DN) (Galer, 1995; MacFarlane et al., 1997). In a literature review,

6 of 13 controlled trials using antidepressants for DN showed significant pain relief using TCAs (McQuay et al., 1996). No differences in the effectiveness of different TCAs have been shown. Current literature also supports TCAs as first-line therapy for the management of postherpetic neuralgia (PHN), and up to 67% of patients respond to TCA treatment (Johnson, 1997). TCAs provide pain relief by independently providing analgesia specific for neuropathic pain, potentiating the effect of opioids, and improving underlying depression and insomnia (Jacox et al., 1994). Although their mechanism of analgesic action has not been clearly defined, TCAs are thought to have an inhibitory effect on nociceptive pathways by blocking the reuptake of norepinephrine. Recently, animal models of peripheral neuropathic pain have shown that TCAs act as sodium channel blockers, similar to local anesthetic/antiarrhythmic agents.

Pharmacokinetic Considerations   Results of small studies conducted to date have revealed conflicting findings, although the majority of data do support a finding of increased steady-state serum/plasma drug concentration (Cp) with age and, perhaps, an increase in Cp of hydroxylated metabolites with age. The consequence of the latter effect is uncertain.

Adverse Effects/Drug-Drug Interactions   The adverse effects of TCAs are well known but their prevalences vary by agent and patient group. In general, older adult patients experience a higher frequency of adverse effects, and slow dose titration is recommended (Rudorfer, Manji, & Potter, 1994). The most common adverse effects of TCAs (e.g., constipation, dry mouth, blurred vision, cognitive changes, tachycardia, urinary hesitation) are associated with anticholinergic effects. Other common adverse effects are orthostatic hypotension, weight gain, and sedation. In general, the secondary amines (e.g., desipramine, nortriptyline) exhibit fewer anticholinergic and sedative effects than the tertiary amines (e.g., amitriptyline, imipramine, doxepin); therefore, the secondary amines are preferable for use in the older adult population (Beers, 1997).

   Additive central nervous system (CNS) depression can be expected when TCAs are concurrently used with ethanol and other sedating medications, whether analgesic or nonanalgesic. These agents can also reduce the hypotensive effects of clonidine and guanadrel and cause potentially fatal reactions when used concurrently with nonselective MAOIs such as phenelzine and tranylcypromine (Hansten et al., 2000).

Contraindications/Drug-Disease-State Interactions/Precautions   TCAs should be used cautiously in patients with narrow-angle glaucoma, benign prostatic hypertrophy, urinary retention, constipation, or cardiovascular disease such as second- or third-degree heart block or other arrhythmias (Beers, 1997; McLeod et al., 1997). TCAs should be avoided in patients with severe liver disease and in patients who have had a recent acute myocardial infarction.

Patients abruptly withdrawn from a TCA may experience withdrawal that manifests as any of a variety of clinical symptoms (e.g., malaise, insomnia, drowsiness, anorexia, muscle aches, apathy, headache, mania, profuse sweating, irritability, abdominal pains, diarrhea, nausea, vivid and terrifying dreams, movement disorders). To avoid a withdrawal syndrome, a slow taper over 2 to 4 weeks (depending on the dose) is recommended.

Dosing and Administration Neuropathic pain generally responds more quickly than depression to TCAs (i.e., 3 to 10 days versus 2 to 4 weeks) and often with one third to one half of the dose used for depression (Table 6.3). Because of their improved adverse effect profiles, therapy should be initiated with one of the secondary amine TCAs in older adult patients. A starting dose of 10 to 25 mg at bedtime is recommended for most TCAs, with dose increments of 10 to 25 mg made no more frequently than every 5 to 7 days. Although the time of administration will not affect a TCA's analgesic activity, bedtime administration is recommended to take advantage of the sedative activity. The TCA dose should depend on the degree of pain relief and emergence of adverse effects. A daily dosage between 50 and 75 mg is usually effective (Galer, 1995). If a patient reaches a dose of 75 mg/day without sufficient pain relief or intolerable adverse effects, a serum drug concentration determination may be reasonable to evaluate whether the patient has abnormally low drug bioavailability or high clearance.

Antiepileptic Drugs

Antiepileptic drugs (AEDs) are considered among the drugs of choice for a variety of neuropathic pain types. The analgesic mechanisms of action for these agents are thought to involve enhancement of membrane stability or GABA-A receptor-mediated inhibition. Traditionally, the most commonly used AED has been carbamazepine (CBZ), whose efficacy is documented for trigeminal neuralgia (TN) (Sidebottom & Maxwell, 1995). Gabapentin may be more useful for painful neuropathies such as DM and PHN (Magnus, 1999), but its cost may be prohibitive.

Pharmacokinetic Considerations Steady-state apparent oral clearance (CL/f) of CBZ falls with advancing age, with reported reductions ranging from 25% to 40% (Bernus, Dickinson, Hooper, & Eadie, 1997; Cloyd,

TABLE 6.3 Recommended Selected Adjunctive Analgesics

Agent	Daily dosing guidelines	Terminal disposition Half-life (hr.)
Carbamazepine[a] (Tegretol,® various)	50–600 mg bid	12–17
Desipramine[b] (Norpramin,® various)	10–75 mg qd	14–25
Gabapentin[b] (Neurontin®)	100–900 mg bid–qid	5–7
Nortriptyline[b] (Pamelor,® various)	10–75 mg qd	15–39

[a] Drug of choice for trigeminal neuralgia
[b] Drug of choice for diabetic neuropathy and postherpetic neuralgia

Lackner, & Leppik, 1994; Graves et al., 1998). Age, by itself, does not affect gabapentin pharmacokinetics although the age-associated decline in renal function would be expected to result in reduced CL/f and renal clearance and increased t $^{1}/_{2}$ (Boyd, Turck, Abel, Sedman, & Bockbrader, 1999).

Adverse Effects/Drug-Drug Interactions The most common adverse effects with CBZ are either dose-dependent or transient, including nystagmus, dizziness, diplopia, lightheadedness, and lethargy. Cognitive impairment, effects on mood and sleep (e.g., agitation, restlessness, irritability, insomnia), syndrome of inappropriate antidiuretic hormone secretion (SIADH), and gastrointestinal (GI) effects can also occur (Troupin, 1996). At higher serum concentrations, headache, diplopia, dysarthria, and ataxia may develop.

Unfortunately, CBZ is associated with a large number of significant drug-drug interactions. As a stimulant of hepatic cytochrome P450 enzyme activity, it can accelerate the hepatic metabolism of several agents, thus potentially reducing their therapeutic effects (e.g., benzodiazepines, corticosteroids, phenytoin [+/–], valproate, estrogen, lamotrigine, quinidine, risperidone, warfarin). Several drugs can reduce the hepatic metabolism of CBZ, potentially resulting in CBZ toxicity (e.g., propoxyphene, valproate, calcium channel blockers, cimetidine, isoniazid, macrolide antimicrobials).

Compared to other AED, gabapentin is subject to few drug-drug interactions and has a lower incidence of adverse effects (Troupin, 1996). Common adverse effects of gabapentin include somnolence, dizziness, ataxia, and fatigue. Less frequently reported adverse effects include nystagmus, tremor, and diplopia (Troupin). These side effects may be avoided or minimized by "starting low and going slow." The only significant pharmacokinetic drug-drug interaction involves a reduction in gabapentin bioavailability with simultaneous administration with magnesium/aluminum–containing antacids.

Contraindications/Drug-Disease-State Interactions/Precautions Contraindications to CBZ include a history of bone marrow depression and hypersensitivity to CBZ or TCA. Baseline evaluation of liver function and a complete blood count should be obtained before implementing therapy. The only contraindication to gabapentin is hypersensitivity to the compound.

Dosing and Administration (Table 6.3) A starting dose of CBZ 50 to 100 mg twice daily should be prescribed, increasing the dose by 100 mg/day on a weekly basis as needed to a maximum of 1,200 mg/day (Guay, 2001). Gabapentin dosing is empirically based on AED dosing recommendations. An initial dose of 100 to 300 mg once daily titrated to three times daily is recommended, increasing the dose as needed to a maximum of 3,600 mg/day (see Case 1 below). Dose adjustment based upon renal function must also be kept in mind.

Local Anesthetic/Antiarrhythmic Agents

Mexiletine, an oral congener of lidocaine, has been reported to be an effective analgesic for neuropathic pain, including diabetic neuropathy and central poststroke pain and it is less toxic than tocainide (Galer, 1995). Like most of the AEDs, this agent blocks sodium channels and thus acts as a membrane stabilizer.

Pharmacokinetic Considerations Most data suggest that the single-dose and steady-state pharmacokinetics of mexiletine are not significantly affected by advancing age (el Allaf, Garlier, & Dresse, 1986; Grech-Belanger et al., 1989). However, one study did report a statistically significant reduction in CL/f of 0.3 percent per year from age 40 years onward (Ueno, Kawaguchi, & Tanaka, 1993).

Adverse Effects/Drug-Drug Interactions Common adverse effects include GI distress, dizziness, tremor, irritability, nervousness, and headache (Irving & Wallace, 1997). GI effects can be minimized by taking the drug with food and by slowly increasing the dose over several weeks. Seizures can occur with very high doses.

Contraindications/Drug-Disease-State Interactions/Precautions   Mexiletine is contraindicated in patients with second- or third-degree heart block. Patients with a history of cardiac abnormalities, an abnormal ECG, or cardiac symptoms should be referred to a cardiologist before mexiletine is prescribed.

Dosing and Administration   A starting dose of 150 to 200 mg one or two times daily should be used, titrated up to a maximum daily dose of 1,200 mg. A dosage between 150 to 300 mg every 8 hours is usually effective.

Baclofen

Baclofen is used predominantly to reduce the spasticity associated with multiple sclerosis, but it is also effective in TN. It achieves its analgesic effect by inhibiting the release of presynaptic excitatory amino acids (Sidebottom & Maxwell, 1995). Baclofen is thought to be generally less effective than CBZ and should be considered as second-line therapy in TN due to its adverse effect profile (Fromm, 1994; Sidebottom & Maxwell, 1995). Baclofen in combination with CBZ may be useful in patients who do not respond to CBZ monotherapy. Since baclofen and CBZ act at different synaptic sites, together they may produce a synergistic analgesic effect (Sidebottom & Maxwell).

Pharmacokinetic Considerations   One study has documented no clinically important effect of advanced age on single-dose baclofen pharmacokinetics.

Adverse Effects/Drug-Drug Interactions   Common adverse effects associated with baclofen include drowsiness, dizziness, ataxia, mental confusion, and gastrointestinal distress (e.g., nausea, vomiting) (Sidebottom & Maxwell, 1995). Approximately 10% of patients cannot tolerate baclofen because of these effects (Fromm, 1994). Unfortunately, combination baclofen/AED therapy may increase the occurrence of some adverse effects, including drowsiness, nausea, and vomiting (Sidebottom & Maxwell, 1995). Slowly increasing the dose can minimize these adverse effects, but pain severity often limits the duration of drug titration (Fromm). As might be expected, baclofen may enhance the sedation caused by other CNS depressants and vice versa.

Contraindications/Drug-Disease-State Interactions/Precautions   Contra-indications to baclofen therapy include the presence of epilepsy, a history of convulsive disorders, and hypersensitivity to the drug. Baclofen should be discontinued gradually after chronic therapy because medication withdrawal may precipitate hallucinations, seizures, anxiety, or tachyarrhythmias up to 2 months after discontinuation. If these symptoms occur, baclofen should be reinstituted at the previous dose and gradually decreased by 5 to 10 mg/day at weekly intervals (Irving & Wallace, 1997).

Dosing and Administration   Baclofen is usually initiated at 5 to 10 mg two or three times daily, increasing the dose by 5 to 10 mg/day every 2 to 3 days to the usual effective range of 50 to 60 mg (Sidebottom & Maxwell, 1995). The maximum daily dose of baclofen is 80 mg.

Corticosteroids

Corticosteroids (CS) are commonly used as adjunctive pain therapy in cancer patients because they can elevate mood, stimulate appetite, decrease nausea and vomiting, and reduce inflammation (Jacox et al., 1994). Diminished capillary permeability and peritumor edema are examples of the beneficial anti-inflammatory effects of CS. Corticosteroids are especially effective for pain caused by soft tissue infiltration, acute nerve compression, visceral distention, temporal arteritis, polymyalgia rheumatica, rheumatoid arthritis and other vasculitides, and increased intracranial pressure (Levy, 1996). Intra-articular corticosteroids should also be considered for the older adult with three or fewer painful joints in the setting of osteoarthritis, rheumatoid arthritis, gout, pseudogout, and other inflammatory arthritides. Joint injections may be repeated every 3 months.

Pharmacokinetic Considerations   Despite widespread usage over several decades, few data exist regarding the effect of aging on corticosteroid pharmacokinetics. One study has documented a 38% reduction in CL/f and a 24% reduction in steady-state volume of distribution of free (non-protein-bound) prednisolone (the active metabolite of prednisone) (Stuck, Frey, & Frey, 1988).

Adverse Effects/Drug-Drug Interactions   Adverse effects seen with short-term CS adminstration include hypertension, hyperglycemia, immunosuppression, psychotic reactions, and cognitive impairment. Adverse effects associated with long-term use include myopathy, Cushing's habitus, and osteoporosis. The benefit of pain relief must be weighed against the occurrence of myopathy, which can greatly impair quality of life. In cases in which myopathy worsens quality of life, CS dose reduction and physical therapy should be considered (Levy, 1994).

Corticosteroids may be involved in numerous drug-drug interactions. Hepatic-enzyme-inducing drugs (e.g., rifampin, barbiturates, phenytoin, carbamazepine) may decrease CS efficacy through enhanced CS metabolism. Concurrent use with potassium-wasting diuretics and amphotericin B enhance CS-associated hypokalemia while concurrent use with sodium-containing medications enhances the risk of edema and hypertension. The efficacy of hypoglycemics may be attenuated by CS.

Contraindications/Drug-Disease-State Interactions/Precautions   Although there are no absolute contraindications to systemic CS, the risks versus benefits of their use should be carefully considered for patients with the following conditions:

- Human immunodeficiency virus (HIV) infection
- Recent intestinal anastomoses
- Cardiac disease (e.g., congestive heart failure)
- Severe renal function impairment
- Current or recent chickenpox (including recent exposure)
- Current or recent measles (including recent exposure)
- Active or latent esophagitis, gastritis, or peptic ulcer disease
- Diabetes mellitus
- Systemic fungal infection
- Ocular herpes simplex infection
- Myasthenia gravis
- Active or latent tuberculosis (TB), including a positive skin test or history of TB

Dosing and Administration   Although there is no consensus about the preferred agent and dosage of corticosteroids, 4 to 8 mg of dexamethasone two or three times daily, 16 to 32 mg of methylprednisolone two or three times daily, or 20 to 40 mg of prednisone two or three times daily are reasonable choices for soft tissue infiltration, acute nerve compression, visceral distention, and increased intracranial pressure. For acute spinal cord compression or acute severe increased intracranial pressure, intravenous administration of 10 to 20 mg of dexamethasone every 6 hours, or 40 to 80 mg of methylprednisolone every 6 hours, is recommended (Levy, 1996). These doses are fairly aggressive for older adult patients, and a lower dose should be considered. After satisfactory pain reduction is achieved, the corticosteroid dose should remain constant for several days, then gradually tapered to the minimum effective dose over the next few weeks to minimize long-term adverse effects (Levy, 1994).

Corticosteroid dosing for inflammatory disorders is variable. For a high index of suspicion of temporal arteritis (i.e., jaw claudication, new onset severe headaches in the setting of shoulder and/or hip girdle morning stiffness), the patient should immediately be placed on high-dose prednisone (1 mg/kg/day) in order to prevent irreversible blindness (Allen & Studenski, 1986, Keltner, 1982), followed by temporal artery biopsy. For less urgent rheumatologic disorders, consultation with a rheumatologist should be sought prior to initiating CS therapy.

Calcitonin

A polypeptide hormone that inhibits osteoclast-induced bone resorption, calcitonin is indicated for treating hypercalcemia and osteoporosis (Jacox et al., 1994; Levy, 1996). Calcitonin is also used to reduce pain from bone metastasis, phantom-limb pain, and vertebral fractures (Levy, 1996). Despite several suggested theories, the mechanism by which calcitonin produces analgesia is still not known (Silverman, 1997). Calcitonin's analgesic properties appear independent of the bone remodeling effect useful in treating osteoporosis. Pain relief has been documented within 1 week of initiating treatment, which is too soon for significant modification of bone turnover. Calcitonin's efficacy in treating bone pain associated with malignancy and postvertebral fracture pain has been demonstrated in clinical trials, although this finding has not been universal. Although the efficacy and the long-term benefits and risks of calcitonin for cancer pain are still not established, a trial of calcitonin may be considered for patients with refractory pain.

Adverse Effects/Drug-Drug Interactions   Most of calcitonin's adverse effects relate to the gastrointestinal system or to local reactions at the site of administration. Nausea with or without vomiting is seen in up to 10% of patients when therapy is initiated, but tolerance to these effects generally develops over time. Local reactions at the site of subcutaneous or intramuscular injection occur in up to 10% of patients, and flushing of the face or hands occurs in 2% to 5% of patients. Local nasal reactions to the intranasal preparation occur in a small percentage of patients (rhinitis 12%, symptoms of the nose 10.6%, and epistaxis 3.5%). Periodic nasal examinations are advised in patients using the intranasal product.

Contraindications/Drug-Disease-State Interactions/Precautions   Since commercially available calcitonin is derived from salmon, allergic reactions can occur; skin testing should be considered before initiating therapy.

Dosing and Administration   Generally, the dose of calcitonin used for treating pain caused by bone metastasis is 200 IU/day for the parenteral and the intranasal product (Levy, 1996). Intranasal calcitonin may be preferred so as to avoid injections and decrease adverse effects. The intranasal product requires careful attention to pump assembly, pump priming, nasal insufflation, and storage.

Summary

For neuropathic pain, tricyclic antidepressants and certain anticonvulsants (especially gabapentin) should be considered the agents of choice. Corticosteroids have a primary role for treating certain rheumatological disorders seen primarily in older adults (e.g., polymyalgia rheumatica and temporal arteritis).

SETTING-SPECIFIC CONSIDERATIONS

The majority of older persons requiring pain medications are likely to be living in the community. Therefore a key consideration is medication adherence. Some general factors to consider in enhancing adherence include (1) modify medication schedules to fit patient lifestyle, (2) consider generics to reduce costs, (3) dispense medications with easy-off caps and use easy to swallow dosage forms, and (4) use larger type direction labels and auxiliary labels (Mallett, 1992; Opdycke, Ascione, Shimp, & Rosen, 1992). Both written and verbal drug information should be provided to the patient and the family. Also, the use of adherence-enhancing aids should be considered (e.g., special packaging, medication record, drug calendar, medication boxes, dose-measuring devices) (Mallett, 1992; Opdycke et al., 1992).

SUMMARY/RECOMMENDATIONS

Adherence to the principles outlined below should result in more optimal analgesic pharmacotherapy for older adults:

1. Learn how to use a few analgesic agents well rather than attempt to learn how to use the entire cadre of available therapies.
2. Maximize the use of acetaminophen for noninflammatory pain prior to exploring further options. Underdosing of this agent is a significant clinical problem.

3. Minimize the use of NSAIDs in noninflammatory pain states, based on their substantial adverse event risk in older adults.
4. Topical agents (e.g., capsaicin) may be helpful in some persistent pain disorders and avoids the systemic side effects seen with oral analgesics.
5. If the patient is committed to long-term opioid therapy, anticipate and preemptively treat opioid-induced constipation, an adverse effect towards which tolerance will not develop.
6. Exercise caution when prescribing opioids for the older adult with dysmobility; nonopioid management is preferable in such cases. If opioids are considered necessary, an assistive device should be considered and the patient monitored very carefully.
7. Use longer acting opioids where possible, to allow for more convenient dosing (e.g., extended-released morphine or oxycodone).
8. Avoid the use of propoxyphene, meperidine, and pentazocine when selecting opioids (Beers, 1997).
9. Opioids do have activity against neuropathic pain. However, secondary tricyclic antidepressants (e.g., desipramine or nortriptyline) and certain anticonvulsants (especially gabapentin) should be considered the agents of choice for pain of this etiology.
10. As-needed dosing of rapid-acting analgesics should not be considered a primary therapeutic strategy in persistent pain. Use of these agents indicates a need to adjust the dose(s) of the scheduled maintenance analgesic agent(s).

CASE STUDIES

Case 1

AH, a 91-year-old male who resides in his own home, developed acute herpes zoster after a bout of "the flu." He was treated with a 7-day course of famciclovir and a tapering dose of oral prednisone. During the acute phase, he required treatment with acetaminophen plus codeine 30 mg, 2 tablets every 4 to 6 hours, to manage his severe pain. It has now been 4 months since his acute illness and he still reports moderate to severe pain of a burning, gnawing nature that requires frequent administration of acetaminophen plus oxycodone in order for him to remain functional. Other concurrent conditions include hypertension, hyperlipidemia, angina pectoris, second-degree heart block, and symptomatic benign prostatic hypertrophy (BPH). His other medications include terazosin, simvastatin, metoprolol, and isosorbide mononitrate.

His estimated creatinine clearance is 32 mL/min. What would be your treatment approach for this gentleman?

Discussion

The patient has developed a moderate to severe case of postherpetic neuralgia, one of the most common neuropathic pain syndromes in older individuals. Although opioids are active in neuropathic pain, they do not constitute the drugs of first choice. Drugs of choice include tricyclic antidepressants and anticonvulsants. Based upon the patient's medical history, specifically his cardiac history and BPH, the use of tricyclic antidepressants would be contraindicated (Beers, 1997). Although CBZ might be a reasonable choice, gabapentin would probably be a better one due to its absence of drug-drug interactions and lack of need for serum drug concentration and laboratory monitoring. This agent could be started in a regimen of 100 mg once daily with slow dose escalation in 100 mg increments at 7 to 10 day intervals to optimum effect. Up to 3,600 mg/day can be used for analgesia. Due to dose-dependent saturable bioavailability, attempts should be made to keep individual doses at or below 600 mg.

Case 2

> JM is an 83-year-old female assisted-living resident with terminal breast cancer metastatic to bone and liver. The hospice team assumes responsibility for her care. Among her problems, severe bone pain is poorly controlled and she suffers from repeated bouts of fecal impaction. Her current medication regimen includes: docusate 100 mg PO qd; meperidine 100 mg PO q 3h while awake; acetaminophen 300 mg/codeine 30 mg, 1–2 tabs q 4–6 h prn (uses 8 tablets/day); morphine elixir 5 mg PO q 4–6 h prn (uses 15 mg/day). What changes would you make to her treatment regimen?

Discussion

Constipation is the major adverse effect of opioids to which tolerance does not develop. Aggressive laxative regimens should be prescribed from the time of opioid initiation. Such regimens should include a combination of a stool softener (like docusate) plus a stimulant laxative (like senna or bisacodyl), with as-needed laxatives available to prevent impaction. After manual disimpaction and use of an oil retention enema followed by an osmotic enema (Fleets®) if needed, the patient should be started on a combination laxative regimen with the dose of the stimulant being titrated to effect.

Bone pain due to metastatic cancer often responds to the addition of a nonsteroidal anti-inflammatory drug (NSAID). Especially useful agents are those with a reduced potential for gastrointestinal or renal adverse effects (e.g., nonacetylated salicylates, rofecoxib). Meperidine should never be used to manage persistent pain, especially in the older adult (Beers, 1997). Its duration of action is short and accumulation of its normeperidine metabolite can lead to central nervous system excitation, including tremors and seizures.

It is appropriate to use an opioid analgesic for chronic malignant pain. In this patient, a conversion chart should be utilized to convert her daily ingestion of the three opioids into "morphine equivalents." In this case, she is receiving the equivalent of 100 mg of morphine orally per day. Due to incomplete cross-tolerance, when converting patients to alternative opioids it is usual practice not to begin at the calculated equivalent dose (i.e., reduce by 33–50%). However, because of her poor pain control, it would be reasonable to start the patient on approximately 75% of the calculated equivalent dose (i.e., approximately oral morphine elixir 15 mg every 4 hours around the clock). An as-needed, immediate-release opioid order is recommended for breakthrough pain. Once JM's pain is controlled, she can be converted to a more convenient maintenance agent such as sustained-release oral morphine.

REFERENCES

Abraham, J. L. (1999). ACP-ASIM End of Life Care Consensus Panel. Management of pain and spinal cord compression in patients with advanced cancer. *Ann Intern Med, 131*, 37–46.

Allen, N. B., & Studenski, S. A. (1986). Polymyalgia rheumatica and temporal arteritis. *Med Clin North Am, 70*(2), 369–384.

American Pain Society. (1992). *Principles of analgesic use in treatment of acute and cancer pain* (3rd ed.). Skokie, IL: Author.

American Pain Society. (1997). The use of opioids for the treatment of chronic pain. *Clin J Pain, 13*, 6–8.

Aronoff, G. R., Berns, J. S., Brier, M. E., Golper, T. A., Morrison, G., Singer, I., Swan, S. K., & Bennett, W. M. (1999). *Drug prescribing in renal failure: Dosing guidelines for adults* (4th ed.). Philadelphia: American College Physicians.

Baillie, S. P., Bateman, D. N., Coates, P. E., et al. (1989). Age and the pharmacokinetics of morphine. *Age Ageing, 18*, 258–262.

Beers, M. H. (1997). Explicit criteria for determining potentially inappropriate medication use by the elderly: An update. *Arch Intern Med, 157*, 1531–1536.

Bellville, J. W., Forrest, W. H., Miller, E., & Brown, B. W., Jr. (1971). Influence of age on pain relief from analgesics. *JAMA, 217*, 1835–1841.

Bernstein, J. E. (1988). Capsaicin in dermatologic disease. *Semin Dermatol, 7*, 304–309.

Bernstein, J. E., Korman, N. J., Bickers, D. R., Dahl, M. V., & Millikan, L. E. (1989). Topical capsaicin treatment of chronic postherpetic neuralgia. *J Am Acad Dermatol, 21*, 265–270.

Bernus, I., Dickinson, R. G., Hooper, W. D., & Eadie, M. J. (1997). Anticonvulsant therapy in aged patients: Clinical pharmacokinetic considerations. *Drugs Aging, 10*, 278–289.

Boyd, R. A., Turck, D., Abel, R. B., Sedman, A. J., & Bockbrader, H. N. (1999). Effects of age and gender on single-dose pharmacokinetics of gabapentin. *Epilepsia, 40*, 474–479.

Brater, D. C. (1999). Effects of nonsteroidal anti-inflammatory drugs on renal function: Focus on cyclooxegenase-2-selective inhibition. *Am J Med, 107*(Suppl. 6A), 65S–71S.

Bruera, E., Fainsinger, R., MacEachern, T., & Hanson, J. (1992) The use of methylphenidate in patients with incident cancer pain receiving regular opiates. *Pain, 50*, 75–77.

Cloyd, J. C., Lackner, T. E., & Leppik, I. E. (1994). Antiepileptics in the elderly. *Arch Fam Med, 3*, 589–598.

Comer, A. M., & Lamb, H. M. (2000). Lidocaine patch 5%. *Drugs, 59*, 245–249.

Crofford, L. J., Lipsky, P. E., Brooks, P., Abramson, S. B., Simon, L. S., & Van de Putte, L. B. A. (2000). Basic biology and clinical applications of specific cyclooxegenase-2 inhibitors. *Arth Rheum, 43*, 4–13.

Davies, K. N., Castleden, C. M., McBurney, A., & Jagger, C. (1989). The effect of ageing on the pharmacokinetics of dihydrocodeine. *Eur J Clin Pharmacol, 37*, 375–379.

Delafuente, J. C. (2000). Arthritis. In J. C. Delafuente & R. B. Stewart (Eds.), *Therapeutics in the elderly* (3rd ed., pp. 499–514). Cincinnati, OH: Harvey Whitney Books.

Divoll, M., Abernathy, D. R., Ameer, B., & Greenblatt, D. J. (1982). Acetaminophen kinetics in the elderly. *Clin Pharmacol Ther, 31*, 151–156.

Drug Facts and Comparisons. (2000). St. Louis, MO: Facts & Comparisons.

el Allaf, D., Carlier, J., & Dresse, A. (1986). Effects of age on the pharmacokinetics of mexiletine. *Int J Clin Pharmacol Res, 6*, 303–307.

Fitzgerald, M. (1983). Capsaicin and sensory neurons—a review. *Pain, 15*, 109–130.

Flanagan, R. J., Johnston, A., White, A. S., & Crome, P. (1989). Pharmacokinetics of dextropropoxyphene and nordextropropoxyphene in young and elderly volunteers after single and multiple dextropropoxyphene dosage. *Br J Clin Pharmacol, 28*, 463–469.

Forman, W. B. (1996). Opioid analgesic drugs in the elderly. *Clin Geriatr Med, 12*, 489–500.

Fromm, G. H. (1994). Baclofen as adjuvant analgesic. *J Pain Symptom Manage, 9*, 500–509.

Galer, B. S. (1995). Neuropathic pain of peripheral origin: Advances in pharmacologic treatment. *Neurology, 45*(Suppl. 9), S17–S25.

Gammaitoni, A., Gallagher, R. M., & Welz-Bosna, M. (2000). Topical ketamine gel: Possible role in treating neuropathic pain. *Pain Medicine, 1*(1), 97–100.

Graves, N. M., Brundage, R. C., Wen, Y., et al. (1998). Population pharmacokinetics of carbamazepine in adults with epilepsy. *Pharmacotherapy, 18*, 273–281.

Gray, S. L., Lai, K. V., & Larson, E. B. (1999). Drug-induced cognition disorders in the elderly—incidence, prevention, and management. *Drug Safety, 21*, 101–122.

Grech-Belanger, O., Barbeau, G., Kishka, P., Fiset, C., LeBoeuf, F., & Blouin, M. (1989). Pharmacokinetics of mexiletine in the elderly. *J Clin Pharmacol, 29*, 311–315.

Griffin, M. R., & Ray, W. A. (2000). Nonsteroidal anti-inflammatory drugs and acute renal failure in elderly persons. *Am J Epidemiol, 151*, 488–496.

Guay, D. R. P. (1995). Analgesics. In J. M. Rippe, R. S. Irwin, J. S. Albert, & M. P. Fink (Eds.), *Intensive care medicine* (Vol. 2, 3rd ed). Boston: Little, Brown.

Guay, D. R. P. (2001). Adjunctive agents in the management of chronic pain. *Pharmacotherapy, 21*, 1070–1081.

Hanlon, J. T., Custon, T., & Ruby, C. M. (1996). Drug-related falls in the elderly. *Top Geriatr Rehabil, 11*, 38–54.

Hanlon, J. T., & O'Brien, J. G. (1989). The pharmacological management of the elderly patient with terminal cancer pain. *J Ger Drug Ther, 3*, 5–30.

Hanlon, J. T., Ruby, C. M., Shelton, P. S., & Pulliam, C. C. (1999). Geriatrics. In J. T. Dipiro, R. L. Talbert, G. C. Yee, G. R. Matzke, B. G. Wells, & L. M. Posey (Eds.), *Pharmacotherapy: A pathophysiologic approach.* (4th ed., pp. 52–69). Norwalk, CT: Appleton and Lange.

Hansten, P. D., Horn, J. R., Koda-Kimble, M. A., & Young, L. Y. (2000). *Drug interactions: A clinical perspective and analysis of current developments.* Vancouver, WA: Applied Therapeutics.

Harati, Y., Gooch, C., Swenson, M., Edelman, S., Greene, D., Raskin, P., Donofrio, P., Cornblath, D., Sachdeo, R., Siu, C. O., & Kamin, M. (1998). Double-blind randomized trial of tramadol for the treatment of the pain of diabetic neuropathy. *Neurology, 50*, 1842–1846.

Herman, R. J., McAllister, C. D., Branch, R. A., & Wilkinson, G. R. (1985). Effects of age on meperidine disposition. *Clin Pharmacol Ther, 37*, 19–24.

Holdsworth, M. T., Forman, W. B., Killilea, T. A., Nystrom, K. M., Paul, R., Brand, S. C., & Reynolds, R. (1994). Transdermal fentanyl disposition in elderly subjects. *Gerontology, 40*, 32–37.

Holmberg, L., Odar-Cederlof, I., Boreus, L. O., Heyner, L., & Ehrnebo, M. (1982). Comparative disposition of pethidine and norpethidine in the old and young patients. *Eur J Clin Pharmacol, 22*, 175–179.

Insel, P. A. (1996). Analgesic, antipyretic and anti-inflammatory agents and drugs employed in the treatment of gout. In J. G. Hardman, L. E. Limbird, P. B. Molinoff, R. W. Ruddon, & A. G. Gilman (Eds.), *Goodman and Gilman's the pharmacological basis of therapeutics* (9th ed., pp. 617–657). New York: McGraw-Hill.

Jacox, A., Carr, D. B., Payne, R., Berde, C. B., Brietbart, W., Cain, J. M., Chapman, C. R., Cleeland, C. S., Ferrell, B. R., Finley, R. S., Hester, N. O., Hill, C. S., Jr., Leak, W. D., Lipman, A. G., Logan, C. L., McGarvey, C. L., Miaskowski, C. A., Mulder, D. S., Paice, J. A., Shapiro, B. S., Silberstein, E. B., Smith, R. S., Stover, J., Tsou, C. V., Vecchiarelli, L., & Weissman, D. E. (1994, March). Management of cancer pain. (Clinical Practice Guideline No. 9. AHCPR Publication No. 94–0592). Rockville, MD: Agency for Health Care Policy and Research, Department of Health and Human Services.

Jaspersen, D. (2000). Drug-induced oseophageal disorders: Pathogenesis, incidence, prevention and management. *Drug Safety, 22,* 237–249.

Johnson, R. W. (1997). Herpes zoster and postherpetic neuralgia: Optimal treatment. *Drugs Aging, 10,* 80–94.

Kaiko, R. F. (1980). Age and morphine analgesia in cancer patients with postoperative pain. *Clin Pharmacol Ther, 28,* 823–826.

Keltner, J. L. (1982). Giant cell arteritis: Signs and symptoms. *Ophthalmology, 89,* 1101–1110.

Leeb, B. F., Schweitzer, H., Montag, K., et al. (2000). A metaanalysis of chondroitin sulfate in the treatment of osteoarthritis. *J Rheumatol, 27,* 205–211.

Levy, M. H. (1994). Pharmacologic management of cancer pain. *Semin Oncol, 21,* 718–739.

Levy, M. H. (1996). Pharmacologic treatment of cancer pain. *N Engl J Med, 335,* 1124–1132.

Lynn, B. (1990). Capsaicin: Actions on nociceptive C-fibres and therapeutic potential. *Pain, 41,* 61–69.

MacFarlane, B. V., Wright, A., O'Callaghan, J., & Benson, H. A. E. (1997). Chronic neuropathic pain and its control by drugs. *Pharmacol Ther, 75*(1), 1–19.

Magnus, L. (1999). Nonepileptic uses of gabapentin. *Epilepsia, 40*(Suppl. 6), S66–S72.

Mallett, L. (1992). Counseling in special populations: The elderly patient. *Am Pharm, NS32,* 71–81.

Matzke, G. R. (1997). Clinical consequences of nonnarcotic analgesic use. *Ann Pharmacother, 31,* 245–248.

McAlindon, T. E., LaValley, M. P., Gulin, J. P., & Felson, D. T. (2000). Glucosamine and chondroitin for treatment of osteoarthritis: A systematic quality assessment and meta-analysis. *JAMA, 283,* 1469–1475.

McLeod, P. J., Huang, A. R., Tamblyn, R. M., & Gayton, D. C. (1997). Defining inappropriate practices in prescribing for elderly people: A national consensus panel. *CMAJ, 156,* 385–391.

McQuay, H. J., Tramèr, M., Nye, B. A., Carroll, D., Wiffen, P. J., & Moore, R. A. (1996). A systematic review of antidepressants in neuropathic pain. *Pain, 68,* 217–227.

Moertel, C. G., Ahmann, D. L., Taylor, W. F., & Schwartau, N. (1972). A comparative evaluation of marketed analgesic drugs. *N Engl J Med, 286,* 813–815.

Odar-Cederlof, I., Boreous, L. O., Bondesson, U., Holmberg, L., & Heyner, L. (1985). Comparison of renal excretion of meperidine and its metabolites in old and young patients. *Eur J Clin Pharmacol, 28,* 171–175.

Opdycke, R. A., Ascione, F. J., Shimp, L. A., & Rosen, R. I. (1992). A systematic approach to educating elderly patients about their medications. *Patient Education and Counseling, 19,* 43–60.

Owen, J. A., Sitar, D. S., Berger, L., Brownell, L., Duke, P. C., & Mitenko, P. A. (1983). Age-related morphine kinetics. *Clin Pharmacol Ther, 34,* 364–368.

Reginster, J. Y., Deroisy, R., Rovati, L. C., Lee, R. L., Lejeune, E., Bruyere, O., Giacovelli, G., Henrotin, Y., Dacre, J. E., & Gossett, C. (2001). Long-term effects of glucosamine sulphate on osteoarthritis progression. *Lancet, 357*, 251–256.

Rindone, J. P., Hiller, D., Collacott, E., Nordhaugen, N., & Arriola, G. (2000). Randomized, controlled trial of glucosamine for treating osteoarthritis of the knee. *West J Med, 172*, 91–94.

Rudorfer, M. V., Manji, H. K., & Potter, W. Z. (1994). Comparative tolerability profiles of the newer versus older antidepressants. *Drug Saf, 10*, 18–46.

Scott, J. C., & Stanski, D. R. (1987). Decreased fentanyl and alfentanil dose requirements with age: A simultaneous pharmacokinetic and pharmacodynamic evaluation. *J Pharmacol Exp Ther, 240*, 159–165.

Shorr, R. I., Griffin, M. R., Daugherty, J., & Ray, W. (1992). Opioid analgesics and the risk of hip fracture in the elderly: Codeine and propoxyphene. *J Gerontol, 47*, M111–M115.

Shorr, R. I., Ray, W. A., Daugherty, J. R., & Griffin, M. R. (1993). Concurrent use of nonsteroidal anti-inflammatory drugs and oral anticoagulants places elderly persons at high risk for hemorrhagic peptic ulcer disease. *Arch Intern Med, 153*, 1665–1670.

Sidebottom, A., & Maxwell, S. (1995). The medical and surgical management of trigeminal neuralgia. *J Clin Pharm Ther, 20*, 31–35.

Silverman, S. L. (1997). Calcitonin. *Am J Med Sci, 313*, 13–16.

Stanski, D. R., Greenblatt, D. J., & Lowenstein, E. (1978). Kinetics of intravenous and intramuscular morphine. *Clin Pharmacol Ther, 24*, 52–59.

Stuck, A. E., Frey, B. M., & Frey, F. J. (1988). Kinetics of prednisolone and endogenous cortical suppression in the elderly. *Clin Pharmacol Ther, 43*, 354–362.

Thompson, J. P., Bower, S., Liddle, A. M., & Rowbotham, D. J. (1998). Perioperative pharmacokinetics of transdermal fentanyl in elderly and young adult patients. *Br J Anaesthesia, 81*, 152–154.

Triggs, E. J., Nation, R. L., Long, A., & Ashley, J. J. (1975). Pharmacokinetics in the elderly. *Eur J Clin Pharmacol, 8*, 55–62.

Troupin, A. S. (1996). Dose-related adverse effects of anticonvulsants. *Drugs Saf, 14*, 299–328.

Ueno, K., Kawaguchi, Y., & Tanaka, K. (1993). Pharmacokinetics of mexiletine in middle-aged and elderly patients. *Clin Pharm, 12*, 768–770.

Vaillancourt, P. D., & Langevin, H. M. (1999). Painful peripheral neuropathies. *Med Clin North Am, 83*, 627–642.

Vane, J. R. (1971). Inhibition of prostaglandin synthesis as a mechanism of action for aspirin-like drugs. *Nature, 231*, 232–235.

Walsh, D. (2000). Pharmacological management of cancer pain. *Semin Oncol, 27*, 45–63.

Walt, R., Katschinski, B., Logan, R., Ashley, J., & Langman, M. (1986). Rising frequency of ulcer perforation in elderly people in the United Kingdom. *Lancet, 1*, 489–492.

Watson, C. P., & Babul, N. (1998). Efficacy of oxycodone in neuropathic pain: A randomized controlled trial in post-herpetic neuralgia. *Neurology, 50*, 1837–1841.

Weiner, D., Hanlon, J. T., & Studenski, S. (1998). CNS drug-related falls liability in community dwelling elderly. *Gerontology, 44*, 217–221.

Invasive Pharmacologic and Nonpharmacologic Modalities

7

Stephen P. Lordon, Doris K. Cope, and Perry G. Fine

Until the mid 1980s, the mainstay of severe persistent pain treatment was oral opioids. For pain from advanced cancer, severe neuropathy, and other long-standing pain syndromes, these agents were often ineffective at doses tolerated by the central nervous system. The excessive sedation and respiratory depression resulting from analgesic doses limited the clinical ability to control pain. In addition, the sometimes exaggerated fear of addiction and government regulation resulted in a significant number of patients with untreated pain. It has been estimated that approximately 28% of cancer patients die in severe untreated pain. The advent of long-term spinal and epidural catheters with both external and internal infusion pumps in the mid 1980s gave pain-medicine physicians the option to more effectively treat severe pain with less than 1/100th the dose of oral opioids and, therefore, limited systemic side effects. When properly regulated, neuroaxial opioid infusion provides continuous and effective analgesia without requiring frequent dosing. In addition, neurolytic blocks specifically targeting pain generators or blocking afferent signal transmission and dorsal column spinal cord stimulation are now available to treat refractory pain. This chapter will review the current knowledge of invasive pharmacological and nonpharmacological options for pain control, including neurolytic techniques and dorsal column stimulation as new alternatives for more effective and safer pain control in older adults. A summary of these invasive modalities is provided in Table 7.1.

EVIDENCE AND PRINCIPLES FOR PRACTICE

Role of the Geriatrician and Pain Management Team in Choosing Invasive Modalities

Conventional medical training has focused on the anatomy of pain systems, physiology of pain transmission, and opioid and nonopioid pharmacology. Even today, pain medicine education is often limited to experiences during a surgical or medical clerkship, in which the practical treatment of cancer and chronic noncancer pain is not commonly incorporated. With the advent of pain fellowships approved by the Accreditation Council for Graduate Medical Education (ACGME), this clinical niche is now being addressed. Also, there have been historical myths and fears about the use of opioids and other controlled substances. In 2001, the Joint Commission on Accreditation of Healthcare Organizations (JCAHO) standards for pain evaluation and treatment mandate a new approach to medical practice in evaluating and treating pain in our patients. In addition to the noninvasive pharmacological modalities of pain management discussed in chapter 6 of this book, there are new and exciting interventional techniques to control refractory pain. Although noninvasive pharmacological modalities, coupled with behavioral and physical therapy techniques, effectively palliate the benign and malignant pain of the majority of patients, there is specialist help available for the most difficult pain problems.

When pain concerns are overwhelming for the geriatrician or primary care physician, referral to a pain management specialist may be necessary. It is important that the patient be fully evaluated in consultation with the pain specialist to ensure all diagnostics and treatments for a specific disease have been explored, and that reasonable conservative treatment for pain has been tried. Physical therapy and/or occupational therapy evaluation may be helpful, especially in patients with myofascial or other musculoskeletal pain syndromes or who have work-related or compensation issues. Psychological factors are often important. Even patients who benefit from improved pain control may continue to experience intense psychological suffering and diminished function. Anxiety, depression, and other forms of psychopathology may magnify pain symptoms, so in many circumstances where these issues prevail, relief of pain per se is not enough to improve patients' overall life functioning. True psychologically induced pain disorders are very rare, but many pain syndromes have a strong contribution from psychological disturbance. Well-defined treatment algorithms are being developed for both noncancer and malignant pain as treatment options are increasing. When conservative approaches fail to control pain, however, selected patients may benefit from the newest invasive modalities, such as intrathecal morphine pumps, neurolytic sympathetic blocks, radiofrequency neurolysis, or dorsal column and deep brain stimulation.

The decision to consider interventional techniques usually occurs after a pain medicine consultation. The primary care physician, pain physician, and patient need to explore risks and benefits in the context of overall goals. For a successful outcome, patient selection requires psychological evaluation, especially for those with long-term nonmalignant pain. Proper patient expectations result in improved patient results, and proper social and family support limits later psychological problems such as drug-seeking behavior.

Psychological Evaluation

First, psychological disturbances and contributors to distress need to be identified and treated. Second, maladaptive behaviors should be examined. These include family support systems that are negatively reinforcing and issues of secondary gain. Psychological interventions such as cognitive-behavioral restructuring, stress management, relaxation therapy, and pain education can be very helpful, and if at all possible, these should be offered. Interdisciplinary treatment plans that include behavioral and rehabilitative therapies may precede, occur concurrently, or follow a given interventional therapy, depending on the clinical circumstances. For instance, excruciating pain or extreme emotional distress can hinder a patient's ability to participate in or concentrate on rehabilitation. Through common sense and experience, criteria have emerged that define which patients should not receive implantable devices (Oakley & Staats, 2000). Relative and absolute contraindications have been developed, including positive Waddell signs (Scalzitti, 1997), unusual pain ratings, noncompliance, inappropriate expectations, and suicidal or homicidal tendencies. Other obstacles to successful intervention include the presence of severe untreated depression and severe personality disorders, creating difficulty in obtaining positive functional outcomes and subjective pain relief. Many clinicians will refrain from implanting an intrathecal pump in individuals with a history of illicit substance abuse. Case reports have documented patients who access their pumps either to obtain drugs or to administer illicit drugs, although these cases are rare.

Perceived disability and dysfunctional behavior also need to be carefully evaluated. Goals for interventional pain modalities need to be appropriate, since return-to-work rates following drug administration systems have been disappointing, with estimates ranging from 7% to 17%. These results, however, are surely biased, as the majority of patients receiving implantable neuroaxial devices have advanced and life-limiting malignancies. In the older adult population, function outcomes, such as ability to perform ADLs, and quality of life would represent more applicable measures.

In summary, truly interdisciplinary assessment of the patient in conjunction with spouse, family, and insurance case managers is needed to make the right decision about the right implantable technology at the right time. In patients with limited life expectancy, it is inappropriate to consider implantable procedures. However, neurolytic blocks and percutaneous neuroaxial catheters may be very appropriate. Excellent further reading on psychological evaluation of pain patients can be found in references that cover this topic in depth (Doleys, 2000; Doleys & Olson, 1997; Loeser, 2001).

Spinal Opioid Administration

History

In 1974, Cavallo et al. demonstrated the effect of morphine analgesia and nalaxone reversible analgesia on the substantia gelatinosa in cats. The first clinical reports of spinal opioids appeared in 1979. Since then, neuroaxial opioid administration of opioids and local anesthetics has become common in treating the perioperative pain patient and now the patient with persistent pain. The term *neuroaxial opioid administration* includes methods that deliver opioids into either the intrathecal or the peridural space; the two most common methods are epidural and direct intrathecal infusion. Systemic opioids do diffuse into the intrathecal space, but with a plasma to cerebrospinal fluid (CSF) concentration gradient of greater than 100:1, leading to negligible spinal effects under most circumstances. Only about 10% of an epidural opioid dose diffuses into the intrathecal space; the balance is absorbed into the systemic circulation. Plasma opioid concentrations of epidurally adminstered opioids approximate systemically administered drug concentrations, leading to a triple site of action for epidural opioid infusions: spinal, supraspinal, and systemic.

Pharmacodynamics and Pharmacokinetics of Neuroaxial Opioids

Spinal opioid receptors that inhibit transduction of nociceptive impulses are located predominately in the substantia gelatinosa of the dorsal horn on pre- and postsynaptic neurons. Selective administration of mu receptor opioid agonists to specific sites proximal to pain signal reception can have a much more potent effect than inhibition at higher central sites (Gourlay, Cherry, & Cousins, 1985; Max et al., 1985). One important physiochemical factor in the pharmacology of spinal opioids is lipid solubility. The more lipid soluble the molecule, the faster it will diffuse across lipid membranes and reach its site of action. Lipophilicity also determines anatomic spread, duration of effect, and likelihood of side effects. Only a certain percentage of hydrophilic and ionized molecules will cross lipid membranes. The percentage of drug that does cross is dependent upon the pH of the drug environment and the pKa of the drug. Only the fraction that is nonioinized or lipophilic will cross the lipid membrane. Sufentanil is a highly lipophilic molecule. It diffuses quickly to the site of action, but it also diffuses quickly away from the site of action. Morphine is hydrophilic and a salt. Only the nonionized lipophilic fraction of morphine will cross lipid membranes.

Epidurally administered opioids appear less potent than intrathecal opioids because these drug molecules must diffuse across several lipid layers, including the dura, and into the cerebrospinal fluid and dorsal horn before the receptor sites are activated. Drugs delivered into the epidural space are absorbed by epidural vessels, fat, and other nonspecific binding sites that reduce the availability of drug diffusion within the central nervous system. Equivalent intrathecal doses of opioids, therefore, only need to be about 10% of the dose required by the epidural route of administration.

Morphine is the prototypic, most frequently administered spinal opioid, and it diffuses readily in the CSF. Besides being a hydrophilic molecule, morphine, is also ionized. Only a small percentage of epidurally administered nonionized morphine passes through the dura and into the CSF. Within the CSF, the nonionized morphine molecules re-ionize, and only a very small fraction of nonionized morphine ever reaches the dorsal horn. Ionized morphine travels rostrally within the CSF circulation, binding to receptor sites throughout the neuraxis, leading to diffuse and multiple levels of analgesia. The slow rostral spread of morphine can cause untoward supraspinal effects that are delayed in onset, such as respiratory depression, nausea, and vomiting. The same factors that cause delayed onset of morphine's actions are also responsible for its extended duration of action. Since morphine is not metabolized in the CSF, it is only the diffusion of the nonionized fraction into the systemic circulation that limits its length of action. Lipophilic opioids like fentanyl and meperidine diffuse across the lipid membranes rapidly, compared to morphine. Also, increased lipid solubility causes increased vascular absorption within the epidural space, with decreased drug available to diffuse into the CSF. However, rostral spread is limited because of decreased ionization within the CSF. It is therefore necessary to deliver lipophilic drugs at the spinal level innervating the site of the pain. Sufentanil has both very high lipid solubility and very high affinity for central mu opioid receptors, but has limited usefulness for epidural long-term infusions because rapid and near-complete vascular absorption limits spinal availability of the drug.

Clinical Applications of Neuroaxial Medications

To date, cancer patients have been the most common pain patients to receive neuroaxial opioids. Increasingly, however, patients with noncancer pain, refractory to other treatments, are being identified as candidates for neuroaxial opioid infusion. Some of these diagnoses include failed back syndrome, complex regional pain syndrome, painful neuropathy, and atypical facial pain. Other plausible indications for intrathecal therapy include osteoporosis with multiple fractures, visceral pain, axial somatic pain, head and neck pain, and painful neurodegenerative diseases such as multiple sclerosis.

The indications for considering intraspinal opioids for chronic noncancer pain are essentially the same as those for cancer pain, namely in those circumstances where pain cannot be controlled adequately by more conservative means or in patients who cannot tolerate high-dose systemic opioids. Clinicians managing intrathecal delivery systems are widely variable in their clinical practice. Clinical guidelines for intraspinal infusions of various medications have been developed (Krames, 1996). Morphine is recommended as the first line of therapy, followed by the addition of bupivicaine (a long-acting local anesthetic), or clonidine (an alpha 2-adrenergic receptor agonist), or alternatively replacing morphine with hydromorphone. Fentanyl or sufentanil can be considered as third-line treatments, alone or in combination with bupivicaine and clonidine. There is little data justifying the use of other intrathecal opioids, such as meperidine or methadone; other local anesthetics, such as ropivicaine; or the variety of agents that have been hypothesized or reported to have some therapeutic benefit, such as neostigmine or ketamine. That is not to say there is not ample room for improvement in spinally mediated analgesia and the necessity for prospective, well-controlled clinical trials of novel agents that have proven safe and effective in phase one trials.

A trial of intraspinal opioids is important before considering a permanent pump implantation. This allows both patient and physician to assess the potential benefit of a permanent procedure as well as approximate the daily opioid requirement. A well-conducted trial can include physical medicine modalities to improve mobility and function as pain control is optimized. In current practice, about 92% of patients are screened before implantation (Paice, Penn, & Shott, 1992). The most common trial methods include continuous epidural infusion (35.3%), followed by bolus intrathecal injection (33.7%) and bolus epidural injection (24.5%). Krames (1996) and Krames and Olson (1997) advocate the use of continuous infusion trials to attempt to mimic the potential long-term infusion. Another advantage is that other drugs, such as local anesthetics, alone or in combination with morphine, can be tested. Risks to this procedure are similar to any implantable device and include wound infection (3–5%), drug intolerance, catheter malfunction, and rapidly escalating pain requiring frequent dose titration.

Absolute contraindications include bleeding diathesis, septicemia, local cutaneous infection, and known allergy to local anesthetics or infused medications. Relative contraindications include patients with compromised immune systems (e.g., diabetes mellitus) and tissue fibrosis at the site of the procedure (e.g., burns or extensive radiation therapy), due to risks of infection and poor wound healing. Also, it is inappropriate to implant an intrathecal pump without postoperative and long-term support and management capability. With both epidural and intrathecal catheters, there is a risk of inflammation and subsequent formation of scar tissue around the catheter, limiting drug delivery, distribution, or absorption.

Many reported clinical series document the successful analgesic effects of continuous intraspinal opioid therapy in excess of 5 years. For short-term use, the overall infection risk of an externalized intrathecal catheter system is extremely low with fastidious placement and if care is taken. Externalized catheters are utilized mostly for diagnostic purposes or in patients who have a limited life expectancy. This less expensive and less invasive method involves a catheter placed in the epidural or intraspinal space that is tunneled subcutaneously and connected to either a subcutaneous or external injection port. The majority of infections, when they occur, are along the catheter's subcutaneous track. Abscesses and meningitis have been very rare. Treatment of infection (catheter removal, antibiotic therapy, surgical debridement) depends upon patient-specific factors, such as prognosis.

Side Effects of Spinal Opioids

Chronic administration of spinal opioids is generally well tolerated. Risk of oversedation is low because most of these patients have already been chronically exposed to opioids and have become tolerant to this common opioid effect. However, with substitution of systemic for spinal opioids, an acute abstinence syndrome can occur. These signs and symptoms are effectively treated with low doses of a benzodiazepine and/or clonidine for a few days to weeks after significant reduction or discontinuation of opioids. Possible side effects of spinal opioids include sedation, nausea, vomiting, urinary retention, decreased gastrointestinal motility, pruritis, and respiratory depression. If these side effects become severe, lowering the infusion rate usually is adequate. Rarely, the opioid needs to be changed. Short-term treatment of specific adverse effects with diphenhydramine, nalaxone, metoclopramide, phenothiazines, or methylphenidate may be required until tolerance to unwanted symptoms develops (days to weeks). Hyperalgesia has been reported with high-dose spinal morphine, greater than 25 mg/day. Similarly, high doses of spinal opioids can result in myoclonic jerks. These are treated by adding baclofen to the pump or changing to another opioid, such as hydromorphone.

Technical Considerations

Totally implantable pumps are expensive, ranging in price from $8,000 to $10,000. Implantation expenses can push the total cost up to $12,000 to $14,000. The cost effectiveness of intrathecal pumps has been well reviewed by Hassenbusch, Paice, Patt, Bedder, and Bell (1997). They found that if a cancer patient's life expectancy exceeds 3 months, the overall cost of intrathecal pain therapy is likely to be less than that of tunneled epidural catheters or external infusion devices, including the personnel necessary to manage the infusions. For patients with chronic noncancer pain, intrathecal therapy has been calculated to be cost-effective at 22 months compared to conventional medical therapy.

Nonopioid Spinal Analgesics

Persistent noncancer pain can be categorized as primarily mechanical, soft tissue, or neuropathic in nature. Often, as with back pain, two if not all three main categories of pain can be operant at the same time. The etiology of the most common chronic soft tissue pain disorder, myofascial pain syndrome, is poorly understood, and unfortunately, opioid therapy by any route is not particularly beneficial in the long run. Contrary to conventional teachings, neuropathic pain (e.g., diabetic neuropathy) often can be improved with opioids in combination with other pain-modulating drugs. Mechanical pain, such as that of osteoarthritis, results from activation of nociceptors, and opioids are usually very effective at interrupting nociceptive pain transmission.

Advances in the understanding of spinal cord physiology have given us the potential to provide pain relief via spinal administered nonopioid drugs that inhibit different mechanisms of pain neurotransmission. Clonidine, baclofen, and ziconitide are examples of nonopioid spinal analgesics. Clonidine is postulated to activate alpha-2 adrenergic receptors on primary afferent and postsynaptic second-order neurons in the dorsal horn. Significant side effects include hypotension and sedation, which can limit the drug's usefulness. There appears to be some cross-tolerance between spinal opioids and spinal clonidine. Animals tolerant to spinal morphine have also been shown to be tolerant to the analgesic effect of clonidine. Baclofen has been shown to activate the beta subset of GABA receptors on the primary afferent and secondary postsynaptic dorsal horn neurons. GABA generally inhibits the release of excitatory neurotransmitters. Oral doses of baclofen are not always effective and have been associated with sedation and weakness. Intrathecal baclofen has been shown to be effective in some cases when oral administration has been ineffective. A single intrathecal bolus of 50–100 ugm is generally used as a diagnostic test dose before proceeding with an implantable, computer-controlled infusion pump. Finding the right dose of intrathecal baclofen is also important. A dose too low will be ineffective, and a dose too high will cause central nervous system depression with sedation, generalized muscle weakness, and possible respiratory arrest. Clinicians who administer this drug intrathecally need to know how to manage these potentially life-threatening complications.

Ziconitide, or SNX-111, a 25 amino acid peptide from a marine snail, is a highly selective N-type voltage-sensitive calcium channel antagonist. Endogenous voltage-sensitive calcium channel antagonists are found in presynaptic primary afferent nerve terminals, and these are thought to block release of pain mediating neurotransmitters. Ziconitide is anticipated to be released for clinical use in the future and will be indicated for the treatment of neuropathic pain, visceral pain, and bone pain. It can only be given intrathecally, and there is no reported development of tolerance. Unfortunately, devastating adverse cerebellar-toxic effects have been reported, including prolonged ataxia and nystagmus. It is difficult to make positive recommendations about this drug at present because of this toxic effect.

Neurolytic CNS Blockade

Permanent destruction of central neural pathways should be reserved for highly select patients with limited life expectancy whose pain has not been well controlled by other reasonable means, and a few other specific but limited cases, for example, trigeminal neuralgia. These blocks are most beneficial in patients with advanced cancer whose pain is unilateral and limited to a few spinal segments. Patients with bilateral, widespread pain are poor candidates for these procedures. The overall goal is to perform a posterior chemical rhizotomy, interrupting the pain pathways of a particular area. Care must be taken not to increase disability through motor weakness, sphincter incompetence, and loss of position sense. When central neurolytic injections are performed properly on well-selected cancer patients, quality of life can dramatically improve with decreased side effects from ineffective systemic medications.

Neurolysis is generally achieved with either ethyl alcohol or phenol. Glycerol is used primarily for trigeminal ganglion blocks. Phenol has local anesthetic properties along with protein denaturing properties, resulting in painless injections. Phenol has to be injected with glass syringes because it reacts with plastic, and it has to be freshly prepared because oxidation occurs rapidly. Accidental intravascular injection, or doses above 1,000 mg, are associated with central nervous depression, convulsions, and cardiovascular collapse. Ethyl alcohol produces dehydration and protein precipitation and has few to no side effects associated with systemic absorption, except typical signs of inebriation in high doses.

Subarachnoid (spinal) neurolytic blocks can offer complete pain relief for up to 3 months in 60% of all cases using either phenol or ethyl alcohol. Central neurolytic blocks are most frequently considered in the thoracic region with unilateral chest wall tumors, and in the sacral region with locally invasive rectal cancer. These two areas have been shown to have few significant disability concerns. Patients with rectal cancer need to have a diverting colostomy along with urinary diversion before they are considered for this block, because sacral nerves 2 through 5 are anesthetized. Occasionally S1 is obliterated with this block, causing foot drop. The excellent pain relief that these blocks provide can be lost when the cancer grows outside the anatomic level of anesthesia. When this occurs, other pain control methods, such as intrathecal opioids, may need to be considered.

Dorsal Column, Central, and Peripheral Nerve Stimulation

History

In 1965 Melzack and Wall introduced the gate control theory of pain transmission that postulated neuromodulation of pain at the dorsal horns of the spinal cord. Based on this theory, Shealy, Mortimer, and Reswick (1967) reported a case study of the treatment of intractable pain in a terminal cancer patient using an internal dorsal column stimulator. Over the past two decades, many technical difficulties have been overcome and refinements have been made so that now this procedure is no longer considered experimental. Presently, over 70,000 spinal cord stimulators have been implanted with an implantation rate increasing by over 30% per year (Barolat & Sharan, 2000).

The currently quoted success rate in properly selected patients is 50–75% pain reduction in about 50% of patients. Prior to permanent implantation, careful psychological assessment and an ample outpatient trial are necessary to determine which patients might have the highest likelihood of benefiting from this therapy.

Clinical Applications

Primary indications for spinal cord stimulation are lumbar and cervical radiculopathy, mononeuropathy, intercostal neuralgia, and peripheral vascular disease. Syndromes that have been reported to respond to dorsal column stimulation (DCS) are complex regional pain syndrome (CRPS) types I and II; failed back surgery syndrome; arachnoiditis; diabetic, alcohol, and AIDS-related neuropathy; stump pain; phantom limb pain; postherpetic neuralgia; spinal cord injury pain; and plexus neuropathies.

Spinal cord stimulation is most commonly applied for the treatment of pain due to failed back surgery syndrome, with CRPS as the second leading indication. Success rates differ widely, but pain relief greater than 50% in at least 50% of patients has been reported in a prospective multicenter study (Burchiel et al., 1996), a longitudinal study (North, Ewend, Lawton, Kidd, & Piantadosi, 1991), and a review of 41 studies from 1966 to 1994 (Turner, Loeser, & Bell, 1995).

Recently, spinal cord stimulation has been shown to be effective in treating chronic refractory angina. DeJongste (2000) reported on the efficacy of DCS in 81 patients with 80% obtaining effective pain control during a period of 4 years. The study group consisted of frequently hospitalized patients with severe coronary artery disease and pain exacerbations that were pharmacologically and surgically unmanageable. Dorsal column stimulators are also being used for ventral sacral root stimulation for bladder control in paraplegic patients. Chronic interstitial cystitis, peripheral vascular disease, and diverse neuropathies are also being treated by spinal cord stimulation.

Mechanisms of Action

Spinal cord stimulators are composed of electrodes that are inserted into the epidural space at the level of spinal nerves affecting the pain and coupled to a pulse generator, which can be an external or internalized (implanted) device. The awake patient is questioned regarding sensations from electrode lead placement and sensations as the physician makes adjustments in electrode positioning until the painful area is "covered" by paresthesias. As would be expected, a discrete regional pain, such as in an extremity, is more appropriately and successfully treated by this modality than is diffuse, poorly localized, or shifting pain.

Multiple mechanisms of action have been proposed for this form of neuromodulation, including sympathetic blockade, increased blood flow, and decreased release of the excitatory amino acids glutamate and aspartate at the dorsal horn. While understanding of the mechanism of spinal cord stimulation is incomplete, some experimental evidence suggests preferential A delta fiber effects plus enhanced release of GABA and attenuated release of glutamate and aspartate at the dorsal horn (Meyerson & Linderoth, 2000).

Supraspinal mechanisms also have been suggested, mediated by adenosine and enkephalin inhibition of nociception. Modulation of descending inhibitory and ascending nociceptive pathways via the release of serotonin and nortriptyline is also postulated. Last, neuromodulation of Substance P, a pain transmitter, has been implicated as a means by which DCS reduces pain (Stiller, 1997).

A variant of DCS, high-frequency (130 Hz) brain stimulation, is being applied to specific thalamic targets as an experimental means of treating dystonia, epilepsy, eating disorders, and Parkinson's disease. The development of new circuits, electrodes, Web-based programmers, and complex waveforms for specific targets are future directions this novel form of therapy is anticipated to take (Benabid et al., 2000).

Radiofrequency and Rhizotomy

History of Radiofrequency Lesions

One of the first clinicians to apply radiofrequency for electrosurgery was Harvey Cushing in the mid 1920s, who developed an experimental model in an early attempt at "electrosurgery" (Cosman & Cosman, 1974). Initially, clinical applications of radiofrequency were used to create lesions in the central nervous system and only in the 1960s was radiofrequency lesioning applied to peripheral nerves. Although the technique has been described in the medical literature since the 1960s, in just the last 10 years, this technique has grown in clinical practice with widespread application and a growing body of supportive medical literature.

Mechanism of Action

The technique of inducing radiofrequency lesions is based on the insertion of an insulated electrode with an uninsulated tip into nervous tissue. If an electrical generator is connected to the insulated needle, the impedance from the surrounding tissue (usually muscle, fascia, or bone) will allow an electrical current to be transmitted to the tissue surrounding the noninsulated tip. Heat is generated in the nervous tissue that equilibrates in temperature with the tip in about 60 sec. This temperature is then relayed back to the generator. The size and location of the coagulated tissue is determined by needle position, size of the uninsulated tip, pulse frequency (usually approximately 500 kilocycles/sec), time duration of stimulation, and pulse modality.

Patient Selection

Kline (1998) recommends the following criteria for selecting patients for radiofrequency procedures:

1. Noninvasive conservative management has failed;
2. Habituating agents, such as opioid analgesics, sedative agents, and alcohol, have been identified and a cessation program has been instituted (cessation of opioid analgesics does not apply to individuals with cancer pain);
3. Psychological factors affecting the pain (e.g., anxiety, depression, anger, secondary gain issues) have been identified and an appropriate behavioral management program has been instituted;
4. The patient has shown an emotional investment in the treatment program by the willingness to make lifestyle changes, address psychological issues, and make good use of the treatment time with physicians, therapists, and psychologists; and
5. Patient expectations regarding the procedures are realistic and procedural risks fully understood.

Applications

Radiofrequency procedures are currently utilized to relieve pain from cervical and lumbar facet arthropathy, to effect multilevel sympathetic or selective intracranial gangliolysis, to treat trigeminal and selective nerve root pain, and to manage otherwise intractable sacroiliac pain. Recently, we have found that L2 bilateral dorsal root ganglionectomy effectively suppresses multiple levels of lumbar discogenic pain (DKC).

Safety Profile

Radiofrequency lesioning is a controlled thermal lesion and much safer than chemical neurolytic procedures, which can be complicated by inadvertent spread of the neurolytic agent through adjacent tissues or vascular absorption. The lesion is made through a percutaneous puncture under fluoroscopic guidance, a technique that is less costly and less invasive than surgical neurolysis. Also, scar tissue formation is usually negligible. However, appropriate training in assessment, modes of management, technical skill building, and extensive experience working with fluoroscopic x-ray guidance are mandatory for safe and optimal results. Recent reviews that include anatomic images are helpful to visualize this technique (Kline, 1998).

Sympathetic Nerve Blockade

Sympathetic blocks can be divided into two basic groups: temporary and permanent (neurolytic). Temporary, or reversible, blocks are used in series to treat progressive but potentially reversible pain syndromes such as sympathetically maintained forms of CRPS or postherpetic neuralgia. Sympathetically maintained shoulder and upper extremity pain often respond to stellate ganglion blockade. This is usually done by a paratracheal injection of a local anesthetic at the level of C6 or C7. Blocking the sympathetic fibers causes increased blood flow to the face and upper extremity, resulting in increased temperature, Horner's syndrome, transient mild swallowing dysfunction, and decreased pain. The pain relief can be significantly longer than the apparent duration of effect of the local anesthetic. Thereby, an increasing interval between blocks is often possible until complete resolution of symptoms occurs. It is generally accepted that reversal of CRPS is easier and much quicker if sympathetic blocks are given early in the course of the syndrome, ideally within days or weeks of onset. It is universally accepted that blocks are less effective in reversing CRPS if symptoms have been sustained over many months or years.

In the lower extremity, lumbar sympathetic blocks are done at L2 or L3 under fluoroscopic guidance because this is where anatomic studies have confirmed most lumbar sympathetic ganglion tissue to reside. Complete reversal of CRPS often occurs after a series of sympathetic blocks, especially in younger, more active patients without long-standing pain. Of course, spontaneous resolution may also be an important factor in recovery of CRPS, but the pain relief afforded by these blocks and the increased ability to comply with rehabilitation efforts appear to be therapy-specific. Controlled studies are difficult for ethical reasons; once the diagnosis is suspected, absence of treatment could lead to intractable disease.

The sympathetic blocks most effective for visceral pain are celiac plexus blocks used to treat upper abdominal pain and superior hypogastric blocks for organic pain in the pelvis. Atypical cystitis and pelvic and scrotal pain can be treated by ganglion impar blocks, lowest in the sympathetic chain. Except in the treatment of hyperhydrosis (increased perspiration), and occasional refractory CRPS patients, neurolytic blocks of the sympathetic nervous system are usually most common in terminally ill patients in whom benefits outweigh risks. The prototypic neurolytic block for cancer pain is the celiac plexus block to treat epigastric pancreatic cancer pain. Since the celiac plexus innervates most of the abdominal viscera including stomach, liver, biliary tract, pancreas, spleen, kidneys, adrenals, omentum, small bowel, and large bowel through the splenic flexure, pain emanating from these organs can be relieved by celiac plexus block. The right and left celiac ganglia and interconnecting nerve fibers form the celiac plexus, located anterolateral to the aorta, immediately caudal to the celiac artery. Blocking the celiac plexus interrupts the efferent sympathetic preganglionic fibers of the synapsing splanchnic nerves and the nociceptive visceral afferents from the upper abdominal viscera. This can result in prolonged and profound pain relief for patients with epigastric and abdominal pain from pancreatic cancer. Various methods have been described, including posterior and anterior approaches, with CT real-time guidance the most recently advanced technique. Fluoroscopic guidance with contrast material injection and position confirmation in multiple planes is also widely utilized. Efficacy is excellent with one meta-analysis reporting good to excellent pain relief in 89% of patients during the first 2 weeks and 90% of the patients reporting significant pain relief at 3 weeks, continuing until death (Eisenberg, Carr, & Chalmers, 1995).

Minor complications include hypotension due to regional splanchnic vasodilation (38%), transient (< 1 day) diarrhea due to unopposed sympathetic tone (49%), and transient (< 1 hour) localized pain (96%). Severe neurological sequelae have been reported in less than 0.1% of the population (Aeschbach & Mekhail, 2000). In a 5-year survey, the incidence of major neurological complications was 0.15% (Davies, 1993). This procedure is similarly efficacious in the treatment of pain from gastric, biliary, hepatic, and other gastrointestinal malignancies.

Other Invasive Procedures: Trigger Point Injections, Facet Blocks, and Epidural Steroid Injections

Trigger point injections

Eighty to 90% of persistent nonmalignant pain patients have myofascial pain on initial evaluation at a pain management center. Myofascial pain is defined as regional muscle pain, associated with a taut palpable band, exquisite point tenderness at a nodule in the taut band, limited range of motion secondary to pain, and the patient's recognition of pain radiation patterns when the examiner applies pressure to the trigger point. Myofascial nodules, or contraction knots, can also be confirmed by visual or tactile identification of a local twitch response, pain or altered sensation in the distribution expected on compression of the nodule, and electromyographic demonstration of spontaneous electrical activity characteristic of active nodules. A twitch response is defined when the affected muscle band spontaneously or actively contracts; the twitch response can be activated by palpation or needle insertion.

The goal of treating myofascial pain is restoration of the affected muscle(s) to normal length and range of motion. Multiple modalities can be used. No one particular treatment has been proven to be better than another. It is common for patients with persistent pain, including myofascial pain, to receive palliative physical therapy modalities such as ultrasound, transcutaneous electrical nerve stimulation (TENS), and/or massage. However, long-term outcomes are greatly improved through a more dynamic rehabilitative focus, with activating therapies such as stretching and strengthening affected muscle groups, changing behaviors with structured activating goals, and ergonomic retraining. Sometimes minimal to moderately invasive treatments, such as trigger point injections or sympathetic or somatic nerve blocks, need to be added to the activating physical therapy in order to alleviate function-limiting pain and interrupt aberrant neuromyogenic reflexes.

The administration of trigger point injections for refractory myofascial pain is quite controversial. The 1999 edition of *Textbook of Pain*, edited by Melzack and Wall, states there is little to no scientific evidence for their usefulness. They also bring up the concern that no definitive studies have shown how many or how often trigger point injections should be performed on an affected muscle. On the other hand, using a randomized, controlled, double-blind methodology, Fine, Milano, and Hare (1988) demonstrated that the therapeutic effects of trigger point injections are naloxone reversible, suggesting a central endorphinergic mechanism of action. Nevertheless, it is true that a major problem in treating myofascial pain is the lack of standardized methods with which to identify and quantify this disorder. Histological studies and experimental electromyography (EMG) have been used to identify contraction knots, but at this time, treatment remains somewhat anecdotal and more of an art than a science. Therefore, from an interventional standpoint, a conservative or minimalist approach, using invasive therapies as adjuncts rather than the sole mode of treatment, seems prudent.

Identification of discrete trigger points prior to injection is fundamental. The taut muscle band on careful palpation often feels nodular and fusiform in shape, with the tender nodule or contraction knot painful to palpation in the middle of the tight band. The practitioner stabilizes the contraction knot with one hand and then aseptically inserts a needle into the muscle with the other hand, stopping when there is a twitch response or referred pain. Sometimes the needle needs to be passed in multiple planes until the proper response is found. The needle is thought to disrupt the neuromuscular junction or the muscle spindle and to allow the contraction knot to release and relax. Some clinicians use a dry needling technique (i.e., no local anesthetic solution) but this may increase discomfort. Most practitioners inject 1–5 milliliters of dilute local anesethetic (to minimize potential myonecrosis), such as 0.25 % bupivicaine, into and around the contraction knot to enhance therapeutic effects and decrease postinjection pain.

Entire groups of muscles affected by this syndrome (e.g., the shoulder and cervical spine) can sometimes be treated effectively with either regional sympathetic or somatic nerve blocks. There is electromyographical evidence that the sympathetic nervous system is involved in maintaining myofascial pain (Hubbard, 1996). In this example, a stellate ganglion block can relax the majority of cervical and upper shoulder muscles to allow a physical therapist to actively stretch the affected muscle group. Sometimes somatic nerve blockade of the muscle group is necessary in order to break the pain-muscle spasm cycle and to facilitate range of motion therapies.

In summary, myofascial pain syndrome is an extremely common cause of muscle pain that is fairly easy to diagnose, but difficult to accurately quantify. The etiology of painful myofascial nodules is unknown. As a guideline, the authors (SPL, PGF) perform a limited number of trigger point injections, no more than four to six, two to four times over a 2- to 3-week period, with the view that this enhances rather than detracts from an active rehabilitation program and minimizes risks of local anesthetic-induced myonecrosis or inflammation. At any point we will stop the injections if they are not clearly therapeutic (decreased pain reports, improved functional measures), the injections are causing the pain to escalate, or the patient is not adhering to the activating physical therapy program. There are relatively few complications with trigger point injections. Pneumothorax has been reported with improperly gauged chest-wall injections. Care must be used when injecting around the neck in order to avoid inadvertent injection of undiluted local anesthetic into cranial arteries, potentially causing loss of consciousness or seizure.

Facet blocks

Facet joints, also known as zygapophyseal joints, are part of the protective bony arch surrounding the spinal cord. Osteoarthritis or traumatically induced arthritis can affect these joints, especially in the cervical and lumbar regions. There is great debate as to whether facet joints can be primary pain generators. The joints and the capsule that surrounds them are well innervated. Facet disease and degenerative disc disease very often occur together, making it difficult to distinguish which is causing the pain. MRI and CT imaging are not reliable means to distinguish pain etiologies because degenerative facet arthritis is seen in 10.4% of asymptomatic patients. Injection of the capsule surrounding lumbar facets with hypertonic saline produces pain in the back, buttocks, and proximal thigh. Injection of other vertebral elements with local anesthesia, however, produces pain patterns that are indistinguishable from those associated with facet joint injection. It is very difficult, therefore, to distinguish facet pain from other potential sources of back pain. If facet injections are going to be considered, a series of injections of either the joint or the nerves innervating the joint is essential. Fluoroscopic guidance is standard practice. There are relatively few complications associated with these injections. Local anesthetic can be used alone, or in combination with a steroid, usually 20 to 40 mg of methylprednisolone acetate or equivalent per facet. The median branch of the dorsal nerve root sends sensory branches to the facet joint above and below a particular nerve level; for example, the L4 median branch nerve divides to innervate the L2/3 as well as the L3/4 facet joint. Controlled studies have shown that in patients without radiculopathy, 38% had relief after injection of the suspected joint, but 25% had similar relief when a randomly assigned median branch block was performed on an unsuspected facet joint. These percentages of pain relief are comparable with a placebo response. Seven percent of patients received total pain relief after facet injection. Carette et al. (1991) performed a controlled trial of steroid facet injections and concluded that facet injections are of little value in the treatment of patients with chronic low back disease. Facet disease can probably be a partial pain generator, but is rarely the major source of pain.

Epidural Steroids

In the 1960s, surgeons reported that nerve roots were swollen in patients undergoing laminectomy for herniated discs. Goebert et al. (1961) reasoned that the inflammation was a key factor in pain generation in patients with herniated discs and began to add hydrocortisone to caudal injections to treat sciatica. They reported that 66% of their patients benefited from this therapy. McCarron, Wimpee, Hudkins, and Laros (1987) demonstrated in dogs that small doses of nucleus pulposus injected epidurally caused marked inflammatory changes of nerve roots and surrounding tissues. It was later learned that PLA-2 is the most likely offending substance in nucleus pulposus extract. Steroids decrease the inflammatory effects of PLA-2, but nonsteroidal anti-inflammatory drugs (NSAIDs) do not. Steroids have also been shown to decrease spontaneous pain from neuromas caused by injury of nerves or nerve roots during back surgery. Placing steroids in the epidural space is thought to treat chemical rather than physical pathology.

The primary indication for epidural steroids is for treatment of radicular pain due to disc herniation. Watts and Silagy performed a meta-analysis in 1995, finding a statistical difference favoring corticosteroids over controls in reducing pain intensity in patients with herniated discs. There continues to be controversy as to whether epidural steroids can effectively relieve symptoms of spinal stenosis. Only a few prospective studies with small numbers have been done. There seems to be clinical consensus, through a considerable body of anecdotal experience, that this technique is worthy of a trial, since some patients who have tried myriad other therapies, and who are not good surgical candidates, experience both pain relief and function improvements from epidural injections.

Complications from epidural steroids, including risks of bleeding, infection, and nerve damage are extremely low. Accumulation of long half-life corticosteroids after repeated injections can lead to Cushing's syndrome or Addisonian crisis. Kay, Findling, and Raff (1994) showed in 14 healthy volunteers receiving three weekly triamcinolone injections that the mean time to return to endogenous steroid production was 1 month, with 5 volunteers taking 3 months. Therefore, spacing injections weeks or months apart will reduce this potential complication.

The decision to perform an epidural steroid injection is not always straightforward. Patients are often referred for a trial of epidural steroids, and although this intervention may be very appropriate, other identifiable contributors to pain, such as psychological factors or a condition that is treatable by entirely different means (e.g., myofascial pain), should be evaluated. In order to determine the efficacy of epidural therapy, the patient should be observed over time for improvement in behaviors and functional capacities concurrent with decreases in pain intensity and, perhaps, medication use. The patient's adherence to rehabilitative therapies should also be monitored.

Future of Invasive Modalities for Pain Management

Development of new drugs and technologies is expensive and takes many years. In 1995 the average cost of new drug development was $280 million and it took an average of 12 years before achieving FDA approval. As a result, drug manufacturers have been looking increasingly at novel drug formulations for existing drugs, such as the transdermal and oral transmucosal fentanyl delivery systems. One approach to improving pharmacotherapeutic specificity is by directing medications to their intended site of action via attachment to monoclonal antibodies or heat-sensitive liposomes. The demand for better and safer pain management products is great, evidenced by the rapid and high utilization of the COX-2 selective inhibitors. The market for invasive pain management modalities, however, is still fairly small, restricted by the need for special training of practitioners and indications for use in a relatively small subset of pain patients. Possibly, the need for invasive therapies will even decrease as improvements are realized in less interventional approaches to pain prevention and treatment. Regardless, in the prevailing market-driven culture, it is reasonable to assume that creative drive, research support, and other incentives will depend on anticipated and perceived need and consumer demand.

One area that is evolving quite rapidly is that of subcategorizing opioid receptors. It was recently discovered that there are at least 7 different subtypes of the mu opioid receptor. The immediate clinical implication of this finding is that not all opioid-responsive pain should necessarily be treated the same way. A patient's response might vary, depending upon the opioid used and the patient's particular opioid genotype. So, knowing what mu receptors to target on whom, where in the body, and for what conditions might be very helpful for clinicians and their patients (Fine, 2001). Currently we can only formulate a best first guess about an individual's potential opioid responsiveness or clinical response to other pain-modulating drugs. It then takes several weeks to months, continually monitoring efficacy and adverse events, to determine the most useful long-term treatment plan, including the indications for, and subsequent benefits of, implantable devices and other invasive therapies.

SETTING-SPECIFIC CONSIDERATIONS

Once a patient has been determined to be an appropriate candidate for one of the various interventional pain therapies, a complete assessment requires consideration of the patient's social setting and comorbidities. All of the procedures described in this text can be performed in an outpatient setting, as long as the facility is equipped to ensure patient safety. This requires safe transport of patients from home or residential care facility and capable caregivers there to provide basic monitoring for adverse events when the patient goes home.

If this is not possible, or if the patient has risk factors that require more skilled monitoring than available at his or her place of residence, then inpatient care is indicated until the patient is determined to be medically stable. For example, a pump or DCS implant patient with a potential for postoperative bleeding, or a celiac plexus block patient who would not tolerate hypotension due to underlying cardiovascular or renal disease, would fall into this category. Each case must be evaluated on individual patient-based issues, rather than pigeonholing the procedures themselves.

Answering the simple question "What can go wrong, and who will be there to prevent further morbidity?" is usually sufficient to determine the best disposition for each patient. In this way, the goals of optimizing positive outcomes while anticipating and minimizing risks can be best accomplished.

SUMMARY/RECOMMENDATIONS

1. Positive results from interventional therapies are highly dependent upon adequate assessment and proper patient selection. This is best accomplished using an interdisciplinary team approach, including physician, psychologist, and physical or occupational therapist.
2. Spinal opioid analgesia is potent, efficacious, and relatively specific compared to systemic opioid therapy. This modality should be considered in patients for whom noninvasive therapies have been ineffective or toxic.
3. Several nonopioid agents, including local anesthetics, clonidine, and baclofen, are available that alone or in combination with opioids can improve spinally mediated pain control, especially in refractory neuropathic pain syndromes.
4. Neurolytic dorsal root blocks (chemical rhizotomy) can be extremely effective in controlling severe cancer pain in patients with limited life expectancy when other means are insufficient or detract from quality of life.
5. Radiofrequency lesions of facet joint afferent innervation (median branch or the dorsal ramus) are becoming increasingly used as a means to treat chronic pain due to spinal osteoarthropathy. Although safe in experienced hands, long-term outcomes of efficacy and cost-benefit analysis are pending prospective study, so this procedure should be considered after other reasonable alternatives.
6. Sympathetic blocks are indicated in cases of neuropathic pain where a sympathetic component is suspected. Confirmation of sympathetically maintained pain in complex regional pain syndromes justifies sympathetic blockade as a component of comprehensive pain treatment and functional rehabilitation.
7. Neurolytic celiac or hypogastric plexus blocks are highly effective in treating abdominal or pelvic visceral pain due to malignant disease. These should be considered very early on in the course of patients with pain syndromes from abdomino-pelvic tumors.

8. Trigger point injections are useful when performed in moderation as an adjunct in the comprehensive treatment of myofascial pain syndromes. All patients with persistent musculoskeletal and visceral pain syndromes should be examined for trigger points since these are a frequent concomitant and amplifier of persistent pain and the myriad diseases and traumas that cause chronic pain.

9. Facet injections with local anesthetic, with or without corticosteroid, are of limited, if any, value in the management of chronic back pain, regardless of presumed etiology.

10. A diagnostic and subsequent therapeutic trial of epidural steroids is indicated in patients with radiculitis that is thought to be caused by a herniated disc. Similarly, patients with pain that is clinically consistent with spinal stenosis might benefit from epidural steroid injections, especially if decompressive surgery poses excessive risks.

CASE STUDIES

Case 1

Mr. Smith is 76 years old and was evaluated by a neurosurgeon for chronic back pain. He was diagnosed as having myofascial pain involving the low back muscles and extensive nonoperable degenerative disc disease throughout his lumbar spine. There was no evidence of spinal stenosis or radiculopathy. He was compliant with a physical therapy program of stretching, lumbar stabilization, and aquatic therapy. Most of his myofascial pain resolved with the physical therapy regimen, but a persistent deep ache remained. A series of lumbar epidural steroid injections were not helpful, nor were NSAIDs. Several different opioids were tried, including a fentanyl patch that helped relieve the pain 50%, but he felt sedated. He was admitted to the hospital for a trial of intrathecal opioids. Morphine at 50 ugm/hour greatly decreased his pain, but he developed marked urinary retention. Hydromorphone at 20 ugm/hour also gave excellent pain relief and resolved his urinary retention. He underwent psychological screening and was found to be appropriate for an intrathecal pump, demonstrating no significant affective or personality disorders. One week later an intrathecal pump was implanted under general anesthesia. His pain became well controlled, and his function markedly increased, without sedation or constipation. He receives medication refills every 3 months.

Discussion

This patient has chronic degenerative disc disease that is neither likely to improve from surgery nor expected to improve over time. He was appropriately given a trial of several opioids, with pain relief limited by CNS effects and urinary retention. It was reasonable to attempt to achieve steady blood levels and avoid serum peaks and troughs with a fentanyl patch, but the dose the patient could tolerate did not relieve his pain or allow him normal functioning. With intrathecal opioids, he can obtain superior pain relief with 1/80th to 1/100th the dose of oral medications, lower blood levels, and less toxicity as the spinal and supraspinal receptors are more directly targeted. His pump can be fine-tuned to give a higher infusion rate to coincide with peak activity level and a lower rate at rest. He still may need occasional breakthrough medication for incident pain but this should be minimal as the pump is better adjusted over time. The necessity for fine-tuning dose adjustments and refills mandates that postprocedure care is arranged prior to implantation for a successful outcome.

Case 2

Mrs. Jones is 67 years old and recently recovered from an L4/5 laminectomy and diskectomy after falling on the ice. After completing a post-surgical physical therapy program, she continued to have pain down the right leg in a L4 distribution pattern; muscle tone, strength, and reflexes in the right leg returned to normal. Repeat lumbosacral MRI revealed no structural lesions around the right L4 nerve root. She was diagnosed with a postlaminectomy pain syndrome. Multiple neuro-pathic pain medications, including amiptriptyline, gabapentin, and oxcarbazepine, were not helpful. A psychological evaluation revealed a mild agitated depression that was successfully treated with sertraline and counseling. Opioids were not helpful because of excessive seda-tion and constipation. She was counseled on undergoing a trial of dorsal column stimulation. She agreed after extensive discussion and grasping the concept that DCS is a reversible procedure. In the oper-ating room the trial electrode was placed in the epidural space over the T10 vertebral body; she obtained over 75% pain relief. Several days later during the follow-up visit, she decided to have the genera-tor implanted. At the 3-month follow-up visit, she was very pleased with the results. Her activity level was starting to improve, and pain scores were 1–2/10.

Discussion

Mrs. Jones has postlaminectomy syndrome, often referred to as failed back syndrome. It is not uncommon to see patients who have undergone multiple surgical procedures with resultant scarring to continue to complain of severe low back and radicular pain. In these patients, careful psychological evaluation is necessary to rule out inappropriate expectations and secondary issues that would result in their dissatisfaction after placement of a dorsal column stimulator. Also, a careful trial period is necessary for the patient to assess the effects of the stimulation on usual pain levels. Caution not to move the electrodes is also necessary, and so in some practices an extended outpatient ("23-hour admission") observation period and surgical binder help assure lead placement. If the patient does not notice marked improvement during the week or more trial period at home, then it is not worth having the generator implanted and the temporary lead is removed. Often, a patient who has had an unsuccessful dorsal column stimulator trial will proceed to an intrathecal catheter trial and pump if pain is severe and refractory to other modalities of treatment.

Case 3

Mr. Carry had intermittent back pain for over 20 years, and it was only after persistent encouragement by his spouse that he consulted his primary care physician. Examination showed moderately tight muscles over the left low lumbar paraspinous region. Back extension increased his pain. He had no radicular symptoms or signs. MRI revealed moderate to severe hypertrophy of the left L4/5 facet. Physical therapy with stretching and lumbar stabilization was only mildly helpful. A series of facet injections with local anesthetic and steroids was helpful, but not long lasting. Local anesthetic injections of the superior and inferior medial branch facet nerves provided temporary pain relief. Radiofrequency rhizotomy of these nerves provided near-complete pain relief.

Discussion

Facet arthropathy is most commonly seen in combination with diffuse degenerative joint disease and spinal stenosis. On physical exam, it is diagnosed by point-specific pain over the facet that is increased by rotation of the spine or hyperextension. If a diagnostic facet or median nerve branch block with local anesthetics under fluoroscopic guidance markedly alleviates the pain for even a short time, a radiofrequency rhizotomy might provide long-lasting relief at minimal risk. When effective, pulsed frequency lesioning provides substantial relief with no period of burn pain or neuritis but may need to be repeated in 1 to 2 years. Constant "burn" lesions theoretically provide permanent relief but may initially exacerbate pain for up to several weeks. Also, permanent motor or sensory deficits do not occur with the pulsed frequency modality but this unfortunate complication, although infrequent, can be a complication of nonpulsed lesioning.

Case 4

Mrs. Burgoyne is 70 years old and was recently diagnosed with pancreatic cancer. She was experiencing mid-thoracic back pain and weight loss. She opted not to undergo chemotherapy or surgery. Pain was initially controlled with acetaminophen and codeine. Constipation was treated with senna and docusate. Several weeks later the pain increased, and she was placed on hydrocodone 5 mg and acetaminophen, up to 12 tablets per day. Sedation became a major concern. A pain management specialist was consulted, and it was decided to proceed with a neurolytic celiac plexus block. Using a continuous CT scanner, the level of the celiac artery was found, and needles were placed on either side of the T10 vertebral body, behind the crura of the diaphragm. Injection of 10 ml 0.25% bupivicaine gave near-complete pain relief. A total of 25 ml 50% ethyl alcohol was injected through each needle. Her blood pressure fell to 90/60, and one-half liter of a balanced salt solution and 5 mg of ephedrine was used to restore her systolic pressure to 110 mm Hg. Diarrhea was transient, and by the following morning, her pain had improved substantially. She remained relatively pain free until her death 3 months later.

Discussion

Pancreatic cancer often results in severe pain and a limited life span. By the time of diagnosis, the disease may be surgically inoperable. Because life span is short, pain relief must be immediate, and there is little time to make medication adjustments over several weeks to months. In this case, a long-acting opioid formulation, oral or transdermal, should be initiated along with a very rapid onset opioid for breakthrough pain. Immediate release oral or transmucosal opioids should supplement the steady blood level of the longer acting analgesic. Hydrocodone and acetaminophen are not the optimal regimen. In the case presented, blood analgesic levels fluctuated as a result of frequent dosing, causing alternating sedation and pain. Neurolysis of the sympathetic pain fibers and sensory afferents to the epigastrium will very likely offer adequate pain relief and diminish the requirement for opioid analgesics. In this type of case, both a lytic block and opioid titration should proceed simultaneously unless comfort is obtained rapidly with analgesics alone. The celiac plexus block will not eliminate pain from distant metastatic lesions or tumor growth outside the deafferented region, so over time additional opioid supplementation for pain control might be necessary. Occasionally, patients "outlive" the effective duration of the neurolytic block, implying that there is regeneration of nerves or development of collateral pain pathways. Repeated diagnostic and neurolytic block can be done. If these blocks fail to provide adequate pain relief, neuroaxial opioids should be considered.

TABLE 7.1 Invasive Pain Management Procedures

Procedure	Indications	Advantages	Disadvantages
Internal intrathecal infusion pump	Pain or muscle spasm unresponsive to systemic medications (e.g., stable cancer pain, spinal osteoarthritis, failed back surgery syndrome, complex regional pain syndrome, peripheral neuropathy, multiple sclerosis, visceral pain)	Improved pain/ muscle spasm control Requires refill only every 3 months	Inpatient trial required Expensive Skilled follow-up care required 3–5% infection risk
External silastic intrathecal catheter	Rapidly changing cancer pain with life expectancy > 1 month	Home health agency able to make changes at bedside	Potential increased infection risk and cost over internalized system External pump Skilled follow-up care required
External nylon intrathecal catheter	Rapidly changing cancer pain with life expectancy < 1 month	Can be easily placed at bedside Low cost	Highest infection risk Skilled hospice care needed
Neurolytic blocks (celiac plexus block)	Gastric, pancreatic, hepatic cancers	Markedly decreased need and side effects of systemic opioids	Transient hypotension and diarrhea Mean length of anesthesia is 3 months

TABLE 7.1 (*continued*)

Subarachnoid block	Locally invasive rectal cancer Unilateral regional thoracic cancer	Markedly decreased need and side effects of systemic opioids	Potential sensory loss Potential motor loss Mean length of anesthesia is 3 months
Dorsal column stimulation	Cervical and lumbar radiculopathy Mononeuropathies Intercostal neuralgia Peripheral vascular disease CRPS I and II Failed back surgery syndrome Arachnoiditis Stump pain Phantom limb pain Postherpetic neuralgia Spinal cord injury pain Plexus neuropathies	Pain control with minimal to no other adjuvant medications	Initial high cost 3–5% infection risk Skilled follow-up required
Peripheral nerve stimulation	Nerve stimulation at a particular damaged peripheral nerve	Localized stimulation Pain control with minimal to no other adjuvant medications	Initial high cost 3–5% infection risk Skilled follow-up required

TABLE 7.1 *(continued)*

Procedure	Indications	Advantages	Disadvantages
Radiofrequency and rhizotomy	Cervical and lumbar arthropathy Sympathetic ganglia Trigeminal and selective nerve root pain Intracranial ganglionectomy Sacroiliac pain syndrome	Pain control with minimal to no other adjuvant medications	Invasive
Sympathetic nerve blockade	Sympathetically maintained pain symptoms Myofascial pain syndrome	Easy Minimally invasive day of procedures	Lumbar sympathetic blockade necessitates fluoroscopy and monitored anesthesia
Trigger point injection	Myofascial pain	Adjunct treatment for myofascial pain syndrome Decrease number of trigger points	Can temporarily increase pain Passive modality
Facet injection	Facet arthritis	Potential to localize pain generator	Facet arthritis is rarely primary pain generator
Epidural steroid injection	Cervical or lumbar herniated nucleus pulposus	Diagnostic or therapeutic decreased pain response to injection	Immunosuppression

REFERENCES

Aeschbach, A., & Mekhail, N. A. (2000). Common nerve blocks in chronic pain management. *Anesthesiol Clin North America, 18*(2), 429–459.

Barolat, G., & Sharan, A. D. (2000). Future trends in spinal cord stimulation. *Neurological Research, 22*(3), 279–284.

Benabid, A. L., Koudsié, A., Pollak, P., Kahane, P., Chabardes, S., Hirsch, E., Marescaux, C., & Benazzouz, A. (2000). Future prospects of brain stimulation. *Neurological Research, 22*(3), 237–246.

Burchiel, K. J., Anderson, V. C., Brown, F. D., Fessler, R. G., Friedman, W. A., Pelofsky, S., Weiner, R. L., Oakley, J., & Shatin, D. (1996). Prospective, multi-center study of spinal cord stimulation for relief of chronic back and extremity pain. *Spine, 21*(23), 2786–2794.

Carette, S., Marcoux, S., Truchon, R., Grondin, C., Gagnon, J., Allard, Y., & Latulippe, M. (1991). A controlled trial of corticosteroid injections into facet joints for chronic low back pain. *N Engl J Med, 325*(14), 1002–1007.

Cosman B. J., & Cosman, E. R. (1974). *Guide to Radiofrequency Lesions Generation in Neurosurgery.* Burlington, MA: Radionics.

Davies, D. D. (1993). Incidence of major complications of neurolytic coeliac plexus block. *Journal of the Royal Society of Medicine, 86*(5), 264–266.

DeJongste, M. J. (2000). Spinal cord stimulation for ischemic heart disease. *Neurological Research, 22*(3), 293–298.

Doleys, D. M. (2000). Psychological assessment for implantable therapies. *Pain Digest, 10*, 16–23.

Doleys, D. M., & Olson, K. (1997). Psychological assessment and intervention in implantable pain therapies. *Medtronic Neurological,* 20.

Eisenberg E., Carr D. B., & Chalmers, T. C. (1995). Neurolytic celiac plexus block for treatment of cancer pain: A meta-analysis. *Anesth Analg, 80*(2), 290–295.

Fine, P. G., (2001). Opiod selection: Plaudits, pitfalls, and possibilities. *The Journal of Pain, 2*(4), 195–196.

Fine, P. G., Milano, R. A., & Hare, B. D. (1988). The effects of myofascial trigger point injections are naloxone reversible. *Pain, 32*, 15–20.

Goebert, H., Jallo, S., et al. (1961). Painful radiculopathy treated with epidural injections of procaine and hydrocortisone acetate: Results in 113 patients. *Anesth Analg, 40*, 130.

Gourlay, G. K., Cherry, D. A., & Cousins, M. J. (1985). Cephalad migration of morphine in CSF following lumbar epidural administration in patients with cancer pain. *Pain, 23*, 312.

Hassenbusch, S. J., Paice, J. A., Patt, R. B., Bedder, M. D., & Bell, G. K. (1997). Clinical realities and economic considerations: Economics of intrathecal therapy. *Journal of Pain and Symptom Management, 14*(Suppl.3), S36–S48.

Hubbard, D. (1996). Chronic and recurrent muscle pain: Pathophysiology and treatment, and review of pharmacologic studies. 4(1/2), 123–143.

Kay, J., Findling, J. W., & Raff, H. (1994). Epidural triamcinolone suppresses the pituitary-adrenal axis in human subjects. *Anesth Analg, 78*, 501.

Kline, M. T. (1998). Stereotactic radiofrequency lesions as part of the management of chronic pain. In R. S. Weiner (Ed.), *Pain management,* (Vol. 2, 5th ed., pp. 563–608). Boca Raton, FL: St. Lucie Press.

Krames, E. (1996). Intraspinal opioid therapy for chronic nonmalignant pain: Current practice and clinical guidelines. *Journal of Pain and Symptom Management, 11,* 333–352.

Krames, E., & Olson, K. (1997). Clinical realities and economic considerations: patient selection in intraspinal therapy. *Journal of Pain and Symptom Management, 14*(Suppl. 3), S3–S13.

Loeser, J. D. (2001). *Bonica's management of pain.* Philadelphia: Lippincott, Williams and Wilkins.

Max, M. B., Inturrisi, C. E., Kaiko, R. F., Grabinski, P. Y., Li, C. H., & Foley, K. M. (1985). Epidural and intrathecal opiates: Cerebrospinal fluid and plasma profiles in patients with chronic cancer pain. *Clinical Pharmacology and Therapeutics, 38,* 631–641.

McCarron, R. F., Wimpee, M. W., Hudkins, P. G., & Laros, G. S. (1987). The inflammatory effect of nucleus pulposus: A possible element in the pathogenesis of low back pain. *Spine, 12,* 760.

Melzack R., & Wall, P. D. (1965). Pain mechanisms: A new theory. *Science, 150*(699), 971–979.

Melzack, R., & Wall, P. D. (Eds.). (1999). *Textbook of pain* (4th ed.). Philadelphia: Churchill Livingstone.

Meyerson, B. A., & Linderoth, B. (2000). Mechanisms of spinal cord stimulation in neuropathic pain. *Neurological Research, 22*(3), 285–292.

North, R. B., Ewend, M. G., Lawton, M. T., Kidd, D. H., & Piantadosi, S. (1991). Failed back surgery syndrome: 5-year follow-up after spinal cord stimulator implantation. *Neurosurgery, 28*(5), 692–699.

Oakley, J., & Staats, P. (2000). The use of implanted drug delivery systems. In P. Prathvi Rej (Ed.), *Practical management of pain* (3rd ed.). St. Louis, MO: Mosby.

Paice, J. A., Penn, R. D., & Shott, S. (1992). Intraspinal morphine for chronic pain: A retrospective, multicenter study. *Journal of Pain and Symptom Management, 11,* 71–80.

Scalzitti, D. A. (1997). Screening for psychological factors in patients with low back problems: Waddell's nonorganic signs. *Physical Therapy, 77*(3), 306–312.

Shealy, C. N., Mortimer, J. T., & Reswick, J. B. (1967). Electrical inhibition of pain by stimulation of the dorsal columns: Preliminary clinical report. *Anesth Analg, 46*(4), 489–491.

Stiller, C. O. (1997). *Neurotransmission in CNS regions involved in pain modulation.* Unpublished master's thesis. Karolinska Institute, Stockholm, Sweden.

Turner, J. A., Loeser, J. D., & Bell, K. G. (1995). Spinal cord stimulation for chronic low back pain: A systematic literature synthesis. *Neurosurgery, 37*(6), 1088–1096.

Watts, R., & Silagy, C. (1995). A meta-analysis of the efficacy of epidural corticosteroids in the treatment of sciatica. *Anaesthesia and Intensive Care, 23,* 564–569.

Exercise Prescription

8

Michael J. Farrell,
Benny Katz, and Max D. Neufeld

Exercise is a viable treatment option for older people with persistent pain. It leads to decreases in pain, improvements in function, and elevation of their mood. Demonstrable impact on the quality of life of older people has elevated exercise from the role of adjunct to a treatment option in its own right. Comprehensive management programs for persistent pain in older people should include exercise as a component of treatment.

The focus of this chapter is upon the interaction of persistent pain and exercise in older people and the use of exercise as a treatment option. The mechanisms and magnitude of exercise required to relieve pain are reviewed and guidelines for prescription suggested. Exercise effects on disability and mood disturbance are also discussed, with emphasis on pain as a factor that could limit the benefit of exercise or necessitate modification of exercise prescription. Case studies are presented to illustrate the principles of exercise prescription in older people with persistent pain.

EVIDENCE AND PRINCIPLES FOR PRACTICE

Exercise Effects on Pain Perception

Exercise has become an accepted component of many cognitive-behavioral programs for persistent pain in old and young alike. Objectives for the prescription of exercise in the management of persistent pain do not invariably include the reduction of pain, sometimes emphasizing functional outcomes. For instance, a program may be considered beneficial if maximum walking distance limited by severe pain increases from 200 meters to 500 meters even if the maximum severity of pain has not altered. However, there are both rationales and empirical evidence for a link between the performance of exercise and the alleviation of pain. There are two general rationales for the presumed effects of exercise on pain intensity and unpleasantness. Exercise may either modify the disease-causing pain or modulate the neural mechanisms that culminate in the experience of pain.

Exercise, Pain, and Disease Modification

Moderate levels of exercise have the potential to modify musculoskeletal disease by increasing the elasticity of connective and contractile tissue; restoring muscle power, endurance, and coordination; reducing the rate of loss of bone density; and influencing the integrity of articular cartilage. Improvements in joint mobility and muscular action translate into enhanced biomechanics and diminished stress on vulnerable tissues adversely affected by disease, changes that presumably reduce nociceptive stimuli. Evidence that links the physiological effects of exercise with reduction of musculoskeletal pain in older people is largely associative. Parallel improvements in pain and musculoskeletal parameters, particularly in osteoarthritis and osteoporosis, are consistent with a causal relationship, but fall short of definitive proof (van Baar, Assendelft, Dekker, Oostendorp, & Bijlsma, 1999). At odds with this line of reasoning is the observation that pain relief is an inconsistent result of exercise among rheumatoid arthritis patients despite contemporaneous decreases in impairment (Stenstrom 1994b). Attempts to identify biologic markers of exercise effects in osteoarthritis have failed to demonstrate any relationship between pain complaints and biochemical indices of cartilage degeneration (Bautch, Malone, & Vailas, 1997). In a study of osteoarthritis, patients' pain and function improved while synovial fluid measures of keratan sulfate and hydroxyproline remained unchanged after a 12-week exercise program. Serial radiological evaluation of osteoarthritis suggests that exercise does not influence this parameter of disease progression. It seems most likely that pain relief after exercise in musculoskeletal disorders is due to enhanced biomechanics rather than any presumed effects on the underlying pathological process.

Exercise has been raised as a potentially deleterious factor in some musculoskeletal conditions. It has traditionally been prescribed very cautiously as a treatment for rheumatoid arthritis for fear of exacerbating joint damage and facilitating disease activity (Ytterberg, Mahowald, & Krug, 1994). Continued reluctance is not supported by the evidence from a growing number of clinical trials of exercise in rheumatoid arthritis (Stenstrom, 1994b; Van den Ende, Vliet Vlieland, Munneke, & Hazes, 1998). The specter of exercise as a risk factor for the onset and exacerbation of osteoarthritis has sprung from epidemiological links between excessive levels of activity and radiological markers of the disease. This association is tenuous, operating primarily in younger men (less than 50 years of age) or as a consequence of high levels of activity before menopause in women (Lane & Buckwalter 1999). Animal studies reporting joint deterioration following exercise also tend to employ extraordinary work rates and/or animals with a genetically engineered predisposition to arthritis (Lapvetelainen et al., 1995; Pap et al., 1998). On balance, it would appear that any reasonable level of exercise is unlikely to have a detrimental affect on disease progression in older people with osteoarthritis.

The impact of exercise on pain associated with activity in peripheral arterial obstructive disease has been ascribed to a range of vascular, rheologic, and metabolic effects. Measures of intermittent claudication bear a significant relationship with some, but not all, attributes of arterial disease. The maximum time to, or maximum distance of, claudication appears to be a function of disease severity, although a substantial degree of variation in claudicant pain is not explained by pathology (Muller-Buhl, Kirchberger, & Wiesemann, 1999).

In neuropathic conditions the potential for exercise to reverse the course of disease is less apparent. However, the proposition that exercise could lead to decreased pain in older people through the process of disease modification is certainly worthy of consideration.

Exercise and Pain Modulation

Exercise may bring about a change in pain sensation by modulating the nociceptive system directly. Individuals engaging in regular strenuous exercises appear less sensitive to pain than those who do not (Janal, 1996). The notion of exercise-induced analgesia has received support from studies of responses of healthy volunteers to painful extrinsic stimuli before and after exercise. The mechanisms for this effect are yet to be elucidated, but may include endogenous opioids and descending influences on dorsal horn neurons (Koltyn, 2000). However, exercise-induced analgesia is of very transient duration and may have little relevance for the changes in sensitivity observed in people who have regularly engaged in vigorous exercise. Exercise-induced analgesia is only evoked by very strenuous activity in younger people and is unlikely to be recruited during the exercise regimens currently prescribed for older people. Furthermore, there is evidence that descending influences are relatively impaired in older people (Washington, Gibson, & Helme, 2000) and are unlikely to contribute to any pain reduction subsequent to exercise. The "stoicism" of athletes could be due to a common response bias that tends to deny unpleasant experiences, including pain (Janal). Cognitive effects may also be the most likely interface between exercise and pain modulation in older people with persistent pain. It seems more likely that exercise, through general effects on levels of fitness and well being, could equip older people with greater reserves to cope with their pain. It is difficult to test for a causal effect of adaptive coping on the experience of pain, although associative evidence supports such a relationship in older people. (Corran, Gibson, Farrell, & Helme, 1994).

Efficacy of Exercise in Reducing Pain in Older People

Clinical trials of exercise in heterogeneous groups of older people with persistent pain have rarely appeared, although preliminary studies have reported favorable outcomes for exercise programs in older groups of mixed diagnoses (Ferrell, Josephson, Pollan, Loy, & Ferrell, 1997). Cross-sectional aging studies of exercise effects on pain have not appeared in the literature. However, a substantial number of reports have demonstrated positive exercise effects on pain report among cases with specific etiologies that predominately affect older people. The following sections summarize this body of research.

Osteoarthritis

The impact of exercise on the clinical presentation of osteoarthritis of the hips and knees has been subject to considerable scrutiny. Improvements in osteoarthritis pain almost invariably occur subsequent to exercise (van Baar et al., 1999). Although the methodological rigor of these studies differs, there appears to be little doubt that exercise achieves genuine benefits in terms of pain relief among subjects completing a program. An important confounding issue, potential increases in analgesics and NSAID among exercise groups, has been ably monitored in several studies and reported as either equivalent across samples or significantly less in exercising groups (Kovar et al., 1992; O'Reilly, Muir, & Doherty, 1999). However, a statistically significant exercise effect on osteoarthritis pain should not be confused with a substantial clinical effect. A recent meta-analysis of exercise trials in osteoarthritis of the hip and knee concluded that the effect of exercise on pain was only small to moderate (van Baar et al., 1999). The average change in pain scores across studies of exercise in osteoarthritis is a reduction of approximately 30%. This falls short of the arbitrary benchmark of 50% that is often instituted in the evaluation of other pain treatments; nevertheless even a 30% average improvement may be considered worthwhile. For additional recommendations on the prescription of exercise for older adults with osteoarthritis, the reader is referred to a recent statement of consensus practice recommendations by the American Geriatrics Society (AGS) Panel on Exercise and Osteoarthritis (2001).

A biomechanical approach to exercise prescription for the relief of pain is warranted in some cases of joint disease. Persistent pain from degenerative tears in the rotator cuff complex is an example of a biomechanical problem that responds to a tailored exercise regimen. Exercises for rotator cuff injuries are designed to reduce tension in the shoulder and neck by repositioning the humerus posteriorly. Agonist scapula muscles are strengthened to improve scapulo-humeral rhythm, reducing stress on the damaged tendons during movement. Regaining active control of the shoulder complex reduces extraneous movements and aberrant postures that act as triggers for nociception.

Back Pain and Lumbar Spinal Canal Stenosis

The relative prevalence of low back pain as a function of age is a matter of dispute. Some epidemiological reports have suggested that low back pain decreases in prevalence after a peak in middle age whereas other studies report a steady rise in low back pain with age (Helme and Gibson, 1999). Regardless of relative levels, spinal disorders are common among older people yet the effects of exercise in low back pain have rarely been assessed in older samples. An uncontrolled trial of isotonic exercise in a convenience sample of older women presenting with persistent back pain appears to be the only report of exercise effects on back pain in subjects of advanced age (Holmes et al., 1996). The benefits of exercise for spinal pain related to osteoporosis are more established, albeit small, and run parallel with decreased rates of loss of bone mineral density (Bravo et al., 1996; Malmros, Mortensen, Jensen, & Charles, 1998; Prior, Barr, Chow, & Faulkner, 1996).

Lumbar spinal canal stenosis associated with spondylosis is more often encountered among older than among younger people. Although back pain is a feature of spinal canal stenosis, leg pain is usually the most disabling symptom. The efficacy of conservative measures in the treatment of spinal canal stenosis has yet to be confirmed, but exercise is frequently advocated as a component of management for this disorder. The symptoms of spinal canal stenosis are exacerbated by lumbar extension, a usual requisite of an upright posture and gait. The rationale for relieving pain with exercise in spinal canal stenosis is to improve dynamic lumbar stability with specific abdominal strengthening and postural adjustment. Adopting a slightly flexed lumbar posture in standing can reduce stenosis and delay the onset of claudicant leg pain.

Rheumatoid Arthritis

Palliation of pain in rheumatoid arthritis is inconsistently reported in trials of exercise. In a recent review of exercise effects in rheumatoid arthritis the prospect of pain relief was not entertained, a common omission that has possibly hindered adequate appraisal of exercise and pain in this clinical group (Van den Ende et al., 1998).

Fibromyalgia

Fibromyalgia is a syndrome of chronic, widespread musculoskeletal pain of unknown etiology. Sufferers often report depression, stiffness, fatigue, poor sleep, and the presence of trigger points. The diagnosis is based on clinical criteria established by the American College of Rheumatology. The prevalence of fibromyalgia in the general population is 2%, with higher rates in females. Prevalence increases with age, with the highest rates of 7% in women aged 60 to 79 years (Wolfe, Ross, Anderson, Russell, & Hebert, 1995). Although pharmacological approaches are the primary mode of treatment there is no evidence to support long-term benefit (Hadhazy, Ezzo, Berman, & Creamer, 2000). Many fibromyalgia patients are deconditioned. An exercise program should be part of the multidisciplinary management approach. Aerobic exercises undertaken three times per week have been demonstrated to reduce tender point tenderness and pain, although sleep problems and fatigue did not improve. The effects of exercise do not appear to be long lasting (Leventhal, 1999). A combined pharmacological and nonpharmacological approach is recommended for the management of fibromyalgia.

Vascular Disorders

Intermittent claudication associated with vascular disease is of particular relevance for the relationship between exercise and pain. The onset of claudicant pain is directly related to activity, and maximum walking distance is a surrogate measure of pain tolerance. From the patient's perspective, exercise is a trigger for pain. However, assiduous compliance with an exercise program can produce substantial benefits for patients with intermittent claudication. A Cochrane review concluded that exercise afforded improvements in walking ability averaging 150% across 10 studies of lower limb vascular pain (Leng, Fowler, & Ernst, 2000). In some instances, exercise effects were superior or comparable to angioplasty and some pharmacological treatments.

Neuropathic Pain Syndromes

No trials of exercise as a treatment for neuropathic pain have appeared in the literature. From a mechanistic viewpoint this is not surprising, given that exercise is unlikely to modify the disorders that commonly cause persistent neuropathic pain in older people, such as postherpetic neuralgia and poststroke pain. If exercise has the capacity to modulate pain in clinical conditions independent of etiology in older people, then this potential treatment option should be elucidated.

Prescribing Exercise to Reduce Pain

It is difficult to be definitive about exercise prescription for the reduction of persistent pain. Comparing different types of exercise across studies is not very enlightening, given that almost all types of exercise appear to have beneficial effects on pain report. Looking for different degrees of effect between two similar treatments when the best possible effect is only small to moderate leaves little room to demonstrate statistically significant and clinically meaningful results. The solution is to design studies that reduce extraneous variance and/or to recruit much larger samples. The cost of studying differential exercise effects may not be warranted. At present, the clinician can reasonably expect that any form of exercise can potentially modify the pain experience and that a varied program including aerobic, flexibility, and strengthening components is the most reasonable approach to take. In cases where pain reduction is one of a number of objectives, other priorities may determine choice of exercise. The elements of a comprehensive exercise program are summarized in Table 8.1.

Individual compliance and the logistics of exercise delivery determine the choice of home exercise versus supervised programs. Similar exercise regimens performed in a domestic or clinical setting do not appear to differ in efficacy. However, the use of specialized equipment, such as isokinetic apparatus, will dictate a clinic-based approach. Ensuring compliance with exercise is problematic irrespective of setting, although one study has reported marginally better results for home-based components of training programs (King, Haskell, Taylor, Kraemer, & DeBusk, 1991). If the choice exists, it may be judicious to offer clinic-based exercise, home-based exercise, or a combination of both, depending on patients' preferences.

Maintaining an exercise program is not easy. Compliance will be less likely if the program is excessively demanding. Conversely, inadequate dosage expends energy without a training effect, reinforcing perceptions

TABLE 8.1 Recommended Elements of an Exercise Program

Mobilizing

Description	Slow stretching movements at end range of major joints and multiarthrodial muscles. Movements should produce subjective sensation of mild resistance.
Duration	Each stretch maintained for 10 to 30 seconds.
Repetitions	Range—from 1 stretch per major joint and muscle group to 10 repetitions.
Frequency	Range—from once a day, three times a week to daily.
Progression	Initiation of a stretching program can be associated with muscle and joint soreness. Superficial heat before stretching facilitates mobilization. Progression should be gradual, depending on associated symptoms. Supervision of mobilizing is required during periods of active joint inflammation.

Strengthening: Isometric

Description	Static contractions of major muscle groups without joint movement, usually performed within the resting range of the muscle.
Intensity	Range—40% to 70% of maximal voluntary contraction.
Repetitions	Range—1 to 10 repetitions.
Frequency	Range—twice daily to five times a day.
Progression	Isometric exercises have limited training effects because muscle strengthening is usually confined to the angle where exercise is performed. Isometric exercises are well-tolerated by patients initiating an exercise program and can be an intermediary step before the introduction of isotonic exercises.

Strengthening: Isotonic

Description	Resisted contractions of major muscle groups through a prescribed joint range.
Intensity	Range—40% to 80% of maximal voluntary contraction.
Repetitions	Range—from 1 to 6 repetitions.
Frequency	Range—2 to 3 times a week. It is preferable to allow a day's rest between bouts of isotonic exercise.
Progression	Resistance can be gradually increased by 5% to 10% per week.

TABLE 8.1 *(continued)*

Aerobic

Description	Sustained repetitive movements of large muscle groups at an intensity that exceeds the usual level of daily activity (i.e., walking, swimming, cycling).
Intensity	Patients should commence aerobic exercise at a low to moderate level of exertion. This level of exertion is consistent with exercise at 50% to 75% of the maximum heart rate. Patients should be able to converse comfortably when exercising at this level.
Duration	Range—initially 4 or 5 brief bouts in succession summing to 20 to 30 minutes of activity, increasing to continuous activity of at least 20 minutes.
Frequency	Range—3 to 4 days per week.
Progression	The intensity or duration of exercise can be increased gradually by 2% to 3% each week.

of the futility of exercise. Fortunately, the level of exercise required to obtain partial relief of pain is not onerous. Low-intensity, thrice-weekly stationary cycling for 25 minutes (Mangione et al., 1999) or 30 maximal knee flexion and extension contractions over 8 to 10 weeks (Schilke, Johnson, Housh, & O'Dell, 1996) have resulted in reduced pain for older people with knee osteoarthritis. To be efficacious in the long term, exercise must become a lifestyle component as the benefits of exercise are lost if the activity is ceased (Morio et al., 2000).

Exercise, Disability, and Mood Disturbance

The symptomotology of common painful disorders in older people is not confined to reports of pain. Physical and psychological morbidity frequently accompanies complaints of pain and constitutes potential targets for the benefit of exercise in their own right. The role of exercise in modifying disability among older people has received substantial empirical support. There have also been encouraging reports of exercise effects on depression in older people. There are two issues to consider when prescribing exercises with the objectives of decreasing disability and improving mood in older people with pain: which exercise is most efficacious and whether an exacerbation of pain can be avoided.

The Risk of Exacerbating Pain with Exercise

Many patients express apprehension about the exacerbation of pain when engaging in exercise. However, the risk of transient discomfort should be weighed against the functional benefits and long-term relief of pain that will accrue after completing an exercise program. Patients with osteoarthritis contemplating an exercise program can be reassured that the risk of exacerbating symptoms is less in reality than they might expect. Coleman, Buchner, Cress, Chan, and de Lateur (1996) carefully monitored adverse events, including pain, during the performance of strength and endurance training programs. In the sample of 105 subjects, 75 of whom had arthritis, minor musculoskeletal injuries resulting in delay or discontinuation of exercise occurred at a rate of 0.48 per 1,000 exercise hours. The majority of these injuries were attributed to factors other than exercise performance (Coleman et al., 1996). Pain was very infrequently worse during or after exercise, an experience replicated in another setting involving osteoarthritis subjects (Mangione et al., 1999). Patients with rheumatoid arthritis are also capable of engaging in a wide variety of exercise regimens without exacerbating their pain (Van den Ende et al., 1998).

Clinicians who design exercise programs must pay deference to those circumstances where there is a biomechanical link between movement and nociception. The objective of increasing aerobic capacity can be complicated by intermittent claudication associated with vascular disease or spinal canal stenosis. If ambulation distance is insufficient to achieve sustained increases in heart rate, then water aerobics may be a suitable alternative. Cycling in a relatively flexed posture may permit the patient with spinal canal stenosis to achieve target heart rates that are unattainable with walking. However, it is probably best to test any assumptions regarding posture, movement, and pain before excluding exercise options. A clinician must be cognizant of the concerns of patients but should be careful not to exclude exercise without an adequate trial.

Prescribing Exercise to Reduce Disability

Many interacting factors influence the nature of disability and impact on choice of exercise. These factors include type of disease, degree of impairment, environment, mood state, and cognition. Exercises are primarily designed to reverse impairment and maximize performance on functional tasks. Common impairments are decreased muscle power, loss of range of movement, and decreased aerobic fitness. Functional objectives of exercise include changes in time or distance walked, enhanced performance of transfers, and improvements in balance and coordination.

The most impressive effect of exercise in reversing impairment in older people with persistent pain is the impact of resisted movement on muscle weakness. Muscle weakness is a common consequence of musculoskeletal disorders and can occur subsequent to any disease or sedentary lifestyle. Improvements in muscle power and endurance of 20% to 40% are frequently cited in reports of clinical trials of exercise among older people with persistent pain. High levels of resistance (i.e., maximum contractions), repeated at low frequency (5 repetitions, 3 times a week) lead to substantial increases in muscle power (Schilke et al., 1996). Muscle endurance is enhanced by submaximal contractions repeated on more frequent occasions (Fisher et al., 1993). Close monitoring of progress is important to advance regimens as power and endurance improve. Even the frailest older patients can benefit from a strengthening program. (See Feigenbaum and Pollock, 1999, for review and details of prescribing.)

Increasing aerobic capacity is a regular objective of exercise programs for older people with persistent pain. Decreased fitness can be a consequence of inactivity or accompany disorders of the cardiovascular and respiratory systems. Sedentary older individuals with severe or unstable medical problems or acutely inflamed joints should not embark on an unaccustomed exercise program. Potential problems are usually detected on routine medical history and physical examination. The risk of precipitating a coronary event or sudden death during an exercise program is small. Even patients with known coronary disease can benefit from graded exercise programs. Exercise stress testing should not be considered a prerequisite before commencing an exercise program; it should be reserved for high-risk patients or those undergoing high-intensity exercise (Ettinger, 1998).

Aerobic capacity can be improved by exercises that achieve target increases in heart rate. The level of heart rate increases required to achieve an exercise effect in older people has not been firmly established under all circumstances. However, among patients with poor exercise tolerance an increase in heart rate of approximately 40% of reserve (heart rate reserve = 220 beats per minute [BPM] – age in years – resting heart rate) sustained for 25 minutes, 3 times a week is sufficient to produce increased fitness (Mangione et al., 1999). If possible, workouts at rates in excess of 80% of VO_2 max for 30 minutes produce superior fitness outcomes in older people generally (Lemura, von Duvillar, & Mookerjee, 2000). The most common form of aerobic exercise for older people with persistent pain is walking. Patients are instructed to walk at their own pace such that they are still able to carry on a conversation. Other exercise options include jogging and stationary cycling, although these more strenuous forms of exercise are no more efficacious than walking in increasing fitness in older people. The duration of exercise is important to achieve a training effect although brief rests are permissible if the heart rate remains near the target range before the exercise is resumed. On balance, an older person with persistent pain can expect an increase in VO_2 max of 10% to 15% after 10 weeks of aerobic exercise.

Flexibility and agility are functions of joint mobility and muscle extensibility. Stretching exercises have not been specifically evaluated in older people with persistent pain, although exercise programs incorporating stretching have produced gains in spinal mobility among women with osteoporosis (Bravo et al., 1996). Small changes in joint mobility have also been reported in response to programs that are either strengthening or aerobic in nature in older people with arthritis (Stenstrom, 1994a; van Baar et al., 1998), although similar evaluations have failed to produce changes in flexibility (Minor, Hewett, Webel, Anderson, & Kay, 1989; Rogind et al., 1998). Among able community-dwelling older people, stretching exercises appear to reduce reports of pain, yet produce inconsistent results for flexibility (King et al., 2000). In the absence of aberrant joint laxity, patients presenting with persistent pain and significant restrictions of movement should be given a trial of mobilizing exercises and their progress closely monitored to establish whether this intervention is of value in individual cases.

Exercises designed to improve muscle power, endurance, and aerobic fitness are likely to produce increases in functional performance. Measures of walking efficacy commonly improve after exercise programs among older people with persistent pain (Bravo et al., 1996; van Baar et al., 1999). Benefits have also been reported for climbing stairs, arising from a chair, lifting and carrying weights, single leg stance, postural sway, and coordination (Bravo et al., 1996; Ettinger, Burns, & Messier, 1997; Maurer, Stern, Kinossian, Cook, & Schumacher, 1999; Messier et al., 2000; Rogind et al., 1998; Stenstrom 1994a). The magnitude of these changes is approximately 5% to 15% of baseline levels. Although a 10% improvement in walking may appear to be a modest change, it can translate into the ability to cross at traffic lights in sufficient time or manage the distance to visit a neighbor.

Current evidence suggests that exercise effects on impairment are associated with decreased levels of disability. Measures of disability and general activity show modest improvements following exercise programs in older people with persistent pain (Ettinger et al., 1997; Kovar et al., 1992; van Baar et al., 1998). Reversing impairments with exercise is an important first step in addressing disability associated with pain, but other issues must also be tackled to ensure that improved functional capacity becomes increased activity.

Exercise and Mood State

Depression and anxiety are common associates of persistent pain in older people. The impact of exercise on their mood state gained initial support from studies of healthy subjects. Older people without psychiatric morbidity report increased positive and decreased negative mood after engaging in exercise (King, Taylor, & Haskell, 1993). Two recent clinical trials have demonstrated impressive effects of exercise in relieving symptoms in older people with moderate and major depression (Blumenthal et al., 1999; Singh, Clements, & Fiatarone, 1997). The effects reported in these two studies were achieved in the absence of any pharmacological intervention. Although pain was not a primary complaint in either study, ancillary reports of pain were common among the subjects. Studies of exercise effects among patients with osteoporosis and osteoarthritis have also demonstrated benefits on levels of anxiety (Minor et al., 1989; O'Reilly et al., 1999; Ross, Bohannon, Davis, & Gurchiek, 1999).

Depression in older people responds to both aerobic and resistance programs of 10 to 16 weeks' duration, seemingly in equal measure (Blumenthal et al., 1999; Singh et al., 1997). A program amalgamating both aerobic and strengthening components may have a wider range of ancillary benefits. A varied program would also be less monotonous and ensure greater compliance. Future studies may determine the relative merits of different exercise regimens for the management of depression in older people.

Ensuring Exercise Compliance

Maximizing compliance is a critical element in the successful management of an exercise program. Exercise, more than any other therapeutic action, requires a substantial commitment of time and energy from the patient. An exercise program will not be adhered to without motivation. In the rarefied atmosphere of a constantly monitored clinical trial, high retention rates can be maintained, although even research-based programs can suffer from dropout numbers that challenge the validity of the results. The clinician does not have access to the same resources as a research team and must rely upon other means to maximize the likelihood of exercise compliance.

The most important thing a clinician can do to facilitate compliance with an exercise program is to assure patients that exercise will be of benefit and that they have the capacity to successfully perform a program. The program should be achievable, relevant, and enjoyable in order to optimize compliance. Older people with persistent pain may have particular concerns about the advisability of exercise and should be reassured that the risk of exacerbating their symptoms during exercise is small and that any acute discomfort will be compensated for by long-term benefits in pain relief and increased function. Self-efficacy contributes significantly to variable performance among older people performing painful tasks (Rejeski, Craven, Ettinger, McFarlane, & Thompson, 1996). Education about the merits of exercise and doses required to gain a training effect will promote a more positive attitude toward a restorative program. When assessing patients for exercise programs the clinician should direct attention to patients' preferred setting for exercise (home versus clinic), previous exercise habits, concerns regarding exacerbation of comorbid disease, and any perceived logistic barriers. A history of compliance is the best predictor of future compliance (Rejeski, Brawley, Ettinger, Morgan, & Thompson, 1997). Consequently, initial efforts to promote adherence are likely to be rewarded with the establishment of exercise as a habit.

Exacerbation of pain during and immediately after exercise does not occur as frequently as patients might expect but does constitute a potential barrier to the benefits of training programs. Commencing an exercise program can give rise to muscle soreness, a contingency that will cause less concern if the prospect is acknowledged beforehand. Patients should also be instructed in suitable warm-up and cool-down protocols to reduce the risk of injury. Monitoring of any adverse events subsequent to exercise will alert the clinician to the need for palliative strategies. The use of a simple analgesic such as acetaminophen or an anti-inflammatory agent taken prior to exercise may ease pain, allowing for a higher level of exercise achievement. Physical strategies, such as local heat, gentle stretches, massage, and TENS, can also help to ease joint and muscle soreness after exercise. Table 8.2 summarizes the strategies that clinicians can use to facilitate compliance with an exercise program.

SETTING-SPECIFIC CONSIDERATIONS

Exercise and Long-Term-Care Residents

The ability of older people with painful persistent conditions to benefit from training is ample evidence that disease is not a barrier to exercise. Indeed, exercise is both feasible and efficacious for frail and institutionalized older people. Beneficial exercise effects have been reported for older patients with chronic heart failure, severe Alzheimer's disease, and among residents of long-term-care institutions (Lazowski et al., 1999; Owen

---

TABLE 8.2 Factors Facilitating Compliance With Exercise Programs

<u>**Communicate**</u>

Evaluate the patient's understanding of the risks and benefits of exercise.

Establish if the patient is motivated to undertake a program.

Assess the patient's level of confidence to complete a program.

<u>**Educate**</u>

Promote the benefits of a regular exercise program.

Acknowledge the potential side effects of exercise and allay negative perceptions of the risks associated with exercise among older people.

<u>**Prescribe appropriately**</u>

Keep the program simple.

Customize the program to patients' needs and abilities.

Prescribe and recommend treatments and actions that will reduce exercise-induced soreness.

Encourage patients to incorporate exercise within their daily routine.

Suggest a setting that is compatible with patients' preferences, (i.e., home versus clinic).

<u>**Monitor and modify**</u>

Set realistic, mutually agreed-on goals for the exercise program.

Regularly assess patients' compliance with the exercise program.

Measure and give feedback on indicators of progress.

Evaluate the patients' perceptions of their progress.

& Croucher, 2000; Rolland et al., 2000). Prescribing exercises for older people with persistent pain and comorbidity should be based on a realistic appraisal of patients' capacities. However, frailty should not exclude the prescription of exercises that are likely to produce training effects. Ideally, a program should include an aerobic component, although this may not be feasible for patients who are not independently ambulant. Strengthening exercises should accompany an aerobic program and, in the absence of the opportunity to perform aerobic exercises, strengthening can be expected to produce favorable functional outcomes among frail older people (Meuleman, Brechue, Kubilis, & Lowenthal, 2000).

SUMMARY/RECOMMENDATIONS

1. Exercise should be considered as a treatment strategy in all cases of older adults with persistent pain.
2. An exercise program is usually combined with pharmacological therapy but can be effective as a single therapy.
3. There are relatively few risks in an exercise program, but many beneficial health effects, in addition to any effect on pain perception.
4. Any type of exercise performed by older adults with persistent pain is likely to have a palliative effect except where specific movements are directly related to the exacerbation of pain.
5. A relatively low level of exercise is adequate to achieve reductions in pain intensity.
6. Exercise designed to achieve functional outcomes can be undertaken without exacerbation of pain in many pain conditions.
7. Prescription of exercise for older people with persistent pain should be guided by the objectives of reducing impairment, increasing functional performance, and reducing disability.
8. Resistance and aerobic exercise regimes are viable adjuncts to the treatment of depression.
9. Older people with significant levels of comorbid disease can comply with exercise programs and achieve significant training effects.
10. Lack of compliance is a major limiting factor for the benefits of exercise, a complication that can be ameliorated by engendering a positive appraisal of the likely outcomes of exercise.

CASE STUDIES

Case 1

A 68-year-old former postman presented to the pain clinic with chronic shoulder, arm, and neck pain, 10 years after undergoing surgery to repair a complete tear in the supra/infraspinatus complex. He complained of poor sleep and experienced difficulty brushing his teeth, combing his hair, getting dressed, and driving a car. He was frustrated that he could not play lawn bowls. Physical examination revealed a typically rounded shoulder (anteriorly displaced humerus), painfully reduced neck and shoulder movement, and associated weakness. Exercise prescription consisted of a graded program in the order of scapular elevation (lifting point of shoulders toward ears), scapula positioning exercises (active protraction, retraction and rotation of the scapula), isometric scapular stabilizing (maintaining scapula in positions that usually occur during normal glenohumeral movements such as scapula rotation during shoulder abduction), neck mobilizing, and isotonic strengthening with light weights in the mid to outer range of the scapular stabilizers and rotator cuff. Pain-free, gentle shoulder mobilizing exercises were introduced late in the program. Graduated aerobic exercises were incorporated to reverse deconditioning associated with reduced levels of general activity. The patient regained a significant degree of active movement of the shoulder with reduced pain, experienced less difficulty with instrumental activities of daily living, and was eventually able to enjoy lawn bowls at a social level but did not return to competition.

Discussion

Impairment and persistent pain associated with a long history of rotator cuff disease can be very disabling. Restoring controlled movement to the shoulder with exercise requires patience and careful prescription to avoid any disincentive for compliance due to exacerbation of pain. A successful program is initiated by exercises that can be performed without pain and lead to decreased stress on the shoulder. Scapular movements and isometric contractions in the early phases of rehabilitation lay the groundwork for more stressful movements to follow. Shoulder flexibility exercises increase pain and are counterproductive early in an exercise program. Pain-free shoulder flexion and abduction exercises in supine should be reserved until after at least 3 weeks of initial stabilizing exercises. Careful monitoring ensures that exercise progression does not occur to the detriment of patients' symptoms and alerts the clinician to the need for pharmacological and other strategies that ameliorate adverse effects.

Establishing short- and long-term goals that are achievable and relevant for the patient increase the probability of compliance. The initial goal in this case was to ease the burden of instrumental activities of daily living. Performing daily rituals with less pain is a very tangible demonstration of progress and provides ample incentive to continue with exercise. Lawn bowls was an important component of the social life of this patient and remaining within the bowling community was a natural long-term goal. Persistent pain can be perceived as a deterrent to social interaction, leading to isolation and increased risk of lowered mood. A sedentary lifestyle precipitates deconditioning and reduces the physical capacity to engage in social activity. In this case, taking advantage of restored shoulder function was facilitated by improved vigor subsequent to a generalized aerobic program.

Case 2

An 82-year-old resident of a hostel was referred to the pain clinic with a 25-year history of low back pain attributed to spondylosis. In the preceding 6 months, she had experienced progressively increasing bilateral leg pain. The history and examination were consistent with lumbar spinal canal stenosis. Her other health problems included osteoarthritis of the left hip and ischemic heart disease. The patient's ambulation distance was restricted by pain to 50 yards and was dependent on the use of a single-point stick. She experienced difficulty with transfers and was receiving assistance with showering. The exercise program prescribed for this case included abdominal strengthening, mobilization exercises for the hips, isotonic strengthening of the major lower limb muscles, and attendance at a seated, general exercise group at the hostel. A wheeled walking frame replaced the walking stick, and gait and postural advice were provided. The patient's ambulation distance increased to 100 yards; transfers from bed and chair remained independent, but she continued to receive assistance with showering. The patient purchased an electric wheelchair and was able to independently visit the local shopping precinct near her hostel.

Discussion

Exercise has a major role to play in ameliorating the impact of spinal canal stenosis, despite the inherent restrictions of movement that characterize this disorder. Abdominal exercises are a very important component for the management of spinal canal stenosis. Initially, exercises for the lumbar spine primary stabilizers (transversus abdominus and multifidus muscles) are taught in varying postures, followed by outer-range isotonic and isometric strengthening of the more superficial abdominal muscles. This is undertaken in association with lumbar and hip flexion exercises to improve flexibility. Strengthening exercises are progressed to include setting the lumbar stabilizers in more functional and dynamic postures. Emphasis is placed on the use of lumbar flexion when standing and walking as an adaptive mechanism.

The short-term goal of abdominal exercises and postural advice is to increase ambulation distance. In this case, increased ambulation distance translated into greater ease in moving within the hostel between the patient's room, other residents' rooms, dining area, and activity hall. Comorbid disease and poor ambulation distance precluded a level of aerobic exercise sufficient to produce a training effect. In the short and long terms, functional transfers were maintained by strengthening the lower limbs. This process was augmented by the generalized exercise program, which had the advantage of a social context. The utilization of suitable aids, notably an electric wheelchair, provides opportunities that would otherwise be beyond the functional capacity of an older person with significant disability.

REFERENCES

American Geriatrics Society Panel on Exercise and Osteoarthritis. (2001). Exercise prescription for older adults with osteoarthritis pain: Consensus practice recommendations. *J Am Geriatr Soc, 49*, 808–823.

Bautch, J. C., Malone, D. G., & Vailas, A. C. (1997). Effects of exercise on knee joints with osteoarthritis: A pilot study of biologic markers. *Arthritis Care Res, 10*, 48–55.

Blumenthal, J. A., Babyak, M. A., Moore, K. A., Craighead, W. E., Herman, S., Khatri, P., Waugh, R., Napolitano, M. A., Forman, L. M., Applebaum, M., Doraiswamy, P. M., & Krishnan, K. R. (1999). Effects of exercise training on older patients with major depression. *Arch Intern Med, 159*, 2349–2356.

Bravo, G., Gauthier, P., Roy, P. M., et al. (1996). Impact of a 12-month exercise program on the physical and psychological health of osteopenic women. *J Am Geriatr Soc, 44*, 756–762.

Christmas, C. (2000). Exercise and older patients: Guidelines for the clinician, *J Am Geriatr Soc, 48*, 318–324.

Coleman, E. A., Buchner, D. M., Cress, M. E., Chan, B. K., & de Lateur, B. J. (1996). The relationship of joint symptoms with exercise performance in older adults. *J Am Geriatr Soc, 44*, 14–21.

Corran, T. M., Gibson, S. J., Farrell, M. J., & Helme, R. D. (1994). Comparison of chronic pain experience between young and elderly patients. In G. F. Gebhart, D. L. Hammond, & T. S. Jensen (Eds.), *Proceedings of the VIIth World Congress on Pain: Vol. 2.* (pp. 895–906). Seattle, WA: IASP Press.

Ettinger, W. H. (1998). Physical activity, arthritis, and disability in older people, *Clin Geriatr Med, 14*, 633–640.

Ettinger, W. H., Jr., Burns, R., & Messier, S. P. (1997). A randomized trial comparing aerobic exercise and resistance exercise with a health education program in older adults with knee osteoarthritis: The Fitness Arthritis and Seniors Trial (FAST). *JAMA, 277*, 25–31.

Feigenbaum, M. S., & Pollock, M. L. (1999). Prescription of resistance training for health and disease. *Med Sci Sports Exerc, 31*, 38–45.

Ferrell, B. A., Josephson, K. R., Pollan, A. M., Loy, S., & Ferrell, B. R. (1997). A randomized trial of walking versus physical methods for chronic pain management. *Aging (Milano), 9*, 99–105.

Fisher, N. M., Gresham, G. E., Abrams, M., Hicks, J., Horrigan, D., & Pendergast, D. R. (1993). Quantitative effects of physical therapy on muscular and functional performance in subjects with osteoarthritis of the knees. *Arch Phys Med Rehabil, 74*, 840–847.

Hadhazy, V. A., Ezzo, J., Creamer, P., & Berman, B. M. (2000). Mind-body therapy for the treatment of fibromyalgia. A systematic review. *J Rheumatal, 27*(12), 2911–2918.

Helme, R. D., & Gibson, S. J. (1999). The epidemiology of pain in older people. In I. K. Crombie, P. R. Croft, S. J. Linton, L. LeResche, & M. V. Korff (Eds.), *Epidemiology of pain* (pp. 103–111). Seattle, WA: IASP Press.

Holmes, B., Leggett, S., Mooney, V., Nichols, J., Negri, S., & Hoeyberghs, A. (1996). Comparison of female geriatric lumbar-extension strength: Asymptotic versus chronic low back pain patients and their response to active rehabilitation. *J Spinal Disord, 9*, 17–22.

Janal, M. N. (1996). Pain sensitivity, exercise and stoicism. *J R Soc Med, 89*, 376–381.

King, A. C., Haskell, W. L., Taylor, C. B., Kraemer, H. C., & DeBusk, R. F. (1991). Group- vs home-based exercise training in healthy older men and women: A community-based clinical trial. *JAMA, 266*, 1535–1542.

King, A. C., Pruitt, L. A., Phillips, W., Oka, R., Rodenburg, A., & Haskell, W. L. (2000). Comparative effects of two physical activity programs on measured and perceived physical functioning and other health-related quality of life outcomes in older adults. *J Gerontol A Biol Sci Med Sci, 55*, M74–M83.

King, A. C., Taylor, C. B., & Haskell, W. L. (1993). Effects of differing intensities and formats of 12 months of exercise training on psychological outcomes in older adults. *Health Psychol, 12*, 292–300.

Koltyn, K. F. (2000). Analgesia following exercise: A review. *Sports Med, 29*, 85–98.

Kovar, P. A., Allegrante, J. P., MacKenzie, C. R., Peterson, M. G., Gutin, B., & Charlson, M. E. (1992). Supervised fitness walking in patients with osteoarthritis of the knee: A randomized, controlled trial. *Ann Intern Med, 116*, 529–534.

Lane, N. E., & Buckwalter, J. A. (1999). Exercise and osteoarthritis. *Curr Opin Rheumatol, 11*, 413–416.

Lapvetelainen, T., Nevalainen, T., Parkkinen, J. J., Arokoski, J., Kiraly, K., Hyttinen, M., Halonen, P., & Helminen, H. J. (1995). Lifelong moderate running training increases the incidence and severity of osteoarthritis in the knee joint of C57BL mice. *Anat Rec, 242*, 159–165.

Lazowski, D. A., Ecclestone, N. A., Myers, A. M., Paterson, D. H., Tudor-Locke, C., Fitzgerald, C., Jones, G., Shima, N., & Cunningham, D. A. (1999). A randomized outcome evaluation of group exercise programs in long-term care institutions. *J Gerontol A Biol Sci Med Sci, 54*, M621–M628.

Lemura, L. M., von Duvillard, S. P., & Mookerjee, S. (2000). The effects of physical training of functional capacity in adults ages 46 to 90: A meta-analysis. *J Sports Med Phys Fitness, 40*, 1–10.

Leng, G. C., Fowler, B., & Ernst, E. (2000). Exercise for intermittent claudication. *Cochrane Database Syst Rev 2*.

Leventhal, L. J. (1999). Management of fibromyalgia. *Ann Intern Med, 131*, 850–858.

Malmros, B., Mortensen, L., Jensen, M. B., & Charles, P. (1998). Positive effects of physiotherapy on chronic pain and performance in osteoporosis. *Osteoporos Int, 8*, 215–221.

Mangione, K. K., McCully, K., Gloviak, A., Lefebvre, I., Hofmann, M., & Craik, R. (1999). The effects of high-intensity and low-intensity cycle ergometry in older adults with knee osteoarthritis. *J Gerontol A Biol Sci Med Sci, 54*, M184–M190.

Maurer, B. T., Stern, A. G., Kinossian, B., Cook, K. D., & Schumacher, H. R., Jr. (1999). Osteoarthritis of the knee: Isokinetic quadriceps exercise versus an educational intervention. *Arch Phys Med Rehabil, 80,* 1293–1299.

Messier, S. P., Royer, T. D., Craven, T. E., O'Toole, M. L., Burns, R., & Ettinger, W. H., Jr. (2000). Long-term exercise and its effect on balance in older, osteoarthritic adults: Results from the Fitness, Arthritis, and Seniors Trial (FAST). *J Am Geriatr Soc, 48,* 131–138.

Meuleman, J. R., Brechue, W. F., Kubilis, P. S., & Lowenthal, D. T. (2000). Exercise training in the debilitated aged: Strength and functional outcomes. *Arch Phys Med Rehabil, 81,* 312–318.

Minor, M. A., Hewett, J. E., Webel, R. R., Anderson, S. K., & Kay, D. R. (1989). Efficacy of physical conditioning exercise in patients with rheumatoid arthritis and osteoarthritis. *Arthritis Rheum, 32,* 1396–1405.

Morio, B., Barra, V., Ritz, P., Fellmann, N., Bonny, J. M., Beaufrere, B., Boire, J. Y., & Vermorel, M. (2000). Benefit of endurance training in elderly people over a short period is reversible. *Eur J Appl Physiol, 81,* 329–336.

Muller-Buhl, U., Kirchberger, I., & Wiesemann, A. (1999). Relevance of claudication pain distance in patients with peripheral arterial occlusive disease. *Vasa, 28,* 25–29.

O'Reilly, S. C., Muir, K. R., & Doherty, M. (1999). Effectiveness of home exercise on pain and disability from osteoarthritis of the knee: A randomised controlled trial. *Ann Rheum Dis, 58,* 15–19.

Owen, A., & Croucher, L. (2000). Effect of an exercise programme for elderly patients with heart failure. *Eur J Heart Fail, 2,* 65–70.

Pap, G., Eberhardt, R., Sturmer, I., Machner, A., Schwarzberg, H., Roessner, A., & Neumann, W. (1998). Development of osteoarthritis in the knee joints of Wistar rats after strenuous running exercise in a running wheel by intracranial self-stimulation. *Pathol Res Pract, 194,* 41–47.

Prior, J. C., Barr, S. I., Chow, R., & Faulkner, R. A. (1996). Physical activity as therapy for osteoporosis. *Canadian Medical Association Journal, 155,* 940–944.

Rejeski, W. J., Brawley, L. R., Ettinger, W., Morgan, T., & Thompson, C. (1997). Compliance to exercise therapy in older participants with knee osteoarthritis: Implications for treating disability. *Med Sci Sports Exerc, 29,* 977–985.

Rejeski, W. J., Craven, T., Ettinger, W. H., Jr., McFarlane, M., & Shumaker, S. (1996). Self-efficacy and pain in disability with osteoarthritis of the knee. *J Gerontol B Psychol Sci Soc Sci, 51,* 24–29.

Rogind, H., Bibow-Nielsen, B., Jensen, B., Moller, H. C., Frimodt-Moller, H., & Bliddal, H. (1998). The effects of a physical training program on patients with osteoarthritis of the knees. *Arch Phys Med Rehabil, 79,* 1421–1427.

Rolland, Y., Rival, L., Pillard, F., Lafont, C., Rivere, D., Albarede, J., & Vellas, B. (2000). Feasibility of regular physical exercise for patients with moderate to severe Alzheimer disease. *J Nutr Health Aging, 4,* 109–113.

Ross, M. C., Bohannon, A. S., Davis, D. C., & Gurchiek, L. (1999). The effects of a short-term exercise program on movement, pain, and mood in the elderly. Results of a pilot study. *J Holist Nurs, 17,* 139–147.

Schilke, J. M., Johnson, G. O., Housh, T. J., & O'Dell, J. R. (1996). Effects of muscle-strength training on the functional status of patients with osteoarthritis of the knee joint. *Nurs Res, 45,* 68–72.

Singh, N. A., Clements, K. M., & Fiatarone, M. A. (1997). A randomized controlled trial of progressive resistance training in depressed elders. *J Gerontol A Biol Sci Med Sci, 52*, M27–M35.

Stenstrom, C. H. (1994a). Home exercise in rheumatoid arthritis functional class II: Goal setting versus pain attention. *J Rheumatol, 21*, 627–634.

Stenstrom, C. H. (1994b). Therapeutic exercise in rheumatoid arthritis. *Arthritis Care Res, 7*, 190–197.

van Baar, M. E., Assendelft, W. J., Dekker, J., Oostendorp, R. A., & Bijlsma, J. W. (1999). Effectiveness of exercise therapy in patients with osteoarthritis of the hip or knee: A systematic review of randomized clinical trials. *Arthritis Rheum, 42*, 1361–1369.

van Baar, M. E., Dekker, J., Oostendorp, R. A., Bijl, D., Voorn, T. B., Lemmens, J. A., & Bijlsma, J. W. (1998). The effectiveness of exercise therapy in patients with osteoarthritis of the hip or knee: A randomized clinical trial. *J Rheumatol, 25*, 2432–2439.

Van den Ende, C. H., Vliet Vlieland, T. P., Munneke, M., & Hazes, J. M. (1998). Dynamic exercise therapy in rheumatoid arthritis: A systematic review. *Br J Rheumatol, 37*, 677–687.

Washington, L. L., Gibson, S. J., & Helme, R. D. (2000). Age-related differences in the endogenous analgesic response to repeated cold water immersion in human volunteers. *Pain, 89*, 89–96.

Wolfe, F., Ross, K., Anderson, J., Russell, I. J., & Hebert, L. (1995). The prevalence and characteristics of fibromyalgia in the general population. *Arthritis Rheum, 38*, 19–28.

Ytterberg, S. R., Mahowald, M. L., & Krug, H. E. (1994). Exercise for arthritis. *Baillieres Clin Rheumatol, 8*, 161–189.

Complementary and Alternative Medicine Modalities   9

Linda A. Gerdner, Nicole L. Nisly,
and Ronald M. Glick

Complementary and Alternative Medicine (CAM) is defined as a wide variety of health care practices that are not an integral part of the Western biomedical system. These practice modalities are usually classified into five major categories: alternative medical systems, mind-body interventions, biologically based treatments, manipulative and body-based methods, and energy therapies. A study conducted in California reported that 41% of seniors used CAM within the previous year (Astin, Pelletier, Marie, & Haskell, 2000). The most frequently sited therapies included herbs (24%), chiropractic (20%), massage (15%), and acupuncture (14%). The most common reasons for seeking a CAM provider were back problems (43%), persistent pain (26%), general health improvement (25%), and arthritis (20%). The majority (58%) of consumers did not discuss the use of these therapies with their physician. Reported reasons that influenced the decision to use CAM therapies were general health improvement, dissatisfaction with conventional medicine, pain management, and fear of drug side effects.

A national telephone survey reported similar findings (Foster, Phillips, Hamel, & Eisenberg, 2000). The total sample was composed of 2,055 adults of whom 311 were 65 years and older. Thirty percent of the older adults had used at least one alternative modality in the past year. Those most commonly used included chiropractic (11%), herbal remedies (8%), relaxation techniques (5%), high-dose or megavitamins (5%), and religious or spiritual healing by others (4%).

Despite the prevalent use of CAM therapies by patients, health care professionals do not receive adequate training to address patients' use of CAM (Wetzel, Eisenberg, & Kaptchuk, 1998) and feel ill-prepared to counsel patients on the efficacy or safety of CAM therapies and on how to integrate their use with traditional medical care. Consequently, this creates the opportunity for a dual, parallel, and uncoordinated system of health care in which patients are at great risk for drug and dietary supplement interactions, unrecognized side effects of supplements or treatments, excessive cost, use of ineffective treatments, or even underuse of effective CAM treatments due to lack of guidance from knowledgeable professionals.

Persistent pain sufferers of all ages are often faced with the message from their health care providers that further treatment options are limited or unavailable. The use of CAM frequently provides the opportunity for patients to restore their hope and the sense of control that their illness has stolen. They become decision makers in their own care, selecting which treatment to seek or which supplement to take. Most CAM practitioners operate in close partnership with patients; patients are viewed as clients and partners, active participants in their own healing. This sense of autonomy, which is frequently lacking in their interaction with the conventional medical system, empowers patients and provides an excellent opportunity for more effective pain management and greater patient satisfaction (Abeles, 1990; Fordyce, 1988).

It would greatly benefit the traditional health care system and academic institutions to adopt a proactive posture in the development of relevant educational curricula on CAM, which requires open-minded collaboration between CAM professionals and educators (National Conference on Medical and Nursing Education in Complementary Medicine, 1996). This educational effort, the implementation of clinical and basic science research, credentialing and referral guidelines for CAM practitioners, and improved quality control of dietary supplements are basic elements for the success of the effort to coordinate and integrate our patients' growing use of CAM and the conventional medical care (Eisenberg et al., 1998).

In 1992, Congress established the Office of Alternative Medicine (OAM) at the National Institutes of Health. In 1998, legislation was enacted to expand its status, mandate, and authority by creating the National Center for Complementary and Alternative Medicine (NCCAM). Its mission is to prevent and alleviate human suffering and promote health through rigorous research on the safety and effectiveness of CAM modalities, research training, and information dissemination for health care providers and consumers. A useful website follows: <http://nccam.nih.gov/nccam/strategic/newleft1.html>.

The purpose of this chapter is to guide the reader on the potential benefits and pitfalls of the most commonly utilized CAM therapies for the treatment of persistent pain in the older adult. Studies including older adults are identified and included when possible.

EVIDENCE AND PRINCIPLES FOR PRACTICE

Alternative Medical Systems

Alternative medicine involves complete systems of theory and practice that have evolved independent of, and often prior to, the conventional biomedical approach. This includes traditional systems that are practiced in individual cultures throughout the world such as Traditional Chinese Medicine and Ayurvedic Medicine. Homeopathy and naturopathy are other examples.

Traditional Chinese Medicine and Acupuncture

Over the last several millennia, prior to the development of modern medicine in the West, the Chinese described a sophisticated understanding of human anatomy and physiology. This system of understanding, evolved into the treatment approach Traditional Chinese Medicine (TCM), which places the greatest emphasis on restoring balance to the system and treating potential problems before they manifest as illness. Historically, the focus of Western medicine has been to understand disease pathology and to treat it. Recently, this focus has been expanded to include prevention of disease.

The TCM approach encompasses a philosophy of health, a unique understanding of pathophysiology, a system of diagnosis, and treatment modalities that include acupuncture, the use of herbs, a well-balanced diet, and mind-body techniques, such as Qi Gong and Tai Chi. The latter two are activities that involve, to varying degrees, physical exercise, breathing techniques, meditation, and focus on energetic flow. Like the TCM approach, these techniques are based on Taoist philosophy utilizing concepts of yin and yang, with the notion that mental and physical health involves maintaining or restoring homeostasis. The gentle movements in Tai Chi are of particular value to older adults, among whom arthritis and osteoporosis may present a problem with more ballistic exercises. Over the last several centuries, schools of acupuncture in Japan, Korea, England, and France have expanded this traditional model.

A key component of this system is the use of acupuncture, which involves the placement of thin solid needles under the skin. Typically, needles are placed in precise points along various organ system meridians, or channels. The number of needles varies. One can tonify the needles or introduce energy into the system. Conversely, one can place the needles without stimulating them, allowing an excess of energy to dissipate. Tonification can be accomplished with manual, thermal, or electrical stimulation of the needles. Traditionally, thermal stimulation is provided with moxibustion or moxa, in which heat is generated by burning herbal preparations containing *Artemisia vulgaris,* or mugwort, to stimulate acupuncture points. In both the West and China, electrical stimulation has become the more common practice.

One's understanding of the mechanism of action of acupuncture depends on the theory underlying one's view. The TCM approach sees pathology as associated with excess, deficiency, or obstruction of the energy flow along one or several organ system meridians. The role of acupuncture is to open the blocked channels and restore balance to the system. While this is reasonable within this system, it is difficult to subject it to a research model along the Western medicine paradigm. The neurophysiologic understanding of the effect of acupuncture involves a mild noxious stimulant of the afferent pathways, with subsequent stimulation of the descending inhibitory systems. This involves endorphinergic and enkephalinergic pathways, as well as stimulation of other neurochemical systems.

Acupuncture interventions can be understood as falling into three main categories. The traditional form of energetic treatment includes the TCM, the French energetic system, and the five-element approach. A second approach does not rely on the traditional acupuncture anatomy of points; rather, it follows the Western anatomic system, focusing on nerve distributions and trigger points. A third system of treatment utilizes reflex somatotopic systems, which involve a representation of the whole body into a microsystem or a part of the human body. Examples include auricular acupuncture, Korean hand acupuncture, and Yamimoto new scalp acupuncture.

Acupuncture is among the most researched and documented of the CAM therapies. The National Institutes of Health 1997 Consensus Conference in Acupuncture reports that there is some evidence for the efficacy of acupuncture in conditions associated with persistent pain such as back pain, osteoarthritis, fibromyalgia, and migraine headaches (Acupuncture NIH Consensus Statement, 1997). As with most CAM therapies, research on the efficacy of acupuncture for the treatment of persistent pain conditions is methodologically limited, largely because of questionable intervention quality, lack of an adequate control group, and/or lack of adequate follow-up (Ezzo et al., 2000).

There are several issues that make acupuncture research difficult to carry out. Western medicine places value on a standard treatment methodology, but this does not allow one to take advantage of the full richness of the TCM approach, which individualizes treatment. It is difficult to develop a placebo or a sham treatment that is comparable to the placebo in medication trials. Needling of nonacupuncture points may have nonspecific antinociceptive effects.

Looking at well-designed studies in the medical literature, we find that for pain conditions pertinent to the older adult population, the use of acupuncture is best examined with osteoarthritis of the knee. Christensen et al. (1992) divided 29 subjects into a treatment group and a no-treatment control group. After the initial study period the control group was treated with the acupuncture protocol. Although they analyzed the two groups separately and found a significant treatment effect, they combined the results of both groups after acupuncture. While this gives them greater numbers, the methodology is not optimal.

Takeda and Wessel (1994) conducted a better-designed study using a similar acupuncture protocol. Forty subjects were randomly assigned to either the experimental group that received acupuncture or the comparison group that received sham acupuncture. The sham group received superficial needling at points around the knee, but 1 inch away from the authentic acupuncture point. Findings revealed a favorable response in both groups, with a trend toward a greater response in the experimental group receiving authentic acupuncture. Although the changes from baseline were statistically significant for both groups, there was no significant difference between the two groups.

The last study was similar in design to that of Christensen and colleagues and included a nontreatment control, which later underwent the active treatment (Berman et al., 1999). This included 73 subjects, 58 of whom completed the protocol. A significant and favorable difference was found between the acupuncture or experimental group and the no-treatment control group. This leaves us in a quandary, as existing studies have been unable to demonstrate that acupuncture has a therapeutic advantage over sham treatment. Both sham and real acupuncture result in a significant improvement from baseline measures.

More recently in the United States, Craig developed a system in which the needles are introduced in the areas of pain, specifically the dermatomes, myotomes, and sympathetic nerve levels affected by the pain syndrome. He found that stimulation of these needles with specific electrical frequencies resulted in significant and lasting changes. This resulted in the development of Craig-PENS (Percutaneous Electrical Nerve Stimulation). Preliminary studies have found this approach to be helpful for low back pain associated with lumbosacral degenerative disc disease, sciatica, diabetic neuropathy, herpes zoster, and pain associated with metastatic bone involvement (Ghoname et al., 1999).

Homeopathy

Homeopathy was developed by Samuel Christian Hahnemann, a German physician, in the latter half of the eighteenth century. There are three main tenets of homeopathy. One is the principle of "similars," which states that patients with specific signs and symptoms can be cured if they are given a drug that produces the same signs and symptoms when given to a healthy individual. The second principle (potentization) is that remedies retain biological activity if they are diluted and shaken (successions) between serial dilutions, and that in fact, the more dilute the remedy, the greater the potency. These serially shaken dilutions are said to produce effects even if diluted beyond Avogadro's number and no original molecules of the original substance remain (Jonas, Linde, & Ramirez, 2000). The last key principle is that the illness is specific to the individual. Furthermore, in classical homeopathy the treatment is not symptom or disease focused, but rather is directed by the patient's unique constitution. Scant empiric evidence is available on the effectiveness of homeopathy and pain (Kleinjen, 1991). Nevertheless there is growing use of homeopathy throughout the world, particularly in Europe (i.e., Germany, England, and France), where more than 20% of physicians use homeopathy in their practices (Fisher & Ward, 1994).

Two styles of homeopathy practice are currently employed: classical and complex homeopathy. Classical homeopathy involves the use of a highly individualized single remedy that takes into account the totality of the patient's symptoms and constitution. Using this model, which has been practiced and studied most frequently, it would be very difficult to recommend to the nonhomeopath health care practitioner a particular remedy for a pain syndrome. For example, several patients with osteoarthritis would receive different remedies, based on the classical homeopath's evaluation of each individual patient. Furthermore, a referral to a well-trained classical homeopath is necessary.

A more modern homeopathic approach is the complex model, which is more adaptable to the Western, disease-oriented model of treatment. It involves a combination of remedies known to be commonly used for a particular disease state. This is in direct contradiction to the classic tenet of homeopathy, which states that the disease is specific to the individual. Thus, it focuses on the diagnosis, instead of on the individual. It is thought to have been developed by the homeopathic pharmaceutical industry in order to bypass the need for an extensive homeopathic evaluation (Chapman, 1999) and to allow self-medication with over-the-counter combination homeopathic remedies. Complex homeopathic formulas are popular among nonhomeopaths and the lay public; yet very few of these formulas have been subjected to controlled trials.

It is important to note that homeopathic remedies are usually inexpensive and that the Homeopathic Pharmacopoeia of the United States was included in the 1938 Food and Drug Act. These remedies are considered drugs; thus they are regulated by the FDA. Because of their high dilution, they will not cause drug–homeopathic-product interactions and are accepted by the FDA as safe drugs. Homeopathic product studies by the National Institutes of Health have been granted an FDA waiver to bypass Phase I and II trials and proceed directly to Phase III trials, demonstrating the overall safety of homeopathic products. The best advice for the nonhomeopath health care practitioner is to refer the patient to a trained and licensed professional who can recommend the remedy that will benefit the individual patient.

A double-blind crossover controlled study of classical homeopathic use of *Rhus toxicodendrum* (poison ivy), in a select group of patients with fibromyalgia syndrome who met the classical homeopathic evaluation criteria for that remedy, found a 25% reduction in the number of painful points (Fisher, Greenwood, Huskisson, Turner, & Belon, 1989). Gipson, Gipson, MacNeill, and Buchanan (1980) conducted a randomized double-blind controlled trial of 46 patients with rheumatoid arthritis who were given classical homeopathic individualized treatment versus placebo. Subjects showed significant benefit from the homeopathic treatment with regard to pain, stiffness, and grip strength.

Naturopathy

Dating back to the latter part of the nineteenth century, naturopathy views disease as a manifestation of alterations in the processes by which the body naturally heals itself, and emphasizes health restoration rather than disease treatment. Licensed in 12 states in the United States, naturopathic physicians may act as primary-care providers after 4 years of postgraduate training. The typical naturopathic practice is characterized by maintenance of health, prevention of disease, patient education, and self-responsibility (Murray & Pizzorno, 1999). It is widely practiced for primary care, including the treatment of pain, and in many cases is covered by insurance companies in the states where licensed. Naturopathy as a system is still lacking in empiric evidence to support its effectiveness in the field of pain, although naturopathic physicians are typically trained in a variety of CAM modalities described in this chapter. These practitioners can serve as advisors to traditionally trained health care practitioners, who have little knowledge of CAM modalities that may be safe and helpful for the older adult with a persistent pain syndrome.

Mind-Body Interventions

Mind-body interventions use a variety of techniques designed to facilitate the mind's capacity to affect bodily functions and symptoms. Examples include prayer, meditation, yoga, and music.

Spirituality and Prayer

Spirituality is a global concept that involves the sense of a "divine intelligence that creates, sustains, and organizes the universe, and an awareness of our inner connection with this higher reality. Through this inner connectiveness comes creative energy and insight, a sense of purpose and direction, an understanding of such events as illnesses, and the knowledge we can gain from them" (Macrae, 1995, p. 8).

Prayer is a mechanism used to enhance spirituality. The focus and manner of expression are primarily determined by religious beliefs. Prayer is perceived by some as an important aspect of healing. It has been defined in numerous ways such as "attuning or joining one's personal self with the consciousness of God" (Macrae, 1995, p. 8). Similarly, Levin (1996, p. 67) defines it as "a form of communion with the deity or Creator." Berg (1980, p. 306) expands this view by stating that prayer is the "process of attunement to God . . . that sends forth a dynamic positive idea which visualizes the condition desired and faith gives thanks in advance."

Importantly, Young (1993) conducted a study to determine the perceived role of spirituality in older adults with chronic illness ($n = 12$; age range, 65 to 89). All participants identified themselves as Christians but stated that spirituality became more important with advanced age and the onset of chronic illness. Participants viewed God as their only hope when traditional medicine could not help. In addition, prayer was identified as the most important spiritual practice. Bearon and Koenig (1990) also found that over half of the 40 subjects (aged 65–75) they interviewed had used prayer in an attempt to alleviate symptom presentation (including pain in joints, bones, and extremities).

A classic study conducted by Byrd (1988) used a double-blind design to evaluate the therapeutic effects of intercessory prayer on hospitalized cardiac patients. Subjects were randomly assigned to either an experimental or control group. Subjects in the experimental group ($n = 192$, mean age = 58) received intercessory prayer by participating Christians praying at another location. The control group ($n = 201$, mean age = 60) did not receive prayer. Interestingly, the experimental group had significantly lower severity scores based on the hospital course. The control group required ventilatory assistance, antibiotics, and diuretics more frequently than the experimental group.

Two studies have focused on the use of prayer to alleviate persistent pain in older adults. The first was conducted by Matthews, Marlowe, and MacNutt (1998) to assess the effects of intercessory prayer in conjunction with standard medical treatment on the clinical course of patients with arthritis ($n = 40$, mean age = 62). Findings revealed a 31% reduction in patient-rated pain.

The second study ($n = 35$; mean age $= 60$) revealed that subjects who identified religion as salient in their coping with pain associated with rheumatoid arthritis reported much higher levels of instrumental, emotional, arthritis-related, and general social support than those who did not. On the days that subjects were able to control and decrease their pain using spiritual/religious coping methods, they were more likely to have a positive mood and higher levels of general support (Keefe et al., 2001).

Matthews (2000) encourages health care professionals to recognize the role that religious beliefs and spiritual practices may have in the care and treatment of many individuals, especially older adults. He emphasizes the need to explore this area with the patient in a dignified and respectful manner. An initial assessment should include inquiry into the patient's religious background and current beliefs and practices. This may include asking questions such as the following:

- Do you consider yourself to be a religious or spiritual person?
- Does your religious faith influence the way you care for yourself or your thoughts about illness?
- Would you like members of the health care team to address these types of issues with you?

Assessing the degree of interest will facilitate the development of appropriate interventions. The health care professional may feel comfortable addressing the patient's spiritual needs in regard to his or her health or request the assistance of an appropriately trained individual such as a priest or shaman. Attention to the patient's spirituality or faith, especially in the setting of a chronic and disabling illness such as persistent pain or cancer, will greatly benefit the patient–health care professional therapeutic relationship and enhance the patient's satisfaction with the treatment.

Meditation

Meditation originated as a spiritual practice within a traditional religious context and was used to promote personal and spiritual growth. Over time, numerous methods have evolved and the role of meditation has been expanded to include relief of stress and physical discomfort. Two of the most popular forms and those with the largest research base are transcendental meditation and mindfulness meditation. A third form, medical meditation, developed by Dharma Singh Khalsa, MD, is gaining popularity and is the focus of developing research.

Transcendental meditation (TM) originated in India and was introduced to the West by Maharishi Mahesh Yogi. Transcendental meditation is performed by sitting with closed eyes and focusing attention on a mantra (i.e., word or syllable). When distraction occurs, attention is focused back on the mantra. This form of meditation has had the most amount of research documented in the scientific literature, primarily in the treatment of cardiovascular disease.

Mindfulness meditation has its roots in Buddhist meditation and was introduced to Western medicine by Jon Kabat-Zinn. Rather than restricting attention to one object or mantra, mindful meditation emphasizes what is referred to as "detached observation." This is initially achieved by concentrating on one primary object, usually the rhythmic flow of breathing, until the focus of attention has become relatively stable. Once this stability has been achieved, the focus or field of attention is gradually expanded, usually by stages, until all physical, mental, and psychological events can be perceived as they occur in time (Kabat-Zinn, 1982).

TM and mindfulness meditation elicit a deep relaxation response. This involves an integrated bodily response that includes increased synchronicity in electroencephalographic patterns; reduction in blood consumption, heart rate, and blood pressure; and increased skin electrical resistance and alterations in blood flow. Many of these changes are consistent with a decreased arousal of the sympathetic nervous system and may represent a decreased responsiveness to norepinephrine (Benson, 1983; Kutz, Caudill, & Benson, 1983).

Medical meditation incorporates the use of kundalini yoga into its protocol. Kundalini yoga uses breathing, movement, and mental focus to bring energy and balance from the lower chakras (centers of energy) of the body to the upper chakras (Khalsa & Stauth, 2001). Khalsa and Stauth report that the therapeutic effects of medical meditation extend beyond the relaxation response. They identify four unique characteristics of this meditation: (1) specific breathing patterns; (2) special posture and movement that include exact positioning of the hands and fingers; (3) mantras that consist of distinct, vibratory sounds; and (4) a unique mental focus.

There is a considerable amount of evidence that details the medical benefits of meditation for use in chronic pain (Caudill, Schnable, Zuttermeister, Benson, & Friedman, 1991; Kabat-Zinn, 1982; Kutz et al., 1983). In 1995, the National Institutes of Health Technology Assessment Conference reviewed the evidence for its use in persistent pain and concluded that the evidence is strong for its reducing persistent pain in a variety of medical conditions (National Institutes of Health Technology Assessment Panel, 1996).

Although most patients with a persistent pain syndrome will likely benefit from a form of meditation training, caution must be exercised when referring patients with certain forms of mental illness (such as psychotic patients), as meditation may worsen symptoms (Walsh & Rauche, 1979).

Yoga

"Yoga is based on an ancient Indian philosophy that uses gentle stretching exercises, breath control, and meditation to gain self-mastery and self-realization" (Jonas & Levin, 1999, p. 584). Very little research has been conducted to evaluate the effect of yoga on persistent pain. A study conducted by Garfinkel and colleagues (1994) found that a supervised yoga program was effective in reducing pain in patients with osteoarthritis of the hands and finger joints. Subjects ranged in age from 52 to 79 years. Although the sample was small ($n = 25$), these findings suggest the potential benefits of yoga as a complementary intervention in pain control of arthritis.

More recently, Garfinkle and colleagues (1998) used a randomized, single-blind controlled trial to evaluate the effects of yoga on carpal tunnel syndrome ($n = 42$; age range, 24–77; median age, 52 years). The experimental group participated in a supervised regimen of 11 yoga postures designed for strengthening, stretching, and balancing joint forces. Sessions were conducted biweekly over an 8-week period. The control group was offered a standard wrist splint. Participants in the experimental group had a statistically significant benefit that included a reduction in pain and an increase in grip strength.

There are a variety of approaches to yoga and significant variation among practitioners. Complications can develop if yoga is done incorrectly or without the proper preparation. A conservative, gradual approach to yoga is most appropriate for older adults and persons with conditions such as arthritis.

Music

Research has shown music to be effective in alleviating symptoms of persistent pain (Beck, 1991; Schorr, 1993; Zimmerman, Pozehl, Duncan, & Schmitz, 1989). Auditory stimulation, such as music, has a physiological effect on the body that may relate to the gate control theory of pain. Intense stimuli through the thalamus, midbrain, and brain stem produce modulating substances (e.g., endorphins and serotonin) that inhibit the release of neurotransmitters, therefore stimulating closure of the gate. Diversion of attention from the pain decreases the adverse nature of the stimulus; thus relaxation occurs that decreases muscle guarding at the painful site (Donovan, 1982). Music also serves to redirect the focus of attention from pain to a more pleasing stimulus (Zimmerman et al., 1989).

Research has shown that listening to preferred music is effective in reducing pain associated with rheumatoid arthritis (Schorr, 1993). Although the sample ($n = 30$) ranged in age from 31 to 81 years, the overwhelming majority ($n = 26$) of these subjects were over 50 years of age, with almost half ($n = 14$) between the ages of 61 and 81.

Zimmerman and colleagues (1989) used a pretest-posttest design to evaluate the effects of music on the intensity of pain assocated with cancer ($n = 40$). Subjects ranged in age from 34 to 79 years (mean = 60 years). Subjects selected their preferred music from ten relaxation tapes, and music was presented for 30 minutes. Findings indicated that music resulted in a decrease in the overall intensity of pain. Similarly, Beck (1991) used an experimental crossover design to measure the effects of therapeutic music on pain in patients with cancer who were receiving scheduled analgesics. Subjects selected their preference from seven types of relaxing music. The effect of music on pain varied by individual; 75% of subjects had at least some response, whereas 47% had a statistically significant, moderate, or great response.

Music therapists, who are familiar with the use of music in the clinical setting, especially in the persistent pain syndromes and psychiatric illnesses, are becoming more available in conventional United States hospitals and are a great asset as members of the treatment team.

Biologically Based Treatments

This category includes natural and biologically based practices, interventions, and products including herbal, special dietary, orthomolecular, and individual biological therapies.

Herbal Remedies

The World Health Organization (WHO) has estimated that 80% of the world's population relies on herbs to address its health care needs. In 1997, the herbal industry constituted a $3.2 billion business, growing at a rate of 25% annually. In the United States it is estimated that one fifth of all adults taking prescription medications are also taking dietary supplements (Eisenberg, 1997). Findings of a national telephone survey reported that 6% of respondents age 65 or older reported taking both herbal compounds and prescription medications simultaneously. Of these individuals, 57% did not report the use of CAM to their physicians (Foster, Phillips, Hamel, & Eisenberg, 2000).

Most health care professionals are not trained to advise patients in the safety and efficacy of herbal remedies as well as potential drug–dietary supplement adverse interactions. Despite the widespread use of dietary supplements by patients with little or no knowledge of their potential risks, few side effects are reported when compared with traditional medications.

This may be due in part to lack of recognition or underreporting of those adverse reactions. In Europe, where surveillance mechanisms have been in place for many years and the reporting of adverse reactions of dietary supplements is a much more common practice, adverse reactions are uncommon, except for cases of accidental or intentional overdoses.

In the United States, herbals are defined as dietary supplements, as per the Dietary Supplement, Health and Education Act of 1984. This act protects them from regulation as food additives unless they are proven unsafe. The manufacturers cannot make therapeutic claims unless they can provide evidence that is acceptable to the FDA. However, companies manufacturing dietary supplements are not regulated by the FDA. Consequently, consumers and health care professionals are left with an unregulated market, where quality control of the growing number of dietary supplements available cannot be assured. Manufacturers interested in high-quality products are beginning to create national standards and self-regulatory and quality control mechanisms that, if successful, will likely improve the standards of the dietary supplement market in the United States.

The Office of Dietary Supplements at the National Institutes of Health provides a database of International Bibliographic Information on Dietary Supplements to assist consumers and health care providers: <http://ods.od. nih.gov/databases/ibids.htm/>. In addition, Table 9.1 provides general guidelines for the use of herbal remedies.

Below we will review agents commonly used for arthritis, a prevalent condition in the older population and a cause of persistent pain.

Ginger   The root of *Zingiber officinale* contains volatile and nonvolatile compounds that have been shown to inhibit platelet aggregation and have anti-inflammatory effects, likely related to prostaglandin, thromboxane, and leukotriene synthesis inhibition. Interestingly, contrary to many anti-inflammatory medications, ginger also has gastroprotective action as well as stimulatory effects on GI motility, similar to that seen with metoclopramide (Yamahara, Hatekeyama, Chatani, Nishino, & Yamahara, 1990). In human studies, it has been found to relieve pain from rheumatoid arthritis and osteoarthritis (Srivastava & Mustafa, 1992). Dose will vary, typically ranging from 500 mg to 1,000 mg of powdered ginger or 1,000 mg of fresh ginger 2 to 4 times a day. It interacts with anticoagulants by increasing the risk of bleeding. Overdose may cause CNS depression and cardiac arrythmias (Fetrow & Avila, 1999).

Capsicum   Derived from a concentrate called oleoresin capsicum formed from dried peppers of the Solanaceae family, capsicum is traditionally used for treating pain associated with rheumatoid arthritis, osteoarthritis,

---

TABLE 9.1 Advising Patients About Herbal Therapies

- All patients should be asked about use of herbal therapies and dietary supplements. Use of these agents (including formulation, brand, dose, and reason for taking the herb/dietary supplement) should be documented in the medical record.

- Respectfully convey to patients that "natural" does not necessarily mean safe (examples: quinine, digoxin).

- Herbal-pharmaceutical interactions do occur; therefore, carefully evaluate (and document in the chart) combined use.

- Lack of standardization of dietary supplements may result in variability in their content and efficacy among manufacturers. Ideally patients should be advised to use the same brand and dose when monitoring for benefits or side effects.

- Dietary supplements should not be used in larger-than-recommended dosages.

- In general, dietary supplements should not be used for more than several weeks because of lack of studies proving long-term safety for most supplements.

- An accurate diagnosis and discussion of proven treatment options are essential prior to the patient's considering use of herbal treatments.

- Adverse effects should be documented in the patient's chart and therapy discontinued.

Note: Adapted from "Advising Patients About Herbal Therapies," by M. Cirigliano and A. Sun, 1998, *JAMA, 289*(18), p. 1566. Adapted with permission of the authors.

diabetic and other neuropathies, as well as postherpetic neuralgia (Bernstein, Bickers, Dahl, & Roshal, 1987; Fetrow & Avila, 1999; Robbins et al., 1998). The analgesic effect may be explained by neuronal depletion of substance P. The typical dose ranges from 0.025% to 0.25%, applied topically 3 to 4 times a day, avoiding eyes and genitalia. Adverse reactions include transient skin irritation, itching, and erythema, which diminishes with repeated use. Typically, relief of pain occurs between 3 and 28 days. If ingested orally, capsicum may cause GI distress and retrosternal discomfort that can be minimized by removing the seeds (Fetrow & Avila, 1999). Caution is advised in patients who are taking monoamine oxidase inhibitors (MAOIs) or centrally acting adrenergic drugs.

Borage   Two small but promising clinical trials have shown beneficial results using gamma-linolenic acid (GLA) found in borage seeds (*Borago officinallis*) for the treatment of rheumatoid arthritis. Leventhal, Boyce, and Zurier (1993) demonstrated significant reduction in symptoms in rheumatoid arthritis patients with active disease who were treated with 1.4 g of GLA as borage seed oil daily for 24 weeks, when compared with the placebo group. A confounding factor was the concomitant use of non-steroidal anti-inflammatory medications and prednisone. A smaller uncontrolled trial conducted by Pullman-Moar and colleagues (1990) treated 14 subjects with 1.1 g of GLA for 12 weeks. Seven of those subjects suffered from rheumatoid arthritis and had an 85% improvement of symptoms. GLA from borage seed oil is converted to dihomogammalinoleic acid, a precursor of monoenoic prostaglandin E1, a potent anti-inflammatory agent (Leventhal et al., 1993). Doses used in human trials are noted above, typically found in capsules of 240–1,300 mg of borage seed oil, containing 20–26% GLA (Fetrow & Avila, 1999). Potentially toxic amounts of pyrrolizidine alkaloids can be found in borage seed oil, so liver function tests should be monitored regularly in patients using this product.

Evening Primrose Oil (EPO)   This biennial herb with yellow flowers (*Oenothera biennis*), regarded by many as a noxious weed, bears seeds containing up to 25% of a fatty acid extract that is another excellent source of gamma-linolenic acid (GLA). It has a better safety profile for long-term use than borage seed oil, as the EPO extract does not contain the toxic pyrrolizidine alkaloids found in borage seed oil (Foster & Tyler, 1999). Among other uses, it has a reported benefit in rheumatoid arthritis by the mechanism of action already described above for borage. Two studies are noteworthy. Belch and colleagues (1988) studied a group of 49 rheumatoid arthritis patients using either EPO, EPO plus fish oil, or a placebo for 1 year. Significant benefit was noted both in the EPO only (73% improved) and the EPO plus fish oil (80% improved) groups when compared with the placebo group (33% improved); patients were able to stop or decrease the amount of nonsteroidal anti-inflammatory drugs they were using for pain control. Other investigators, however, were unable to demonstrate any difference between an EPO-treated group and a placebo (olive oil) group in patients with rheumatoid arthritis (Brzeski, Madhok, & Capell, 1991). Adverse effects include nausea, indigestion, headaches, and softened stools, but no serious effects have been reported. Dose varies from 500 mg to 6 grams per day.

Feverfew   Research supports the use of feverfew (*Tanacetum parthenium*) as a prophylactic treatment for migraine headaches (Johnson, Kadam,

Hylands, & Hylands, 1985; Murphy, Heptinstall, & Mitchell, 1988; Palevitch, Earon, & Carasso, 1997). Dosages in these studies have ranged from 50 to 100 mg daily. The *PDR for Herbal Medicines* (1998) identifies feverfew for the treatment of migraine, arthritis, and rheumatic diseases with a recommended dosage of 50 mg daily. The medicinal portion of the plant acts by slowing platelet aggregation, prostaglandin synthesis, and the release of histamines. It also reduces the release of serotonin from thrombocytes and polymorphonuclear leukocytes (*PDR for Herbal Medicines*, 1998, p. 1171).

Turmeric   Turmeric is a member of the ginger (Zingiberaceae) family that grows in tropical Asian countries and India. Relief from the pain of arthritis is among the many reported uses for turmeric. Few clinical studies have been published that demonstrate the benefits of turmeric among patients with arthritis (Klepser & Nisly, 2000). Although turmeric has also been suggested for use in osteoarthritis, there are no published trials evaluating its efficacy in this setting. Curcumin is the yellow pigment and major active component of turmeric (Werbach & Murray, 1994). Deodhar, Sethi, and Srimal (1980) evaluated the effects of 400 mg of curcumin three times a day, versus phenylbutazone, 100 mg three times a day for 2 weeks in 18 patients with rheumatoid arthritis in a randomized, double-blind, crossover study. All anti-inflammatory agents were discontinued 4 days prior to study initiation. Both agents demonstrated statistically significant subjective improvement in morning stiffness, walking time, and joint swelling. There was no improvement, however, in any of the objective measures. Both agents resulted in significant overall observer-rated general improvement but only phenylbutazone resulted in overall patient-perceived improvement. It is worth mentioning that due to its poor side-effect profile, phenylbutazone has been removed from the United States market by its manufacturer. Side effects such as heartburn and peptic ulcer disease can occur following extended use or overdose.

Curcumin has been reported to induce abnormalities in liver function tests in rats. Sharp, transient hypotensive effects have been noted to occur in dogs following curcumin administration. This effect has yet to be reported in humans. CNS effects potentially linked to curcumin include mild, transient giddiness. There are two cases of turmeric-induced allergic contact dermatitis in the literature. Turmeric should not be used in patients with bile duct obstructions or gallstones. No drug interactions have been reported in the literature. However, turmeric may possess anticoagulation properties via its inhibition of thromboxane A_2, B_2 or both. Therefore, turmeric may increase the risk of bleeding among patients taking anticoagulants such as warfarin, or antiplatelet drugs such as aspirin, or other nonsteroidal anti-inflammatory drugs. Because some of the active ingredients of turmeric are hepatically metabolized, caution should be exercised when using turmeric concurrently with agents that are metabolized via the cytochrome P450 system. The average daily dose is 1.5 to 3 grams of turmeric powder divided into two or three doses and taken between meals (Klepser & Nisly, 2000).

Other Modalities

Prolotherapy

Prolotherapy is an injection technique that is useful for treating localized somatic dysfunction. It has been practiced for over 50 years. The rationale for this treatment is based on the idea that much musculoskeletal pain is associated with ligamentous injury. For example, an acute musculoskeletal injury can result in a tear or a shearing of ligaments. Particularly among older adults, for whom healing may be slow and incomplete, chronic strain can result and the dysfunction can be compounded by osteoarthritic changes in the area. The laxity of ligaments can result in further deformity and muscles will compensate for the lack of stability with compensatory spasm. The injection of a mildly noxious agent such as 12% glucose solution creates an inflammatory reaction. This is followed by tightening of collagen bonds, renewed stability, resolution of muscular spasm, and decrease in pain (Hackett, Hemwall, & Montgomery, 1991; Reeves, 1995).

In the older adult population, prolotherapy can be of benefit for both acute injuries and chronic conditions. A common scenario may include the combination of a valgus deformity at the knee associated with osteoarthritis and pronation of the foot. A series of two or three sets of injections may be needed. Areas injected may include the knee joint, medial collateral ligament, pes anserinus bursa region, and tibio-talar joint. A small ($n = 38$) randomized clinical trial of prolotherapy versus a placebo injection for knee osteoarthritis revealed some benefit at 1 year (Reeves & Hassanein, 2000). Larger studies are needed to confirm benefits and safety.

Prolotherapy can be used for other musculoskeletal conditions particularly affecting the lumbosacral spinal region. Chronic dysfunction of the sacroiliac joint is often associated with chronic ligamentous strain. For such difficulties, one commonly considers corticosteroid injections into the spring ligament joint. However, these injections often result in only transient improvement. The improvement from prolotherapy is often lasting. Only qualified health care professionals who have been trained in this technique should perform it.

Physical Manipulation Techniques

This category includes methods that are based on manipulation and/or movement of the body, also known as hands-on treatments. Although these treatments were initially considered as alternative approaches and have not always been accepted by Western medicine as valid, there has been a growing body of research supporting their efficacy. They are discussed in this chapter because historically they have been considered CAM techniques. Additionally, studies exploring the use of CAM treatments include chiropractic and other manual modalities. As a sign of integration into the Western approach, physical therapists commonly use similar manual techniques.

Chiropractic   Chiropractic is a widely used therapy in this category, licensed in all 50 states and covered under most insurance policies. This profession focuses on the relationship between structure (primarily the spine) and function, and how that relationship affects the preservation and restoration of health, using manipulative therapy as an integral treatment tool. Chiropractic is generally indicated in managing conditions affecting the neuromuscular skeletal system such as strains, sprains, disc disease or herniation, tendinitis, bursitis, headache, spondylolisthesis, whiplash injury, osteoarthritis, myofascial pain, and disorders of the cervical, thoracic, and lumbar spine and pelvis (Lawrence, 1999).

Older adults with osteoporosis are at increased risk of complications as a result of chiropractic manipulation, particularly when forceful thrust or high-velocity techniques are employed. Rib cage manipulation in those with osteoporosis should also be performed cautiously. Low-force techniques should be used in patients at risk for fracture. In addition to osteoporotic fractures, cervical manipulation in the older adult may be associated with a risk of vertebrobasilar insufficiency. Absolute contraindications to chiropractic manipulation include osteomyelitis, tumor, and aneurysm of the area that is symptomatic (Lawrence, 1999).

A modicum of empiric evidence supports chiropractic manipulation for the treatment of back pain, acute back pain in particular (Bigos et al., 1994). Patients with low back pain seem to prefer chiropractic treatment over traditional medical management and physical therapy (Koes et al., 1992).

Osteopathy   Osteopathy encompasses a holistic approach to patient care. Integrated in the training of an osteopathic physician is the use of manual techniques. Although they are facile in the use of high-velocity or thrust techniques, osteopaths also use indirect techniques that can be advantageous in the older adult population. For example, the muscle energy technique takes advantage of the relaxation phase that occurs after an isometric contraction to enhance range of motion in a restricted area. This can be used for restriction of spinal mobility or for other joint restrictions such as a frozen shoulder. Additionally, gentler mobilization strategies have greater appeal than high-velocity techniques for the older adult with cervical spine disease because of the risk of precipitating vertebral artery insufficiency. As a CAM modality, osteopathic manipulation is still lacking in scientific evidence for effectiveness in persistent pain syndromes. Nevertheless, osteopathic manipulation is usually practiced as part of a whole therapeutic approach by osteopathic physicians licensed in all 50 states.

Massage Therapy   An ancient treatment recorded in many classic texts such as the Bible, the Vedas, and ancient records from China and Japan, massage therapy is defined as hand manipulation of body tissues to promote wellness and to reduce stress and pain. This therapy comprises several techniques that are usually used in combination, depending on the client's needs. These are Swedish massage (stroking and kneading), shiatsu (pressure points), and neuromuscular massage (involving deeper pressure applied to certain areas of the body such as connective tissues, tendons, ligaments, and nerves). A massage session is usually enhanced by soft music and aromatic oils and essences (Field, 1999).

Research ($n = 50$ adults) shows immediate beneficial effects such as improved mood, decreased stress hormone levels such as salivary cortisol, and increased alertness as documented by EEG tracings (Field et al., 1996). Changes have been noted even after 4 to 6 weeks posttreatment and include a decrease in depression; improved sleep; lowered stress as measured by urinary cortisol, norephinephrine, and epinephrine levels (Field, 1992); and enhanced immune function as demonstrated by an increase in natural killer cells (Ironson et al., 1996). Other indications for massage include low back pain, cancer pain, pressure ulcers, and reduction of pain and stress in intensive care units (Field, 1999). Massage therapy is regulated in approximately half of the states with varying requirements for training.

Energy Therapies

Energy therapies focus either on energy fields originating within the body (biofields) or those from other sources (electromagnetic fields).

Therapeutic Touch, Healing Touch, Reiki   Therapeutic touch was developed by Delores Krieger, PhD, RN, and Dora Kunz in 1972. It is a contemporary interpretation of several ancient healing practices. There are four basic assumptions underlying the use of therapeutic touch. These assumptions include the following: A human being is an open energy system, the anatomical human being is bilaterally symmetrical, illness is an imbalance in an individual's energy field, and human beings have natural abilities to transform and transcend their conditions of living. The practice of therapeutic touch involves learned skills for consciously directing or sensitively modulating human energies (Krieger, 1986, 1993, 1997) as a means of healing by restoring energy balance.

Krieger (1986, 1993, 1997) has written extensively on the procedures involved in therapeutic touch. Simply stated, the practitioner begins by centering him- or herself both physically and psychologically. This is achieved by finding the inner peace within oneself for the purpose of becoming integrated, unified, and focused. Centering oneself is finding the "inner reference of stability" (Krieger, 1986). The natural sensitivity of the hands is then used to symmetrically scan the energy field of the client to assess differences in the quality of energy flow. The practitioner then mobilizes areas of the energy field that are perceived as nonflowing (i.e., congested, static, or sluggish). The practitioner proceeds by directing and modulating the transfer of human energy in an effort to rebalance and restore energy flow.

There is a growing body of research to support the use of therapeutic touch (TT) for a variety of conditions involving persistent pain. Two studies have focused their efforts on the effects of TT in older adults. Lin and Taylor (1999) found that TT was effective in reducing chronic musculoskeletal pain in older adults ($n = 90$; mean age, 78 years). Subjects were recruited from retirement communities, nursing homes, adult day-care centers, and community senior centers. Another study conducted by Eckes-Peck (1997) found TT to be effective in reducing the persistent pain of degenerative arthritis in 82 subjects, ranging in age from 51 to 90 years (mean = 72 years). Subjects were recruited from senior housing complexes, a senior citizens' center, a seniors' meal site, and local churches.

Older adults were included in three other studies that measured the effects of TT on persistent pain. However, the samples in these studies included a broad age range. The use of TT for tension headaches (Keller & Bzdek, 1986) was supported in a sample of 60 subjects ranging in age from 18 to 59, with a mean age of 30. Therapeutic touch was also shown to be effective in reducing pain associated with terminal cancer (Giasson & Bouchard, 1998) in 20 subjects ranging in age from 38 to 68. A larger study ($n = 99$, ranging in age from 38 to 68) conducted by Turner, Clark, Authier, and Williams (1998) found that TT resulted in a significantly greater reduction in pain, as measured by the McGill Pain Questionnaire, and a greater reduction in anxiety on the Visual Analogue Scale for Anxiety compared to subjects receiving sham therapeutic touch. In addition, Heidt (1991) published a case study that supported the use of TT in relieving the "unrelenting" pain associated with herpes zoster in a 56-year-old woman.

Similarly, healing touch (Hover-Kramer, Mentgen, & Scandrett-Hibdon, 1996) incorporates a variety of therapeutic interventions (including many of those developed by Krieger) as a means of repatterning and aligning the energy field for the purpose of healing. Reiki is another systematic energy-based approach to healing that is gaining popularity (Jarrell, 1990). However, there is as yet very little research to support the use of these interventions.

Electromagnet therapy Electromagnet therapy is gaining popularity in the United States, for treatment of persistent pain associated with a wide variety of musculoskeletal conditions. Electromagnetic-field therapeutic methods are generally classified into four groups: pulsed electromagnetic fields (PEMFs), pulsed radiofrequency (PRF), low-frequency magnetic waves, and static magnetic fields. The latter is generally found in two basic types, unipolar and bipolar. These terms refer to the magnetic poles facing the skin. Unipolar magnet therapy usually refers to the use of several individual magnets aligned with the same magnet pole toward the skin. Bipolar magnet therapy usually uses a flexible plasalloy wheel of magnet material that has impressed upon it an alternating spatial pattern of north and south magnetic domains (Collacott, Zimmerman, White, & Rindone, 2000).

Experimental and clinical data suggest that magnetic fields can have an analgesic action (through enhancement of endorphin production) as well as anti-inflammatory and spasmolytic activities. Most of the data on the effectiveness of therapeutic magnetic fields in the treatment of a variety of pain syndromes come from experiments using the PRF and PEMFs devices (Markov & Pilla, 1995; Rhodes, 1981). A randomized pilot trial of static MF on patients with pain due to polio ($n = 50$) revealed significant benefit (Vallbona, Hazelwood, & Jurida, 1997). Little data are available on the effectiveness of static MFs. Furthermore, the use of static magnets, pillows, and mattresses is still nonevidence-based. While harmless, these practices may be financially costly. Pulsed electromagnetic energy treatment is an emerging and promising field in the therapy of pain. It will likely be available through physical therapy departments in the traditional health care setting. Professionals caring for an older adult with a persistent pain syndrome for whom surgery is not an option (e.g., low back pain) may wish to contact the physical therapy department and inquire specifically about the availability of such therapies for their patients.

How to Counsel Patients on the Use of CAM

When a health care professional chooses to participate in a patient's decision to use CAM, the most important step is to ask regularly about current CAM practices. We know that most patients will not spontaneously reveal their use of CAM to their health care practitioner (Eisenberg et al., 1993; Eisenberg et al., 1998). Furthermore, "if you do not ask, they will not tell." Guiding patients on the use of CAM typically will occur under two conditions. First, the patient may verbalize an interest in or preference for CAM. Second, the primary care provider may recognize the limitations of the conventional medical treatments available for that particular patient's condition and the potential benefits of CAM, when used in place of, or (more commonly) as a complement to, the patient's standard care.

As with any other treatment, the first step is to identify the goals and endpoints. For example, the goal for an older adult with osteoarthritis might be to decrease pain and improve function. Therefore, the practitioner could advise oral administration of glucosamine and chondroitin (see chapter 6) in conjunction with nonsteroidal or pain medications (or in place of those medications, if by patient preference or intolerance to those medications) and physical therapy. Careful follow-up and endpoints need to be established for CAM treatments as well as for traditional care. After 3 to 6 months of glucosamine and chondroitin use in an appropriate dose, the health care professional would recommend stopping that therapy if no improvement was observed. Patients need to be made aware of the current status of the dietary supplement market, as it is not regulated or supervised by the FDA. The health care professional should be able to discuss with the patient the currently known information on the CAM treatment's benefits and safety issues and how it compares with the standard treatment approach, which should always be offered. Careful documentation of that discussion should always take place.

A second issue is the justification for the use of CAM approaches in these modern days of evidence-based medicine, standards of care, and legal concerns. As a condition becomes more chronic and disabling and conventional medical approaches have less to offer, one becomes more willing to pursue alternative or complementary approaches, especially if these treatments have demonstrated reasonable evidence for effectiveness and safety and are not costly.

The practitioner may be concerned that by utilizing CAM treatments, the patient may reject appropriate conventional treatments. Here is the opportunity to explore the partnership and open communication between the health care professional and the patient. A knowledgeable and open-minded health care professional should be able to hear patients' preferences and concerns regarding their care and should be able to discuss the known (or unknown) evidence for safety and efficacy on available conventional treatments as well as CAM therapies. Then, a joint decision on which treatment option(s) to choose should be made. Careful follow-up and support strengthen the health-care professional–patient relationship and allow patients to be active participants in their own healing. Obviously, this is less of a concern when there is no standard medical or surgical approach that can ameliorate the condition. In our experience, with open communication, respect, and education, a patient will rarely choose against using a valuable and well-proven conventional therapy or elect to use a dangerous or toxic CAM therapy.

It is important to weigh the impact of the placebo effect on a patient's response to treatment. In interpreting research studies, the clinician wants to know to what extent the placebo effect has been factored in before recommending the treatment. This is less of a consideration for the individual patient. The clinician cannot quarrel when the individual is doing better with a nontoxic treatment, the costs are not onerous, and the patient does not reject other appropriate interventions.

Finally, health care professionals need to advise patients to seek treatment from licensed CAM professionals. If they know the CAM professionals in their community they may make a direct referral, as with any other health care referral. If not, they should try to be aware of their state's laws regarding licensing of CAM professionals, as different CAM modalities may or may not be regulated and licensed in their state. This is easily done by consulting the state's medical board. It is desirable to maintain an open and courteous communication with the patient's CAM provider if possible and to obtain information on treatment goals, endpoints, and cost, and provide patient follow-up to identify benefits or risks of the CAM treatment. See the summary (Table 9.2) of the most promising therapies for persistent pain syndromes in older adults, based on scientific evidence that is currently available.

SETTING-SPECIFIC CONSIDERATIONS

Older-adults are at a higher risk of experiencing adverse drug reactions, drug-drug interactions, and anesthetic and surgical complications than younger individuals. The integration of CAM and conventional medicine has the potential for decreasing the risk of polypharmacy and invasive procedures in this population (O'Brien, 1996) across all settings of care. Several CAM interventions have important implications for residents in long-term-care facilities. For example, the use of prerecorded music is relatively inexpensive, requires minimal time expenditure, and can easily be implemented by trained nursing personnel (Gerdner & Buckwalter, 1999). Therapeutic touch and massage therapy require special training, but as noninvasive modalities, they offer particular appeal for the demented nursing-home resident in whom fear associated with any type of intervention that utilizes foreign materials (e.g., acupuncture, prolotherapy)

TABLE 9.2 Most Promising CAM Modality for Persistent Pain in Older Adults

Modality	Medical problem	Evidence
acupuncture	musculoskeletal pain	moderate
capsicum herb	diabetes, RA, neuropathy	moderate
chiropractic	back pain	strong
homeopathy	fibromyalgia, RA	limited
massage therapy	pain, stress, immunity	moderate
meditation	chronic pain	strong
music therapy	RA, cancer	moderate
prolotherapy	musculoskeletal pain	limited
therapeutic touch	musculoskeletal pain	moderate
yoga	DJD, carpal tunnel	limited

may be limiting. In general, modalities that require concentration in order to facilitate their therapeutic efficacy (e.g., yoga, meditation) are probably not appropriate for many nursing home residents or for cognitively frail older adults living in the community. Clearly, additional research is needed in order to determine the effectiveness of the CAM modalities presented in this chapter. Only then will it be possible to properly target these treatments toward the wide array of older adults who might benefit from their implementation.

SUMMARY/RECOMMENDATIONS

1. Health care professionals treating persistent pain syndromes in the older population should become familiar with commonly utilized Complementary and Alternative Modalities (CAM) described in this chapter. The main reasons for this recommendation are as follows:
   - A large and growing number of patients are utilizing CAM, mostly unsupervised and without the guidance of a trained health care professional. This uncoordinated use of CAM and traditional medical treatments increases the risk of side effects and adverse interactions.
   - CAM therapies have, in many cases, a long tradition of use by many cultures throughout the world with demonstrated benefits in the treatment of pain. Many CAM modalities have an excellent safety profile and low cost. They emphasize active patient partic-

ipation in their treatment and are perceived by patients as very empowering.

2. The knowledgeable health care provider can help guide patients in their choice of CAM treatments that can, in many cases, complement and expand the therapeutic options available to treat older patients with persistent pain syndromes.

3. The ultimate goal is to facilitate the merger of safe, effective, evidence-based CAM with conventional approaches into a practice of integrative medicine, in which multiple health care professionals work as an interdisciplinary team to expand the repertoire of ways to achieve and maintain health.

CASE STUDIES

Herbs

Case

Mrs. Schulz is a 68-year-old woman with breast cancer and persistent pain secondary to metastases. She consults her physician regarding the use of CAM treatments for these problems. She has been followed by oncology since her initial diagnosis 5 years ago. Treatment included surgery, radiation, chemotherapy, and a later stem cell transplant, now with widely metastatic disease to her bones that causes great pain.

During the first encounter, the physician reviews her chart and learns that she is using tamoxifen, opioid pain medications, and "multivitamins." Asked to list by name all of the dietary supplements she is presently using, including herbs, vitamins, and homeopathy, she surprisingly provides a four-page list of dietary supplements at a cost of approximately $1,000 a month. An appointment is made for the following week to review the list of dietary supplements, allowing the physician time to carefully study the list for safety, drug interactions, and efficacy.

At the follow-up visit, the review of vitamin use shows that Mrs. Schultz is using several vitamins in duplication, with nearly identical content, increasing the cost and the risk for excessive vitamin intake. Suggestions are provided for safe vitamin dosage and decrease of vitamin intake by 70%. Mrs. Schulz is told that the majority of the herbs she has chosen are safe, but there is concern about the use of chaparral and comfrey, as they may cause severe hepatic toxicity. Mrs. Schulz agrees to stop taking these herbs and to complete liver-function tests. The remainder of the supplements appear safe. Mrs. Schulz is queried about her reasons for taking each of the supplements. Known data on the efficacy of the herbs she has chosen for pain, depression, and cancer treatment are then reviewed, along with recommended dosage for each herb, using standardized preparations.

Discussion

Most patients do not reveal their use of CAM unless asked. Maintaining an open and respectful attitude for the patient's choice of using CAM and presenting evidence of knowledge in your discussion with the patient are key elements to successfully guide patients in their use of dietary supplements and other CAM treatments. Setting up an appointment time to specifically review the patient's use of dietary supplements may be necessary if the medical problem is complex and the number of supplements and medications is large. The help of a knowledgeable clinical pharmacist or drug information staff can be invaluable to assist in identifying potential drug–dietary supplement adverse interactions and potential side effects.

Percutaneous Electrical Nerve Stimulation

Case

Mrs. Smith is a 77-year-old woman with lumbar spinal stenosis. She has been told that she requires surgery, but is at high risk due to coronary artery disease and chronic obstructive pulmonary disease. Pain is localized in her low back, left buttocks, and posterior thigh. The pain is constant, aching, and moderate in intensity. When Mrs. Smith is standing for more than 5 minutes the pain becomes severe, extending into her calf.

Mrs. Smith has been treated with Percutaneous Electrical Nerve Stimulation (PENS), with needle placement in the low back, buttocks, and left hip and thigh twice per week for the first 5 weeks. There was fluctuation in her symptoms during this time, but she showed consistent and steady improvement with subsequent visits. Treatment was reduced to weekly sessions for 2 months and then every 2 to 4 weeks, depending on her symptoms. She notes that at rest her pain is improved from 6/10 initially to 3/10, which she feels is tolerable. She has cut back on the periodic hydrocodone/acetaminophen used for sleep and now rarely uses it. She can stand for 15- to 20-minute intervals, has been more active, and can complete her physical therapy program without exacerbation of her pain.

Discussion

Although acupuncture or PENS may be a temporizing measure for a patient with severe spinal stenosis, most clinicians would not advocate it as an alternative treatment in the scenario of intractable pain and progressive motor or sensory loss. However, because this patient is a poor surgical risk, it makes sense to pursue this complementary approach. In light of the symptomatic improvement, surgery in this high-risk patient may be deferred. It is important to provide and document careful informed consent by the patient, an explanation of why this approach was chosen, potential risks and benefits, and regular follow-up.

Acupuncture

Case

Mr. Davis is an 81-year-old male with the primary complaint of lower abdominal pain associated with the diagnosis of diverticulitis. A review of Mr. Davis's history and a thorough medical evaluation indicate that he most likely has had irritable bowel syndrome and mild lumbar degenerative disease. He now has episodic acute flares superimposed on this chronic abdominal discomfort. He is vigilant about a high-fiber diet and takes a spasmolytic agent, both of which have decreased the frequency of his flares. He is a semiretired owner of a small tool and dye manufacturing company and he and his wife would like to travel. However, he never knows when his pain, which can be disabling, will flare. He recently changed his primary care physician to a doctor of osteopathy who is trained in acupuncture. Mr. Davis indicated that he had a trip to Europe planned in 6 weeks and hoped to be able to travel without interference from his pain.

Given the time constraints, treatments were initiated two to three times per week. Acupuncture included a meridian-based approach directed towards problems with the large intestine, and electrical stimulation for points in the lumbar region. Osteopathic manipulation was also performed in the lumbosacral spine. The patient noted moderate improvement in discomfort and confessed that he ate without any ill effects a meal that normally would have resulted in discomfort. The use of relaxation techniques was discussed, but the patient indicated that he has always been too hyper to engage in them. However, given his earlier interest in the martial arts, Mr. Davis was quite amenable to participating in a Tai Chi class.

Discussion

This patient has had an extensive evaluation and the diagnosis is well known. He is compliant with the traditional treatment proposed, but it does not completely relieve his symptoms. Although the symptoms are not life-threatening, they are limiting and the patient would benefit from adding a CAM treatment for better symptom control. The TCM approach includes the use of acupuncture and lifestyle changes focused on restoring balance to the system. The treatment may focus on an anatomic organ in the Western medicine sense or organ function in the TCM view. In this case both were used. Additionally, the well-trained and licensed practitioner integrated this approach with manual techniques.

Osteopathy

Case

Mrs. Johnson is a 68-year-old woman who works part-time as an administrative secretary. She had a prior right shoulder strain at work and after the acute pain resolved she continued to have restricted range of motion. She was seen by an orthopedic surgeon, diagnosed with frozen shoulder or adhesive capsulitis, and received a shoulder injection and referral for physical therapy. She continued to have pain on abduction, resulting in more splinting. Mrs. Johnson declined manipulation under anesthesia.

An osteopathic physician specializing in physical medicine and rehabilitation was consulted. Physical examination was notable for restriction of shoulder and cervical spine motion and mild C5 pain. Tissue texture changes in the right lower cervical paraspinal region were also noted.

Given the patient's guarding with passive motion, the physician performed a posterior shoulder joint injection with bupivicaine and a small amount of corticosteroid. The next week he performed one injection with local anesthetic and followed it with a stretching program. At these visits, the physician utilized osteopathic techniques (muscle energy, functional-indirect) to increase abduction and external rotation. The patient was also seen in a physical therapy program that started with passive range of motion and progressed to active range of motion. The physician focused his treatment on her shoulder girdle and cervical spine, using muscle energy mobilization and myofascial release for restriction in her levator scapulae, upper trapezius, and cervical spine. After 3 weeks of the initial therapy, her shoulder abduction improved from 85° to 120°. This subsequently improved to 150° and she was discharged to continue her home program. The patient mentioned incidentally that her daily headaches, which had predated her shoulder injury, were now rare.

Discussion

Given the patient's history of a thorough medical evaluation that resulted in a definite diagnosis and the failure of a standard conservative approach, the physician utilized an alternative approach developed by the British physician, James Cyriax. This approach included injections, passive mobilization, and progression to an active program (Cyriax & Cyriax, 1993). The manual techniques, which are a standard part of the osteopathic physicians repertoire, are described by Philip Greenman (1996).

REFERENCES

Abeles, R. P. (1990). Schemas, sense of control and aging. In J. Rodin & K. W. Schaic (Eds.), *Self-directedness: Causes and effects through the life course*. Hillsdale, NJ: Erlbaum.

Acupuncture NIH Consensus Statement. (1997, November 3–5). *15*(5), 1–34. (Also available online: <http://consensus.nih.gov/cons/107/107_statement.htm>)

Astin, J. A., Pelletier, K. R., Marie, A., & Haskell, W. L. (2000). Complementary and alternative medicine use among elderly persons: One-year analysis of a Blue Shield Medicare Supplement. *Journal of Gerontology: Medical Sciences, 55A*(1), M4–M9.

Bearon, L. B., & Koenig, H. G. (1990). Religious cognitions and use of prayer in health and illness. *Gerontologist, 30*(2), 249–253.

Beck, S. L. (1991). The therapeutic use of music for cancer-related pain . . . crossover study. *Oncolology Nursing Forum, 18*(8), 1327–1337.

Belch, J. F., Ansell, D., Madhok, R., O'Dowd, A., & Sturrock, R. D. (1988). Effects of altering dietary essential fatty acids on requirements for non-steroidal anti-inflammatory drugs in patients with rheumatoid arthritis: A double-blind, placebo-controlled trial. *Annals of the Rheumatic Diseases, 47*, 96–104.

Benson, H. (1983, May–June). The relaxation response and norepinephrine: A new study illuminates a mechanism. *Integrative Psychiatry*, 15–23.

Berg, E. P. (1980). Faith healing. *Australian Family Physician, 9*, 303–307.

Berman, B. M., Singh, B. B., Lao, L., Langenberg, P., Li, H., Hadhazy, V., Bareta, J., & Hochberg, M. (1999). A randomized trial of acupuncture as an adjunctive therapy in osteoarthritis of the knee. *Rheumatology, 38*(4), 346–354.

Bernstein J., Bickers, D. R., Dahl, M. V., & Roshal, J. Y. (1987) Total capsaicin relieves chronic post-herpetic neuralgia. *Journal of the American Academy of Dermatology, 17*, 93–96.

Bigos, S., Bowyer, O., Braen, G., Brown, K., Deyo, R., Haldeman, S., Hart, J. L., Johnson,

E. W., Keller, R., Kido, D., et al. (1994, December). *Acute low back pain in adults.* (Clinical practice guideline No. 14, AHCPR Publication No. 95–0642). Rockville, MD: Agency for Health Policy and Research, Public Health Service, U.S. Department of Health and Human Services.

Brzeski, M., Madhok, R., & Capell, H. (1991). Evening primrose oil in patients with rheumatoid arthritis and side-effects of non-steroidal anti-inflammatory drugs. *British Journal of Rheumatology, 30,* 370–372.

Byrd, R. C. (1988). Positive therapeutic effects of intercessory prayer in a coronary care unit population. *Southern Medical Journal, 81*(7), 826–829.

Caudill, M., Schnable, R., Zuttermeister, P., Benson, H., & Friedman, R. (1991). Decreased clinic use by chronic pain patients: Response to behavioral medicine intervention. *Clinic Journal of Pain, 7*(4), 305–310.

Chapman, E. H. (1999). Homeopathy. In W. B. Jonas & J. S. Levin (Eds.), *Essentials of complementary and alternative medicine* (pp. 472–489). Philadelphia: Lippincott, Williams & Wilkins.

Christensen, B. V., Iuhl, I. U., Vilbek, H., Bulow, H. H., Drijer, N. C., & Rasmussen, H. F. (1992). Acupuncture treatment of severe knee osteoarthrosis: A long-term study. *Acta Anaesthesiologica Scandinavica, 36*(6), 519–525.

Cirigliano, M., & Sun, A. (1998). Advising patients about herbal therapies, *JAMA, 289*(18), 1565–1566.

Collacott, E. A., Zimmerman, J. T., White, D. W., & Rindone, J. P. (2000). Bipolar permanent magnets for the treatment of chronic low back pain: A pilot study. *JAMA, 283*(10), 1322–1325.

Cyriax, J. H., & Cyriax, P. J. (1993). *Cyriax's illustrated manual of orthopaedic medicine* (2nd ed.). Boston: Butterworth-Heinemann.

Deodhar, S. D., Sethi, R., & Srimal, R. C. (1980). Preliminary study on antirheumatic activity of curcumin (deferuloyl methane). *Indian Journal of Medical Research, 71,* 632–634.

Donovan, M. (1982). Cancer pain: You can help. *Nursing Clinics of North America, 17*(4), 713–728.

Eckes-Peck, S. D. (1997). The effectiveness of therapeutic touch for decreasing pain in elders with degenerative arthritis. *Journal of Holistic Nursing, 15*(2), 176–198.

Eisenberg, D. M. (1997). Advising patients who seek alternative medical therapies. *Annals of Internal Medicine, 127*(1), 61–69.

Eisenberg, D. M., Davis, R. B., Ettner, S. L., Appel, S., Wilkey, S., Van Rompay, M., & Kessler, R. C. (1998). Trends in alternative medicine use in the United States, 1990–1997: Results of a follow-up national survey. *JAMA, 280,* 1569–1576.

Eisenberg, D. M., Kessler, R. C., Foster, C., Norlock, F. E., Calkins, D. R., & Delbanco, T. L. (1993). Unconventional medicine in the United States: Prevalence, costs, and patterns of use. *New England Journal of Medicine, 328*(4), 246–252.

Ezzo, J., Berman, B., Hadhazy, V. A., Jadad, A. R., Lau, L., & Singh, B. B. (2000). Is acupuncture effective for the treatment of chronic pain? A systematic review. *Pain, 86,* 217–225.

Fetrow, C., & Avila, J. (1999). *Professional's handbook of complementary and alternative medicines.* Springhouse, PA: Springhouse.

Field, T. (1992). Massage reduces anxiety in child and adolescent psychiatric patients. *Journal of the American Academy of Child and Adolescent Psychiatry, 31*(1), 125–131.

Field, T. (1999). Massage therapy. In W. B. Jonas & J. S. Levin (Eds.). *Essentials of complementary and alternative medicine* (pp. 383–391). Philadelphia: Lippincott, Williams, & Wilkins.

Field, T., Ironson, G., Scafidi, F., Nawrocki, T., Gonclaves, A., Burman, I., Pickens, J., Fox, N., Schanberg, S., & Kuhn, C. (1996). Massage therapy reduces anxiety and enhances EEG pattern of alertness and math compuations. *International Journal of Neuroscience, 86*, 197–205.

Fisher P., Greenwood A., Huskisson E. C., Turner, P., & Belon, P. (1989). Effect of homeopathic treatment on fibrositis (primary fibromyalgia). *British Medical Journal, 299*, 365–366.

Fisher, P., & Ward, A. (1994). Complementary medicine in Europe. *British Medical Journal, 309*, 107–111.

Fordyce, W. (1988). Pain and suffering: A reappraisal. *American Psychologist, 43*(4), 276.

Foster, D. F., Phillips, R. S., Hamel, M. B., & Eisenberg, D. M. (2000). Alternative medicine use in older Americans. *Journal of the American Geriatric Society, 48*, 1560–1565.

Foster, S., & Tyler, V. E. (1999). *Tyler's honest herbal: A sensible guide to the use of herbs and related remedies* (4th ed.). New York: Hawthorn Herbal Press.

Garfinkel, M. S., Schumacher, H. R., Husain, A., Levy, M., & Reshetar, R. A. (1994). Evaluation of a yoga based regimen for treatment of osteoarthritis of the hands. *Journal of Rheumatology, 21*(12), 2341–2343.

Garfinkel, M. S., Singhal, A., Katz, W. A., Allan, D. A., Reshetar, R., & Schumacher, H. R. Jr. (1998). Yoga-based intervention for carpal tunnel syndrome. *JAMA, 280*, 1601–1603.

Gerdner, L. A., & Buckwalter, K. C. (1999). Music therapy. In G. M. Bulechek & J. C. McCloskey (Eds.), *Nursing interventions: Effective nursing treatments* (3rd ed., pp. 451–468). Philadelphia: W. B. Saunders.

Ghoname, E. A., Craig, W. F., Wite, P. F., Ahmed, H. E. Hamza, M. A., Henderson, B. N., Gajraj, N. M., Huber, P. J., & Gatchel, R. J. (1999). Percutaneous electrical nerve stimulation for low back pain: A randomized crossover study. *JAMA, 281*(9), 818–823.

Giasson, M., & Bouchard, L. (1998). Effect of therapeutic touch on the well-being of persons with terminal cancer. *Journal of Holistic Nursing, 16*(3), 383–398.

Gipson, R. G., Gipson, S. L. M., MacNeill, A. D., & Buchanan, W. W. (1980). Homeopathic therapy in rheumatoid arthritis: Evaluation by double-blind clinical therapeutic trial. *British Journal of Clinical Pharmacology, 9*, 453–459.

Greenman, P. E. (1996). *Principles of manual medicine* (2nd ed.). Baltimore: Williams & Wilkins.

Hackett, G. S., Hemwall, G. A., & Montgomery, G. A. (1991). *Ligament and tendon relaxation treated by prolotherapy* (5th ed.). Oak Park, IL: Gustav A. Hemwall.

Heidt, P. R. (1991). Helping patients to rest: Clinical studies in therapeutic touch. *Holistic Nursing Practice, 5*(4), 57–66.

Hover-Kramer, D., Mentgen, J., & Scandrett-Hibdon, S. (1996). *Healing touch: A resource for health care professionals.* New York: Delmar.

Ironson, G., Field, T., Scafidi, F., Hashimoto, M., Kumar, M., Kumar, A., Price, A., Goncalves, A., Burman, I., Tetenam, C., Patarca, R., & Fletcher, M. A. (1996). Massage therapy is associated with enhancement of the immune systems cytotoxic capacity. *International Journal of Neuroscience, 84,* 205–218.

Jarrell, D. G. (1990). *Reiki plus: First degree* (3rd ed.). Celina, TN: Reiki Plus Institute.

Johnson, E. S., Kadam, N. P., Hylands, D. M., & Hylands, P. J. (1985). Efficacy of feverfew as prophylactic treatment of migraine. *British Medical Journal, 291,* 569–573.

Jonas, W. B., & Levin, J. S. (1999). *Essentials of complementary and alternative medicine.* Philadelphia: Lippincott, Williams & Wilkins.

Jonas, W. B., Linde, K., & Ramirez, G. (2000). Homeopathy and rheumatic disease. *Rheumatic Disease Clinics of North America, 26*(1), 117–123.

Kabat-Zinn, J. (1982). An outpatient program in behavioral medicine for chronic pain patients based on the practive of mindfulness meditation. *General Hospital Psychiatry, 4,* 33–37.

Keefe, F. J., Affleck, G., Lefebvre, J., Underwood, L., Caldwell, D. S., Drew, J., Egert, J., Gibson, J., & Pargament, K. (2001). Living with rheumatoid arthritis: The role of daily spiritualiting and daily religious and spiritual coping. *journal of Pain, 2*(2), 101–110.

Keller, E., & Bzdek, V. M. (1986). Effects of therapeutic touch on tension headache pain. *Nursing Research, 35*(2), 101–104.

Khalsa, D. S., & Stauth, C. (2001). *Meditation as medicine: Activate the power of your natural healing force.* New York: Pocket Books.

Kleinjen, J. et al. (1991). Clinical trials of homeopathy. *Br Med Journal, 302,* 316–323.

Klepser, T., & Nisly, N. (2000). Turmeric (*Curcuma longa*) as an anti-inflammatory for arthritis. *Alternative Medicine Alert, 3*(4), 44–47.

Koes, B. W., Bouter, L. M., Van Mameren, H., Essers, A. H. M., Verstegen, G. M. J. R., Hofhuizen, D. M., Houben, J. P., & Knipschild, P. G. (1992). Randomized clinical trial of manipulative therapy and physiotherapy for persistent back and neck complaints: Result of one year follow-up. *British Medical Journal, 304,* 601–605.

Krieger, D. (1986). *The therapeutic touch: How to use your hands to help or to heal.* New York: Prentice-Hall.

Krieger, D. (1993). *Accepting your power to heal: The personal practice of therapeutic touch.* Sante Fe, NM: Bear & Company.

Krieger, D. (1997). *Therapeutic touch inner workbook.* Sante Fe, NM: Bear & Company.

Kutz, I., Caudill, M., & Benson, H. (1983). The role of relaxation in behavioral therapies for chronic pain. *International Anesthesiology Clinics, 21*(4), 193–200.

Lawrence, D. J. (1999). Chiropractic medicine. In W. B. Jonas & J. S. Levin (Eds.), *Essentials of complementary and alternative medicine* (pp. 275–288). Philadelphia: Lippincott, Williams & Wilkins.

Leventhal, L. J., Boyce, E. G., & Zurier, R. B. (1993). Treatment of rheumatoid arthritis with gamma-linolenic acid. *Annals of Internal Medicine, 119,* 867–873.

Levin, J. S. (1996). How prayer heals: A theoretical model. *Alternative Therapies in Health and Medicine, 2*(1), 66–73.

Lin, Y.-S., & Taylor, A. G. (1999). Effects of therapeutic touch in reducing pain and anxiety in an elderly population. *Integrative Medicine, 1*(4), 155–162.

Macrae, J. (1995). Nightingale's spiritual philosophy and its significance for modern nursing. *IMAGE, 27*(1), 8–10.

Markov, M. S., & Pilla, A. A. (1995). Electromagnetic field stimulation of soft tissues, *Wounds, 7,* 143.

Matthews, D. (2000). Prayer and spirituality. *Rheumatic Disease Clinics of North America, 26*(1), 177–187.

Matthews, D. A., Marlowe, S. M., & MacNutt, F. S. (1998). Intercessory prayer ministry benefits rheumatoid arthritis patients. *Journal of General Medicine, 13*(Suppl. 1), 17.

Murphy, J. J., Heptinstall, S., & Mitchell, J. R. A. (1988). Randomized double-blind placebo-controlled trial of feverfew in migraine prevention. *Lancet, 2*(8604), 189–192.

Murray, M., & Pizzorno, J. (1999). Naturopathic medicine. In W. B. Jonas and J. S. Levin (Eds.), *Essentials of complementary and alternative medicine* (pp. 304–321). Philadelphia: Lippincott, Williams & Wilkins.

National Conference of Medical and Nursing Education in Complementary Medicine (1996, June 5–7). Jointly Sponsored by the Office of Alternative Medicine at the National Institutes of Health. Bethesda, Maryland.

National Institutes of Health Technology Assessment Panel. (1996). Integration of behavioral and relaxation approaches into the treatment of chronic pain and insomnia. *Journal of the American Medical Association, 276*(4), 313–318.

O'Brien, M. E. (1996). Integrative geriatrics: Combining traditional and alternative medicine. *North Carolina Medical Journal, 57*(6), 364–367.

Palevitch, D., Earon, G., & Carasso, R. (1997). Feverfew (*tanacetum parthenium*) as a prophylactic treatment for migraine: A double-blind placebo-controlled study. *Phytotherapy Research, 11,* 508–511.

PDR for Herbal Medicines (1998). Montvale, NJ: Medical Economics.

Pullman-Moar S., Laposata, M., Lem, D., Holman, R. T., Leventhal, L. J., DeMarco, D., & Zurier, R. B. (1990). Alterations of the cellular fatty acid profile and the production of eicosanoids in the human monocytes by gamma-linolenic acid. *Arthritis and Rheumatology, 33,* 1526–1533.

Reeves, K. D. (1995). Technique of prolotherapy. In T. A. Lennard (Ed.), *Physiatric procedures in clincal practice* (pp. 57–70). Philadelphia: Hanley & Belfus.

Reeves, K. D., & Hassanein, K. (2000). Randomized prospective double-blind placebo-controlled study of dextrose prolotherapy for knee osteoarthritis with or without ACL laxity. *Alternative Therapies in Health & Medicine, 6*(2), 68–74, 77–80.

Rhodes, C. (1981). The adjunctive utilization of Diapulse (pulsed high peak power electromagnetic energy) in accelerating tissue healing in oral surgery. *Q Nat Dent Assoc, 39,* 166.

Robbins, W. R., Staats, P. S., Levine, J., Fields, H. L., Allen, R. W., Campbell, J. N., & Pappagallo, M. (1998). Treatment of intractable pain with topical large-dose capsaicin: Preliminary report. *Anesthesia and Analgesia, 86,* 579–583.

Schorr, J. A. (1993). Music and pattern change in chronic pain. *Advances in Nursing Science, 15*(4), 27–36.

Srivastava, K., & Mustafa, T. (1992). Ginger (*Zinziber officinale*) in rheumatism and musculoskeletal disorders. *Medical Hypothesis, 39,* 342–348.

Takeda, W., & Wessel, J. (1994). Acupuncture for the treatment of pain of osteoarthritic knees. *Arthritis Care & Research, 7*(3), 118–122.

Taylor, G. (1998). A nurse-directed interdisciplinary center for the study of complementary therapies. *Journal of Emergency Nursing, 26*(6), 486–487.

Turner, J., Clark, A. J., Authier, D., & Williams, M. (1998). The effect of therapeutic touch on pain and anxiety in burn patients, *Journal of Advanced Nursing, 28*(1), 10–20.

Vallbona, C., Hazelwood, C. F., & Jurida, G. (1997). Response of pain to static magnetic fields in post polio patients: A double-blind pilot study. *Archives of Physical Medicine & Rehabilitation, 78,* 1200–1203.

Walsh, R., & Rauche, L. (1979). The precipitation of acute psychoses by intensive meditation in individuals with a history of schizophrenia. *American Journal of Psychiatry, 138*(8), 185–186.

Werbach, M. R., & Murray, M. T. (1994). *Botanical influences on illness: A sourcebook of clinical research.* Tarzana, CA: Third Line Press.

Wetzel, M., Eisenberg, D., & Kaptchuk, T. (1998). Courses involving alternative medicine at US medical schools. *JAMA, 280,* 784–787.

Yamahara J., Hatekeyama, S., Chatani, N., Nishino, Y., & Yamahara, J. (1990). Gastrointestinal motility enhancing effects of ginger and its active constituents. *Chemistry and Pharmacology Bulletin, 38,* 430–431.

Young, C. (1993). Spirituality and the chronically ill Christian elderly. *Geriatric Nursing, 14*(6), 298–303.

Zimmerman, L., Pozehl, B., Duncan, K., & Schmitz, R. (1989). Effects of music in patients who had chronic cancer pain. *Western Journal of Nursing Research, 11*(3), 298–309.

Persistent Pain and Neuropsychological Function

10

Lisa Morrow, Judith Saxton, and Eric G. Rodriguez

One of the most disabling features of pain is the common report that it interferes with concentration and memory, which in turn may lead to difficulty in performing everyday activities such as reading, watching television, or completing even simple household tasks (Jamison, Sbrocco, & Parris, 1988) resulting in a reduced overall quality of life. Although these complaints are commonly heard in clinical settings, very little research has been conducted on the neuropsychological concomitants of persistent pain, especially as they relate to older adults who have the added burden of normal age-related cognitive decline and the possibility of comorbid age-related medical disorders. Even less research has addressed the complex issue of pain in patients with dementia and other disorders of cognition, although it might be expected that neuropsychological consequences of persistent pain might be magnified by coexisting cognitive impairment. Conversely, if pain symptoms were treated, cognitive symptoms may show improvement with reduction of pain. Pain and cognitive symptoms may therefore be bidirectional: Pain may exacerbate reductions in neuropsychological function by lowering a person's cognitive resources, and alleviating pain may then improve mental status.

This chapter describes neuropsychological function related to persistent pain in older adults. An introduction to neuropsychology is provided, followed by a brief review of the literature on the cognitive changes of normal aging. We then review the fairly limited research literature related to cognitive changes in older pain patients and we describe several clinically relevant case studies of older adults with pain.

EVIDENCE AND PRINCIPLES FOR PRACTICE

Introduction to Neuropsychology

Over the past two decades, the field of neuropsychology has grown faster than any other area in psychology. Neuropsychology, by definition, is the evaluation of a person's mental and behavioral status in relation to brain function. Much of the foundation of clinical neuropsychological assessment has stemmed from the study of war-injured patients during and following World War II (Luria, 1980; Newcombe, 1969). Early research focused on developing tests that could localize damage to a certain area of the brain. Using neuropsychological tests to localize damage was considerably easier and less invasive than medical procedures available at that time (e.g., pneumoencephalogram). Neuropsychological tests were found to be predictive of location of injury. For example, lower performance on verbal tests was associated with left hemisphere lesions, while poorer performance on spatial and nonverbal tests was associated with right hemisphere lesions. Likewise, certain tests were associated with more frontal lesions while others were associated with more parietal lesions.

Neuropsychological tests provide an objective determination of behavior and thus can help determine whether the brain is impaired or functioning normally. A neuropsychological examination may be of use when diagnosing developmental, degenerative, and acquired disorders of brain function. Any of the myriad medical and behavioral conditions that alter brain function will measurably affect neuropsychological performance. Central nervous system (CNS) disorders such as multiple sclerosis, Alzheimer's disease, stroke, tumor, and epilepsy are among the most common causes of altered function. In addition, head injury, developmental disorders, neonatal complications, exposure to neurotoxins (e.g., lead, alcohol) and genetic alterations (e.g., Down's syndrome) are known to affect neuropsychological test performance. Other disorders, such as untreated hypertension, diabetes mellitus, and systemic lupus erythematosus have also been shown to be associated with lower performance on neuropsychological tests (Tarter, Butters, & Beers, 2001). Likewise, behavioral factors may impede neuropsychological function. That is, alteration in mood, such as depression or anxiety, can affect performance, as can fatigue and reduced motivation. As detailed below, research over the last two decades has also shown that both acute and persistent pain, not surprisingly, can result in lower neuropsychological test performance as well (Hart, Martelli, & Zasler, 2000).

Referral for Neuropsychological Assessment

A neuropsychological assessment is indicated if a patient reports alterations in cognitive function, such as a decline in attention and concentration, memory impairment, changes in language or learning ability, difficulty with spatial awareness, or problems with organizing and planning. Neuropsychological tests typically assess these areas of cognitive function using paper-and-pencil tests, although some tests are now administered by computer. Like the paper-and-pencil tests, computerized tests still require the presence of an examiner during the testing. Most assessments entail extensive history taking, along with several hours of testing. If the case is complex, for example, an older patient with a complicated medical history, persistent pain, and possible early signs of dementia, the patient may require up to 4 or 5 hours of testing.

Neuropsychological Test Batteries

Neuropsychological test batteries are frequently either "fixed" or "flexible." Fixed batteries, as the name implies, use a specific group of tests that are administered to all patients, regardless of injury or referral questions. The two most common fixed batteries are the Halstead-Reitan Neuropsychological Test Battery (HRNTB) (see Reitan & Wolfson, 1992) and the Luria-Nebraska Neuropsychological Battery (LNNB) (see Golden, Purisch, & Hammeke, 1985). The HRNTB is a fairly extensive battery and may take up to 8 hours to administer. It was originally developed to localize lesions and has been shown to provide a valid way to discriminate brain-injured from nonbrain-injured patients. The HRNTB consists of 13 core tests that range from motor speed and grip strength to problem solving, attention, auditory discrimination, and language function. The LNNB is much shorter and provides a summary of performance in 11 domains of function. The domains tapped by the LNNB range from motor function to receptive speech, spatial orientation, reading, arithmetic, and memory.

Brain lesions are localized more readily today with the use of advanced technological neuroimaging methods such as Computerized Tomography (CT), Magnetic Resonance Imaging (MRI) and Positron Emission Tomography (PET). Neuropsychological testing may be used in conjunction with neuroimaging to provide information on the cognitive and behavioral consequences of the anatomic lesion(s). For this purpose, neuropsychologists are likely to use a more "flexible" approach to testing. Flexible batteries, as the name implies, utilize different tests depending on the clinical referral question. Thus, different tests would be used if the patient was being evaluated for dementia than would be used if the patient was being evaluated for traumatic brain injury. A dementia evaluation would typically include orientation, language, and memory measures, while assessment of head injury would include similar measures but might also include complex information-processing tests as well as personality measures.

Frequently Encountered Tests

Adequate neuropsychological evaluation should always assess a wide array of cognitive functions. The most common areas included in an evaluation are general intelligence, learning and memory, attention and mental flexibility, visualspatial ability, language, sensory function and motor speed, and executive function and abstract reasoning.

Tests of *general intelligence* provide an estimate of IQ or general knowledge. Typically, these tests are more resistant to cerebral insult and are often used as a marker for premorbid function. The Wechsler Adult Intelligence Scale, now in its third edition (WAIS-III) (Wechsler, 1997a), is probably the most widely used measure of intelligence, though some subscales are more indicative of premorbid function (e.g., vocabulary) than others (e.g., digit span).

The most common indication of CNS alteration is a change in *learning and memory*. A neuropsychological evaluation will generally include measures of both verbal and nonverbal memory as well as short-term recall (recall after several seconds or minutes), delayed recall (recall after 30 to 60 minutes), and remote memory (early-life events). Typically, short-term recall is assessed by asking patients to recall a list of items or repeat back a short story that was read to them. Nonverbal memory may be tested by asking the patient to look at designs or faces and to recall them. Working memory, where one has to hold information in memory and at the same time perform an alternate task, is another type of memory that is commonly evaluated in neuropsychological exams. Some of the more widely employed measures of learning and memory include the Wechsler Memory Scale (Wechsler, 1997b), the California Verbal Learning Test (Delis, Kramer, Kaplan, & Ober, 1987), the Wide Range Assessment of Memory and Learning (Adams & Sheslow, 1990), and the Memory Assessment Scales (Williams, 1991).

Assessing for changes in *attention and mental flexibility* is particularly important, as deficits in attention will affect other cognitive tasks, such as learning. Attention is often categorized into several areas: sustained attention, divided attention, and focused attention. One of the most widely used tests of attention and mental flexibility is the Trail Making Test (Reitan & Wolfson, 1992). In Part B of this test the patient is asked to draw a line connecting a series of numbers and letters in alternating sequence (e.g.,

1–A, 2–B) as quickly as possible. Not only is this one of the most frequently used tests, it has also been shown to be one of the most sensitive tests to CNS damage.

Deficits in *visualspatial ability* are more common following damage to the right cerebral hemisphere. Tests of visualspatial function typically ask the patient to manipulate objects, copy line drawings, or arrange sticks or blocks to match a pattern. Alternatively, the patient may be asked to negotiate a maze or to imagine how an object would look if rotated. Common tests in this domain include subtests from the WAIS-III, such as Block Design and Object Assembly. Not infrequently, persons with right hemisphere damage will manifest a "unilateral neglect syndrome." That is, patients will fail to notice objects or material on the left side. For example, they may read only from the middle of the page or fail to eat food on the left side of their plate. In extreme circumstances they may not dress the left side of their body.

Measures of *language function* include assessment of spontaneous speech, naming objects, reading comprehension, and fluency. Tests that are commonly used to measure language function include the Reitan-Indiana Aphasia Screening Test (Reitan & Wolfson, 1992), the Boston Naming Test (Kaplan, Goodglass, & Weintraub, 1983) and the Boston Diagnostic Aphasia Exam (Goodglass & Kaplan, 1983).

Tests of *sensory function* and *motor speed* are often used to compare the left and right sides of the body. Sensory tests ask patients to recognize material presented in the auditory, visual, and tactile modalities. Motor tests, such as the Grooved Pegboard (Rourke, Yanni, MacDonald, & Young, 1973), ask the patient to place pegs in holes as quickly as possible.

Tests of *problem solving* and *abstract reasoning* measure behaviors that are thought to be subserved by the frontal lobes. These tests typically involve having the patient try to discern how to solve a problem with only limited cues, make deductive reasoning judgments, or come up with abstract concepts. Common measures of problem solving include the Wisconsin Card Sorting Test (Heaton, 1981), the Tactual Performance Test, and the Category Test (Reitan & Wolfson, 1992).

Cognitive Functioning in Normal Aging

There is considerable evidence that some otherwise healthy, normally aging individuals experience a deterioration in memory as they grow older (Kaszniak, Poon, & Riege, 1986; Poon, 1985). Difficulties with learning and remembering new information are reported as people enter middle age. Indeed, many individuals note a change in memory as early as their 40s. However, older adults typically report that the most notable changes begin in the 60s and 70s and consist of a generalized forgetfulness and an inability to hold information in mind (Craik, Anderson, Kerr, & Li, 1995).

The literature of experimental psychology has suggested that the pattern of forgetfulness in aging is typically associated with decline in secondary memory, also known as long-term memory or recent memory, more than primary (short-term or immediate) memory or tertiary (remote) memory (Schacter, Kaszniak, & Kihlstrom, 1991). However, contrary to what many older individuals believe, memories from childhood are not easier to remember: older individuals just spend more time reminiscing (Craik et al., 1995). The memory deficits of aging are also said to occur in "episodic" rather than "semantic" memory. Tulving (1972) was the first to distinguish between episodic memory, by which he meant, for example, remembering an episode or event that occurred the previous evening; and semantic memory, by which he meant the store of facts of knowledge about the world. However, the most substantial changes of memory with aging appear to involve "working memory" (Baddeley, 1986). In working memory the individual not only has to hold information in mind for a short time, but has to perform some mental operation on that information or perform another task simultaneously (Bromley, 1958; Craik, 1977; Dobbs & Rule, 1989; Salthouse, 1996).

The relationship between age-related memory changes and the executive functions subserved by the frontal lobes has also been highlighted. The frontal lobes may be particularly vulnerable to aging both structurally (Coffey et al., 1992) and functionally. Frontal lobe functions have been reported to be impaired in individuals with age-associated memory impairment (Crook et al., 1986; Hanninen et al., 1997) and, indeed, some organizational aspects of memory test performance in older adults resemble those of younger individuals with frontal lobe lesions (Stuss, Craik, Sayer, Franchi, & Alexander, 1996). Reduced speed of information processing has also been held to play a major role in the memory changes associated with aging and accounts for a substantial proportion of age-related variance in memory tasks (see Luszcz, Bryan, & Kent, 1997; Salthouse, 1996).

However, it is not clear that all cognitive abilities decline with aging, or at least all abilities may not decline at the same rate. There remains considerable disagreement regarding the extent of decline that can be attributed to aging per se. It has been suggested that overlearned, well-practiced, and familiar skills conceptualized as "crystallized" abilities can be preserved well into the 70s and 80s (Horn, 1982). In contrast, activities requiring "fluid" intelligence, such as reasoning and problem solving for which familiar solutions may not be readily available, can show evidence of gradual decline through middle age into old age (Horn, 1982). Successful completion of activities requiring fluid intelligence probably involves adequate executive functioning, working memory capacity, and adequate speed for information processing, all of which may be compromised in an older patient.

Cognitive Deficits in Acute Pain

Acute pain in older adults typically results from surgery, injury, or the exacerbation of chronic diseases such as arthritis. Arthritis is one of the major disorders of aging, with up to 80% of older individuals suffering from some type of the disorder (Davis, 1988). The treatment of arthritis has typically focused on controlling the inflammation that leads to pain, and only recently have physicians focused more directly on management of the pain itself (Clark, 2000). In one of the few direct studies of acute pain and its impact on cognition in hospitalized older adults, Duggleby and Lander (1994) investigated the impact of postoperative pain and use of analgesics on mental status. In their sample of patients aged between 50 and 80 undergoing hip replacement surgery, they found that pain, rather than medication use, predicted mental status decline.

Confounding the identification of acute pain in postoperative patients is the increased risk of delirium in older patients (Williams et al., 1985). Delirium is a disorder of cognition and behavior characterized by acute onset with fluctuating course, disorganized thinking, and altered level of consciousness and inattention. It is a serious and frequently undetected disorder that is particularly common among older adults following surgery but is also seen frequently in nonsurgical hospitalized patients as well as in residents of long-term-care facilities. Delirium, especially when it goes unrecognized, may be associated with increased morbidity and mortality (Gottlieb, Johnson, Wanich, & Sullivan, 1991; Levkoff, Besdine, & Wetle, 1986; Parikh & Chung, 1995). When the altered cognition and behavior of a delirious patient are noted, they are often mistakenly assumed to indicate dementia. Such failure to correctly ascribe alterations in mental status to delirium may result in failure to seek, discover, or treat significant medical conditions responsible for the delirium. Few studies have investigated the impact of pain on the development of delirium and even fewer have investigated the problem in older patients. In a series of 361 older patients (mean age 67 years) undergoing elective noncardiac surgeries, 34 patients developed delirium within the first 3 postoperative days (Lynch et al., 1998). After controlling for known preoperative risk factors for delirium such as age, alcohol abuse, cognitive function, physical function, serum chemistries, and type of surgery, the authors found that higher pain scores were associated with increased risk of delirium. The authors suggest that better control of postoperative pain may reduce the incidence of delirium and thus reduce the misdiagnosis of dementia.

It is important to note that not only in the postsurgical patient, but all delirium in older adults persists much longer than is generally believed. Many clinicians assume that postsurgical delirium resolves within a relatively short period of time, that is, a few days. However, it has been our experience that postsurgical delirium can persist for months. One reason the true duration of delirium in older adults is not widely appreciated may be the discontinuities in care related to moves from unit to unit within the hospital and from facility to facility as the patients are discharged from acute care to rehabilitation and long-term-care facilities. Clinicians unfamiliar with patients' prehospitalization cognitive status may assume that such patients are experiencing a prodromal dementia. Despite the insistence of families that they were "fine before the surgery," these delirious patients are labeled with dementia, and further investigation to discover potential causes of delirium may not be undertaken.

Cognitive Deficits in Persistent Pain

Almost all studies of neuropsychological impairment in persistent pain sufferers have focused on individuals in middle age, around 45 years. These studies have shown significant decrements in cognitive function, particularly in the areas of attention, memory, and mental flexibility/executive function, with a dose-response relationship (Eccleston, 1994, 1995; Eccleston, Crombez, Aldrich, & Stannard, 1997; Kewman, Vaishampayan, Zald, & Han, 1991). The impact of persistent pain in older individuals is confounded by the increased incidence of other medical and neurologic-neuropsychiatric conditions concomitant with age.

The risk of dementia increases exponentially with increasing age, with a prevalence of 1.4% in individuals in their 60s, rising to over 25% in individuals aged over 85 (Jorm & Henderson, 1993; Jorm, Kortem, & Henderson, 1987). Dementia is characterized by a progressive decline in a wide range of cognitive functions that interfere with the individual's ability to carry out his or her usual activities. Such a global decline in functioning would be expected to affect the individual's perception of pain (Farrell, Katz, & Helme, 1996) as well as the ability to report pain symptoms accurately. The most obvious impact on demented patients is the inability to communicate distress in ways that might direct the attention of caregivers and clinicians to discovering and treating pain. Patients who simply evidence generalized distress through disruptive verbalizations or behaviors may be wrongly assumed to require behavioral modifications or tranquilizing medication when what they need is treatment of a painful condition. To date, there have been very few empirical studies of the impact of persistent pain on individuals with dementia. This is not surprising as the lack of objective measures of pain means that patients must be relied on to rate the severity and intensity of their pain using various pain-rating tools. The reliability of such ratings in individuals with cognitive impairment is, of course, questionable (Nikolaus, 1997; Parmelee, 1996). A number of pain rating scales are available, such as the visual analogue scale and the verbal descriptor scale. Weiner, Peterson, and Keefe, (1998) have demonstrated that a "pain thermometer," in which patients rate the level of their pain, is a reliable indicator in older adults who have moderate levels of dementia. Hurley, Volicer, Hanrahan, Houde, and Volicer (1992) also developed an objective scale for measuring discomfort in noncommunicative patients with advanced Alzheimer's disease. Although reliable measures of pain perception may be difficult to establish, especially with very old and/or cognitively impaired patients, clinical observation suggests that fewer episodes of acting-out behavior occur when the individual's pain is under control.

Psychiatric Comorbidity

The evaluation and treatment of pain in older individuals and research into its effects may be confounded by the increased risk of depression in older individuals with persistent pain and, conversely, the increased sensitivity to pain in older adult depressed patients. Patients with persistent low back pain are three times more likely to experience depression than the general population (Sullivan, Reesor, Mikail, & Fisher, 1992); conversely, almost 60% of patients with depression report pain symptoms (Magni, Schifano, & DeLeo, 1985; Von Knorring, Perris, Eisemann, Eriksson, & Perris, 1983). It has long been recognized that depression alone, without other comorbidity, can be associated with cognitive deficits (Emery, 1988; Folstein & McHugh, 1978; Kiloh, 1961; Stoudemire, Hill, Gulley, & Morris, 1989). It has been suggested that approximately 20% of older depressed patients may exhibit severe cognitive deficits (LaRue, D'Elia, Clark, Spar, & Jarvik, 1986). The neuropsychological deficits of depression can be varied and include impaired attention and concentration leading to poor encoding of information, impaired retrieval of previously learned information, impaired verbal fluency, difficulties with visualconstructional functioning, and impaired executive abilities (Butters, Salmon, & Butters, 1994). Thus, complaints from patients with depression are very similar to those of persistent pain patients and include forgetfulness and difficulty with concentration. Furthermore, depression is a common occurrence in disorders such as Parkinson's disease, vascular dementia, and stroke among others, and, as discussed above, patients with these disorders may also experience significant pain. It is reasonable to assume that pain exacerbates depression, which exacerbates cognitive impairment, leading to impaired functioning, difficulty with decision making, and perhaps poor judgment, resulting in poor compliance with medications and thus in increased morbidity and mortality.

Some patients report experiencing pain for which no objective medical cause can be identified. More often, patients report more severe levels of pain than would typically be expected for a given illness or disease state. In some cases these patients can be described as preoccupied with the experience of the pain or fixated on their physical symptoms. Older patients with dementia may also appear to dwell on their pain. The underlying cause of the preoccupation in dementia may be a perseverative behavior secondary to progressive deterioration of executive functions, which is part of the dementing disorder. Alternatively, it may simply be a learned behavior: Expressions of pain lead to increased attention from staff and family, thus reinforcing the likelihood of the patients' continuing to express feelings of pain. The preoccupation sometimes leads the individual and/or family members to believe that the pain is a medical mystery and to seek more and more medical opinions in order to solve the problem. As the number of medical evaluations increases so does the number of potential diagnoses and with this the possibility of inappropriate treatment interventions (Clark, 2000; Katon et al., 1991; Kouyanou, Pither, Rabe-Hesketh, & Wessely, 1998). Such patients are in general more likely to exhibit irrational thinking (Katon et al., 1991; Kouyanou et al., 1998), which can be further confounded by the possibility of medication interactions. Thus, identification and appropriate pharmaceutical management of psychiatric disorders is critical to the effective treatment of pain in these older patients. These concepts are addressed more fully in chapter 3.

Medical Comorbidity

Increasing age is associated with increasing risk for comorbid medical conditions, especially chronic disorders. Many chronic disorders commonly seen in older adults cause pain, for example, arthritis (joint pain), peripheral arterial disease (claudication or rest pain), and diabetes mellitus (neuropathic pain.) Some disorders may be associated with both persistent pain and cognitive deficits. As many as 80% of older adults suffer from some type of arthritis (Davis, 1988). As many as 5% of stroke victims suffer intractable pain (Bowsher, 1995) in addition to the potential neurologic (e.g., hemiplegia) and cognitive sequelae of the stroke, notably difficulties with speech, language, and executive functioning. Pain is also reported in approximately 50% of individuals with Parkinson's disease (Goetz, Tannen, Levy, Wilson, & Garron, 1986; Koller, 1984; Starkstein, Preziosi, & Robinson, 1991). Up to 40% of Parkinson's patients exhibit cognitive deficits amounting to dementia (Ebmeier et al., 1991; Mayeux et al., 1992).

In such disorders, the coexistence of pain and dementia complicates the management of each. Patients with dementia may be, for example, especially vulnerable to adverse effects of analgesic medications. Opioids in particular frequently produce delirium in patients with dementia, and delirium, especially in hospitalized patients, is associated with poor outcomes. Nonetheless, given the adverse effects of pain on cognitive function, any intent to optimize cognition in persons with dementia mandates vigorous efforts to treat pain. Judicious trials of analgesic medications may reduce pain and enhance cognition, but the clinician must be prepared to adjust medication dose and schedule and to try various categories of medications to maximize benefit while minimizing adverse effects.

Treating pain in persons with dementia is particularly difficult because afflicted patients may be incapable of providing information on their subjective experience to guide evaluation and management. Basic information such as location, duration, relieving and exacerbating factors, associated symptoms, and response to treatment may be unobtainable, even from persons with moderately advanced dementia. Clinicians treating such patients must rely heavily on observations made during the clinical encounter and on the reports of caregivers.

Mechanism for Impaired Cognitive Functioning in Older Adult Pain Patients

One of the most disturbing features of pain is the report that it interferes with attention and concentration and prevents individuals from performing their usual daily activities. One possible neuropsychological mechanism by which pain may do this is via working memory. As discussed above, in working memory the individual must not only hold information in mind, but must also manipulate and reorganize it, or combine it with other incoming information in an ongoing fashion. We suggest that attention to the pain occupies working memory capacity and thus uses up attentional capacity, which is necessary for the successful completion of other activities. Thus, there is not enough capacity left for thinking and processing of everyday activities. The net result is that patients report that they cannot concentrate.

The cumulative burden on cognitive processing resulting from multiple diseases could be overwhelming. While the impact of impaired cognition in younger individuals is clear, (i.e., an inability to return to lucrative employment), the impact of impaired cognition for older individuals is sometimes less obvious but nonetheless potentially devastating. For example, impaired concentration and memory in an older stroke patient could impact the person's ability to take advantage of physical rehabilitation. Impaired concentration and memory undoubtedly result in poor compliance with medication regimens. As mentioned above, cognitive difficulties cause problems with everyday activities, many of which involve the use of complex machinery, such as operating a lawn mower and an automobile. Finally, impaired cognition could result in difficulties with complex decision making, raising questions of overall competence to manage one's own affairs.

SETTING-SPECIFIC CONSIDERATIONS

Most neuropsychological assessments are completed in an outpatient clinic setting, where the patient typically spends 3 to 5 hours undergoing testing with a selection of the tests outlined above. However, it is not always practical to conduct assessments at an outpatient clinic, as some patients may require testing before being discharged from a hospital or while residing in a rehabilitation institute or nursing home. In a hospital or nursing home setting, testing may be restricted to the bedside. In these instances, testing is often limited to asking the patient to draw a clock or a Greek cross or to complete a cognitive screening test such as the Mini-Mental State Exam (Folstein, Folstein, & McHugh, 1975), the Dementia Rating Scale (Mattis, 1988), or the Rivermead Behavioural Memory Test (Wilson, Cockburn, & Baddeley, 1991). These types of cognitive screening tests provide an overall index of general function and require relatively little time to administer. In addition, they sample responses to questions dealing with language, orientation, memory, and simple construction. While these screening tests provide a quick assessment of overall ability, they do not provide a satisfactory assessment of subtle changes in cognitive function. If lower than expected scores are found on a screening assessment and the reasons are not apparent (e.g., Alzheimer's disease), a referral for a more comprehensive neuropsychological evaluation should be made. Most comprehensive evaluations can still be done in inpatient settings, although testing will likely be spaced out over several days so as not to fatigue the patient.

SUMMARY/RECOMMENDATIONS

1. The presentation, assessment, and management of pain in older adults is complicated by the cumulative burden of medical and psy-

chiatric conditions interacting with the cognitive changes of both normal aging and disease.

2. Attention to pain may interfere with normal cognitive function by occupying "working memory," thereby reducing the amount of cognitive resources available for the performance of everyday activities.

3. Pain, particularly persistent pain, which is undertreated in general, is neglected as a potentially remediable contributor to cognitive impairment. Apart from the imperative to reduce suffering, relief of persistent pain may confer additional benefit by reducing excess cognitive dysfunction.

4. Even when persistent pain is recognized and efforts are made to treat it, clinicians are confronted by substantial challenges in gathering reliable information, in treating without causing new harm, and in assessing the response to treatment.

CASE STUDIES

Case 1

An 81-year-old man with mild dementia (Folstein Mini-Mental State Examination 6 months earlier was 24) was unusually restless over a 2-day period. He was pacing, rarely sitting for more than a few minutes, and seemed confused. He had frequent awakenings at night. He ate very little. On the second day, his wife noted blood-stains in his underpants. On questioning, he seemed to endorse difficulties urinating.

In the emergency department, he was oriented to person and place but gave the year as 1957. He was described as agitated and confused. Physical exam was remarkable for hypertension and a distended bladder. He was immediately less restless after 1,700 cc of grossly bloody urine was drained from his bladder, and was able to give the year as 1998 (in 2000).

In the hospital, he had two episodes of obstruction of the bladder catheter with blood clots. As in the initial episode, he became restless, confused, and disoriented with each episode. He became promptly more calm and less disoriented on relief of the catheter obstruction. During none of his three episodes did he indicate that he sensed a need to void, although on relief of the obstruction, he was able to say that he experienced much relief of a previous discomfort.

Discussion

This patient with mild dementia appeared to suffer acute delirium related to bladder obstruction, with prompt resolution of confusion and disorientation on relief of the obstruction and the attendant pain. Interestingly, while he never complained of pain or any localizing symptom during his acute episodes, relief of the pain resulted in immediate improvement, not only in his restlessness, but also in his cognition. Delirium, as this case suggests, was the chief manifestation of pain in this patient. The presence of dementia increases the risk for delirium, lowering the threshold for the severity of the provoking cause. In this case, assessment was complicated by the patient's inability to report, much less localize, pain.

Case 2

A 73-year-old female homemaker was brought to clinic by her husband for consultation regarding disabling back pain. She had had intermittent low back pain over three decades, but in the past year, the pain had become more severe. The husband noted that she cited pain as a reason to avoid social events and for more general inactivity. Pain did not disrupt her sleep. The patient offered a vague account of the pain and was unable on direct questioning to offer specific information, for example, on precipitating or relieving factors. Her husband reported offering her acetaminophen and several over-the-counter NSAIDs with equivocal results. Her past medical history included osteoarthritis in both knees and well-controlled hypertension. The review of systems was positive for urinary incontinence, two falls, and short-term memory loss. On physical examination, the patient was in no evident discomfort. She was able to get out of a chair and onto the exam table unassisted. There was no tenderness to palpation or percussion in the low back. Straight leg raising produced bilateral discomfort in the ipsilateral hamstrings. She had moderately limited spinal flexion and extension. Lower extremity deep tendon reflexes were symmetric and normally brisk. Lumbosacral radiographs revealed moderate changes of osteoarthritis. Folstein Mini-Mental State Examination score was 19/30. On further questioning, her husband reported that he had assumed responsibility for cooking and shopping over the past year, in part because the patient cited her back pain as causing too much discomfort, and in part because she seemed less able to manage.

Discussion

This woman was unable to give a specific account of her pain. The apparent coincident worsening of her pain and the onset of a cognitive disorder complicates the assessment of her pain and raises questions about potential interactions between the two disorders. Was persistent pain interfering with her ability to attend to and register new information? Was a depressive disorder related to the persistent pain causing the so-called pseudodementia syndrome? Was the complaint of pain serving as her rationalization for her inability, which actually derived from progressive cognitive impairment? Over a series of visits and several discussions with the husband, the latter effect seemed likely to account for a significant proportion of her complaint of pain.

Case 3

An 85-year-old woman with hip fracture was treated with meperidine following open reduction and internal fixation of the fracture. Prior to her injury the patient was cognitively intact. On the 2nd postoperative day, her daughter reported that the patient was agitated and seeing flying cats and long-dead relatives in her hospital room. When questioned by the physician, the patient denied pain, but the nurses' notes documented pain on all movement. Physical examination and a complete blood count revealed no acute medical problem. The meperidine was thought to be contributing to the patient's delirium, so it was discontinued on the 3rd postoperative day and acetaminophen was used for pain relief. The patient remained delirious, and a physical therapist reported that she was not participating in rehabilitation. On the 5th postoperative day, a urinalysis indicated a urinary tract infection and ciprofloxacin was started. Over the following 3 days, she became gradually less delirious.

Discussion

This patient suffered a postoperative delirium. Opioid analgesics, and especially meperidine, are associated with delirium in older patients. Discontinuation of meperidine did not result in prompt resolution of her delirium, suggesting that there may have been other contributory factors. In fact, a urinary tract infection was diagnosed and she became less delirious after the antibiotic was started. The meperidine, however, may have continued to cause symptoms after it was discontinued, in part because it has a long-acting metabolite (normeperidine), which is itself deliriogenic. The patient's pain may have been inadequately treated with acetaminophen, and pain may also have contributed to her delirium. The abrupt discontinuation of an opioid may produce a withdrawal syndrome with features of delirium. Thus, pain, efforts to treat pain, and efforts to ameliorate delirium may all contribute to the complex causation of altered cognition, especially in older patients.

REFERENCES

Adams, W., & Sheslow, D. (1990). *Wide range assessment of memory and learning.* Wilimington, DE: Jastak Associates.

Baddeley, A. D. (1986). *Working memory.* Oxford, England: Clarendon Press.

Bowsher, D. (1995). The management of central post-stroke pain. *Postgrad Medical Journal, 71,* 598–604.

Bromley, D. B. (1958). Some effects of age on short-term learning and memory. *Journal of Gerontology, 13,* 398–406.

Butters, M. A., Salmon, D. P., & Butters, N. (1994). Neuropsychological assessment of dementia. In M. Storandt & G. R. VandenBos (Eds.), *Neuropsychological assessment of dementia and depression in older adults: A clinician's guide.* Washington, DC: American Psychological Association.

Clark, M. R. (2000). Pain. In C. E. Coffey & J. L. Cummings (Eds.), *Textbook of geriatric neuropsychiatry* (2nd ed.). Washington, DC: American Psychiatric Press.

Coffey, C. E., Wilkinson, W. E., Parashos, I. A., Soady, S. A., Sullivan, R. J., Patterson, L. J., Figiel, G. S., Webb, M. C., Spritzer, C. E., & Djang, W. T. (1992). Quantitative cerebral anatomy of the aging human brain: A cross-sectional study using magnetic resonance imaging. *Neurology, 42*(3, Pt. 1), 527–536.

Craik, F. I. M. (1977). Age differences in human memory. In J. E. Birren & K. W. Schaie (Eds.), *Handbook of the psychology of aging.* New York: Van Nostrand Reinhold.

Craik, F. I. M., Anderson, N. D., Kerr, S. A., & Li, K. Z. H. (1995). Memory changes in normal aging. In A. D. Baddeley, B. A. Wilson, & F. N. Watts (Eds.), *Handbook of memory disorders.* New York: Wiley.

Crook, T. H., Bartus, R. T., Ferris, S. H., Whitehouse, P., Cohen, G. D., & Gershon, S. (1986). Age-associated memory impairment: Proposed diagnostic criteria and measures of clinical change—report of a National Institute of Mental Health work group. *Developmental Neuropsychology, 2*(4), 261–276.

Davis, M. A. (1988). Epidemiology of osteoarthritis. *Clinical Geriatric Medicine, 4,* 241–255.

Delis, D. C., Kramer, J. H., Kaplan, E., & Ober, B. A. (1987). *California Verbal Learning Test: Adult Version.* San Antonio, TX: The Psychological Corporation.

Dobbs, A. R., & Rule, B. G. (1989). Adult age differences in working memory. *Psychology and Aging, 4,* 500–503.

Duggleby, W., & Lander, J. (1994). Cognitive status and postoperative pain: Older adults. *Journal of Pain and Symptom Management, 9*(1), 19–27.

Ebmeier, K. P., Calder, S. A., Crawford, J. R., Stewart, L., Cochrane, R. H., & Besson, J. A. (1991). Dementia in idiopathic Parkinson's disease: Prevalence and relationship with symptoms and signs of parkinsonism. *Psychological Medicine, 21,* 69–76.

Eccleston, C. (1994). Chronic pain and attention: A cognitive approach. *British Journal of Clinical Psychology, 33,* 535–547.

Eccleston, C. (1995). Chronic pain and distraction: An experimental investigation into the role of sustained and shifting attention in the processing of chronic persistent pain. *Behaviour Research and Therapy, 33*(4), 391–405.

Eccleston, C., Crombez, G., Aldrich, S., & Stannard, C. (1997). Attention and somatic awareness in chronic pain. *Pain, 72,* 209–215.

Emery, V. O. B. (1988). *Pseudodementia: A theoretical and empirical discussion.* Cleveland, OH: Western Reserve Geriatric Education Center.

Farrell, M. J., Katz, B., & Helme, R. D. (1996). The impact of dementia on the pain experience. *Pain, 67,* 7–15.

Folstein, M. F., Folstein, S. E., & McHugh, P. R. (1975). Mini-Mental State: A practical method for grading the cognitive state of patients for the clinician. *Journal of Psychiatric Research, 12,* 189–198.

Folstein, M. F., & McHugh, P. R. (1978). Dementia syndrome of depression. *Aging, 7,* 87–93.

Goetz, C. G., Tannen, C. M., Levy, M., Wilson, R. S., & Garron, D. C. (1986). Pain in Parkinson's disease. *Movement Disorder, 1*(1), 541–549.

Golden, C. J., Purisch, A. D., & Hammeke, T. A. (1985). *Luria-Nebraska Neuropsychological Battery: Forms I and II manual.* Los Angeles: Western Psychological Services.

Goodglass, H., & Kaplan, E. (1983). *Boston Diagnostic Aphasia Examination.* Philadelphia: Lea & Feiberger. Distributed by Psychological Assessment Resources, Odessa, FL.

Gottlieb, G. L., Johnson, J., Wanich, C., & Sullivan, E. (1991). Delirium in the medically ill elderly: Operationalizing the *DSM-III* criteria. *International Psychogeriatrics, 3,* 181–196.

Hanninen, T., Hallikainen, M., Koivisto, K., Partanen, K., Laakso, M. P., Riekkinen, P. J., & Soininen, H. (1997). Decline of frontal lobe functions in subjects with age-associated memory impairment. *Neurology, 48*(1), 148–153.

Hart, R. P., Martelli, M. F., & Zasler, D. (2000). Chronic pain and neuropsychological functioning. *Neuropsychology Review, 10,* 131–149.

Heaton, R. K. (1981). *Wisconsin Card Sorting Test (WCST).* Odessa, FL: Psychological Assessment Resources.

Horn, J. L. (1982). The theory of fluid and crystallized intelligence in relation to concepts of cognitive psychology of aging in adulthood. In F. I. M. Craik & S. Trehub (Eds.), *Advances in the study of commuication and affect: Vol. 8. Aging and cognitive processes.* New York: Plenum.

Hurley, A. C., Volicer, B. J., Hanrahan, P. A., Houde, S., & Volicer, L. (1992). Assessment of discomfort in advanced Alzheimer patients. *Research in Nursing and Health, 15,* 369–377.

Jamison, R. N., Sbrocco, T., & Parris, W. C. (1988). The influence of problems with concentration and memory on emotional distress and daily activities in chronic pain patients. *International Journal of Psychiatry in Medicine, 18*(2), 183–191.

Jorm, A. F., & Henderson, A. S. (1993). *The problem of dementia in Australia.* Canberra: Australian Government Publishing Service.

Jorm, A. F., Kortem, A. E., & Henderson, A. S. (1987). The prevalence of dementia: A quantitative integration of the literature. *Acta Psychiatrica Scandinavica 76,* 465–479.

Kaplan, E. F., Goodglass, H., & Weintraub, S. (1983). *The Boston Naming Test* (2nd ed.). Philadelphia: Lea & Feiberger.

Kaszniak, A. W., Poon, L. W., & Riege, W. (1986). Assessing memory deficits: An information processing approach. In L. W. Poon (Ed.), *Clinical memory assessment of older adults* (pp. 168–188). Washington, DC: American Psychological Association.

Katon, W., Lin, E., Von Korff, M., Russo, J., Lipscomb, P., & Bush, T. (1991). Somatization: A spectrum of severity. *American Journal of Psychiatry, 148*(1), 34–40.

Kewman, D. G., Vaishampayan, N., Zald, D., & Han, B. (1991). Cognitive impairment in musculoskeletal pain patients. *International Journal of Psychiatry in Medicine, 21*(3), 253–262.

Kiloh, L. G. (1961). Pseudo-dementia. *Acta Psychiatrica Scandinavica, 37,* 336–351.

Koller, W. C. (1984). Sensory symptoms in Parkinson's disease. *Neurology, 34,* 957–959.

Kouyanou, K., Pither, C. E., Rabe-Hesketh, S., & Wessely, S. (1998). A comparative study of iatrogenesis, medication abuse, and psychiatric morbidity in chronic pain patients with and without medically explained symptoms. *Pain, 76*(3), 417–426.

LaRue, A., D'Elia, L. F., Clark, E. O., Spar, J. E., & Jarvik, L. F. (1986). Clinical tests of memory in dementia, depression and healthy aging. *Journal of Psychology and Aging, 1,* 69–77.

Levkoff, S. E., Besdine, R. W., & Wetle, T. (1986). Acute confusional states (delirium) in the hospitalized elderly. *Annual Review of Gerontology and Geriatrics, 6,* 1–26.

Luria, A. R. (1980). *Higher Cortical Functions in Man* (2nd ed., revised and expanded). New York: Basic Books.

Luszcz, M. A., Bryan, J., & Kent, P. (1997). Predicting episodic memory performance of very old men and women: Contributions from age, depression, activity, cognitive ability and speed. *Psychology and Aging, 12,* 340–351.

Lynch, E. P., Lazor, M. A., Gellis, J. E., Orav, J., Goldman, L., & Marcantonio, E. R. (1998). The impact of postoperative pain on the development of postoperative delirium. *Anesthesia and Analgesia, 86,* 781–785.

Magni, G., Schifano, F., & DeLeo, D. (1985). Pain as a symptom in elderly depressed patients: Relationship to diagnostic subgroups. *European Archives of Psychiatry and Neurological Sciences, 235,* 143–145.

Mattis, S. (1988). *Dementia Rating Scale* (DRS). Odessa, FL: Psychological Assessment Resources.

Mayeux, R., Denaro, J., Hemenegildo, N., Marder, K., Tang, M. X., Cote, L. J., & Stern, Y. (1992). A population-based investigation of Parkinson's disease with and without dementia. Relationship to age and gender. *Archives of Neurology,* 42, 492–497.

Newcombe, F. (1969). *Missile wounds of the brain: A study of psychological deficits.* London: Oxford University Press.

Nikolaus, T. (1997). Assessment of chronic pain in elderly patients. *Therapeutische Umschau,* 54, 340–344.

Parikh, S. S., & Chung, F. (1995). Postoperative delirium in the elderly. *International Anesthesia Research Society,* 80, 1223–1232.

Parmelee, P. A. (1996). Pain in cognitively impaired older persons. *Clinics in Geriatric Medicine,* 12, 473–487.

Poon, L. W. (1985). Differences in human memory with aging: Nature, causes and clinical implications. In J. E. Birren & K. W. Schaie (Eds.), *Handbook of the psychology of aging* (2nd ed., pp. 427–462). New York: Van Nostrand Reinhold.

Reitan, R. M., & Wolfson, D. (1992). *The Halstead-Reitan Neuropsychological Test Battery: Theory and clinical interpretation* (2nd ed.). Tucson, AZ: Neuropsychology Press.

Rourke, B. P., Yanni, D. W., MacDonald, G. W., & Young, G. C. (1973). Neuropsychological significance of lateralized deficits on the Grooved Pegboard Test for older children with learning disabilities. *Journal of Consulting and Clinical Psychology,* 41, 128–134.

Salthouse, T. A. (1996). General and specific speed mediation of adult age differences in memory. *Journal of Gerontology: Series B, Psychological Sciences & Social Sciences,* 51(1), 30–42.

Schacter, D. L., Kaszniak, A. W., & Kihlstrom, J. F. (1991). Models of memory and the understanding of memory disorders. In T. Yanagihara & R. C. Petersen (Eds.), *Memory disorders: Research and clinical practice* (pp. 111–134). New York: Marcel Dekker.

Starkstein, S. E., Preziosi, T. J., & Robinson, R. G. (1991). Sleep disorders, pain, and depression in Parkinson's disease. *European Neurology,* 31, 352–355.

Stoudemire, A., Hill, C., Gulley, L. R., & Morris, R. (1989). Neuropsychological and biomedical assessment of depression-dementia syndromes. *Journal of Neuropsychiatry and Clinical Neurosciences,* 1, 347–361.

Stuss, D. T., Craik, F. I., Sayer, L., Franchi, D., & Alexander, M. P. (1996). Comparison of older people and patients with frontal lesions: Evidence from word list learning. *Psychology of Aging,* 11(3), 387–395.

Sullivan, M. J., Reesor, K., Mikail, S., & Fisher, R. (1992). The treatment of depression in chronic low back pain: Review and recommendations. *Pain,* 50(1), 5–13.

Tarter, R. E., Butters, M., & Beers, S. R. (2001). *Medical neuropsychology* (2nd ed.). Kluwer Academic/Plenum.

Tulving, E. (1972). Episodic and semantic memory. In E. Tulving & W. Donaldson (Eds.), *Organization of memory* (pp. 382–403). New York: Academic Press.

Von Knorring, L., Perris, C., Eisemann, M., Eriksson, U., & Perris, H. (1983). Pain as a symptom in depressive disorders II. Relationship to personality traits as assessed by means of KSP. *Pain,* 17(4), 377–384.

Wechsler, D. (1997a). *Wechsler Adult Intelligence Scale* (3rd ed.). New York: The Psychological Corporation.

Wechsler, D. (1997b). *Wechsler Memory Scale (3rd ed.).* New York: The Psychological Corporation.

Weiner, D., Peterson, B., & Keefe, F. (1998). Evaluating persistent pain in long term care residents: What role for pain maps? *Pain, 76,* 249–257.

Williams, J. M. (1991). *Memory Assessment Scales: Professional manual.* Odessa, FL: Psychological Assessment Resources.

Williams, M. A., Campbell, E. B., Raynor, W. J., Musholt, M. A., Mlynarczyk, S. M., & Crane, L. R. (1985). Predictors of acute confusional states in hospitalized elderly patients. *Research in Nursing and Health, 8,* 31–40.

Wilson, B. A., Cockburn, J., & Baddeley, A. (1985). *The Rivermead Behavioural Memory Test.* Reading, England: Thames Valley Test Coland; and Gaylord, MI: National Rehabilitation Services.

Pain and Suffering in Older Adults Approaching the End of Life

11

Linda King and Robert Arnold

Changes in medical technology and in society over the last half century have altered the face of dying persons—death more frequently occurs at an older age, typically after a chronic, progressive illness, and often in institutions. Recently, increasing interest in the role of palliative care in improving the quality of remaining time for dying patients has developed (Field & Cassel, 1997). Palliative care is directed at alleviating suffering and maximizing quality of life, not only for patients for whom death is very near but also for individuals facing the earlier stages of a serious or life-threatening illness.

Defining when a person is dying has become more difficult as more individuals die as a result of chronic conditions. Individuals often live decades with an incurable illness. One definition of dying states, "People are considered to be dying when they have a progressive illness that is expected to end in death and for which there is no treatment that can substantially alter the outcome" (American Geriatrics Society Ethics Committee, 1998). This broad definition applies along a continuum that may last decades, from the time of diagnosis of a serious, progressive illness until death.

Increased attention to the dying experience of older adults reveals many deficits in the management of pain and suffering. Patients with a life-limiting illness often suffer from uncontrolled pain and other distressing physical symptoms. These symptoms result from the life-threatening disease itself, the treatments used to manage the disease, and coexisting chronic medical conditions (osteoarthritis, peripheral neuropathy, etc.). Suffering at the end of life also stems from psychological, spiritual, and existential distress, as well as unmet practical, financial, and social needs.

Optimal end-of-life care requires careful pain and symptom management throughout the disease course. Health care providers working with patients with life-threatening illness need to recognize and address all aspects of suffering to improve the dying experience of older adults. The goal of this chapter is to highlight current deficits in the management of pain and suffering in older adults living with chronic, progressive illnesses and to provide strategies for recognizing and managing suffering.

EVIDENCE AND PRINCIPLES FOR PRACTICE

Deficits in Pain and Symptom Management at the End of Life

A growing evidence base confirms that many older adults die in pain while also suffering from other unrelieved symptoms. Two large, concurrent prospective studies—the Study to Understand Prognoses and Preferences of Outcomes and Risks of Treatments (SUPPORT) and the Hospitalized Elderly Longitudinal Project (HELP)—examined the end-of-life experience of several thousand hospitalized patients. The median age of patients enrolled in the SUPPORT trial was 65 and the HELP trial looked at hospitalized persons aged 80 or older. As many as 50% of patients experienced moderate or severe pain during the last 3 days of life (SUPPORT Principal Investigators, 1995). One quarter of cancer patients experienced severe pain in the 3–6 months before death and more than 40% were in serious pain during their last 3 days of life (McCarthy et al., 2000). Over 40% of patients dying with congestive heart failure experienced severe pain during the 3 days before death and 63% were severely short of breath (Levenson et al., 2000). During the last 6 months of life, one quarter of patients with chronic obstructive pulmonary (COPD) experienced severe pain and two thirds had severe dyspnea (Lynn et al., 2000). Inadequate symptom management has been observed in patients dying in various settings. Outpatients with cancer, especially those over age 70, commonly experience uncontrolled pain that limits their ability to function. They receive inadequate analgesics (Cleeland et al., 1994) despite published guidelines for cancer pain management. A study of symptom prevalence in the hospital during the last 48 hours of life revealed high rates of multiple symptoms, including severe pain, dyspnea, restlessness, agitation, fatigue, nausea, anorexia, and incontinence across a large variety of terminal diagnoses (Goodlin et al., 1998). A study in a nursing home setting revealed that 70% of patients experienced severe pain, 56% severe or moderate dyspnea, and 61% other distressing physical symptoms during the last 3 months of life. Family members often felt that symptom management was inadequate for their dying loved ones (Baer & Hanson, 2000).

A large study of older adults living with cancer in nursing homes revealed that over a quarter of patients experienced daily pain (Bernabei et al., 1998). Many of these patients received no analgesics, especially those over age 85 and those with cognitive impairment. Unrelieved symptoms have been shown to correlate with declines in patients' perceived quality of life. Maximizing quality of life requires optimal management of physical symptoms.

Barriers to Pain and Symptom Management at the End of Life

Many of the barriers to effective pain and symptom management at the end of life relate to deficits within the health care system. A number of studies reveal that health care providers consistently underestimate patients' level of pain. In addition, providers harbor attitudes that inhibit good pain management—views regarding the frequency of drug-seeking behaviors in patients with pain and worries that pain medicine will hide illness. Studies also reveal that health care providers lack sufficient knowledge regarding the basics of pain management including appropriate dosing, conversions, and side effects of medications. Finally, prior to the recent passage of Joint Commission on Accreditation of Healthcare Organizations (JCAHO) regulations regarding pain management, many health care institutions have not required attention to patients' pain. The result of these inadequacies has been suboptimal pain management.

In addition to flaws in the health care system, patient-related barriers contribute to inadequate symptom control (Jacox et al., 1994). Many patients expect to have worsening pain as their disease progresses. They may not report new or worsening pain to their loved ones or physicians because of concern about distracting physicians from treating the underlying disease, fear that pain means the disease is worsening, and concern about becoming addicted or not having enough pain medicine as death approaches. Even if pain is optimally assessed and an appropriate treatment plan developed, patients may not follow through with treatment recommendations. Taking regularly scheduled medications can serve as an ongoing reminder of advanced disease. Denial and fears regarding tolerance, dependence, and side effects may result in poor compliance with medications. These patient-related barriers can be minimized by actively exploring these concerns with patients.

The meaning a patient attributes to pain and other physical symptoms also affects how the neural inputs are perceived and how well a patient responds to treatment. Any degree of pain (e.g., the input from damaged tissues or nerves), even a fairly minor discomfort, may cause great suffering (the experience of the nerve transmission) when the source of the pain is unknown, when the meaning of the pain is very serious, when the pain is chronic, or when the patient feels out of control and overwhelmed. In contrast, even if pain is quite severe, if the cause of the pain is known and treatment is available and the patient believes it will be effective, then the pain may be less overwhelming and the patient may not report suffering as greatly with the pain. Suffering can be relieved while working to relieve persistent pain by making the source of the pain known, by changing its meaning for the patient, and by demonstrating that it can be controlled and that an end is in sight (Cassell, 1982). Explicitly discussing these often unaddressed concerns may allow for better pain control.

A particularly salient fear in the last weeks of life is that the use of opioids will kill the patient by causing respiratory depression. Health care providers, patients, and families may mistakenly equate the appropriate use of drugs to manage terminal symptoms (including pain and dyspnea) with euthanasia or assisted suicide. The use of these drugs is ethically appropriate and necessary as long as the intent is to relieve distress rather than shorten life. This principle, termed *the rule of double effect*, states that an action (such as giving opioids to relieve symptoms) is ethically justifiable if the intent is to achieve a positive effect (symptom relief), even with the risk of *foreseen* but *unintended* consequences (respiratory depression, sedation, and death) (Sulmasy, 1999). The intent of the intervention (to relieve symptoms) distinguishes it from euthanasia and assisted suicide in which the intent is to hasten death. Withholding of appropriate symptomatic therapy is never justified on ethical, moral, legal, or professional grounds (see chapter 12 for further discussion). Open and ongoing communication with family and other caregivers regarding the intention, risks, and benefits of prescribed therapies is essential to avoid misunderstandings. In reality, with careful dose titration, symptom control can almost always be achieved without causing respiratory depression or excessive sedation. When a balance between symptom relief and sedation is difficult to achieve, individual patient values can guide therapy. Some patients will accept some degree of sedation to assure maximal symptom relief, while others will tolerate persistent symptoms to avoid sedation. Explicit discussion of goals of treatment with patients can guide management decisions.

General Principles of Pain and Symptom Management at the End of Life

Assessment and management of pain and other physical symptoms at the end of life rely on the same general principles of pain management described throughout this text, but several specific points are worth noting. Patients with life-threatening illness often have multiple pains and other physical symptoms. Each symptom should be prioritized and assessed fully. Because multiple symptoms are commonly experienced simultaneously in advanced disease, symptom assessment tools have been developed to assess and follow multiple symptoms, including pain, over time. Examples include the Edmonton Symptom Assessment Scale and the Memorial Symptom Assessment Scale (Bruera et al., 1991; Portenoy et al., 1994).

Patients approaching the end of life often have a rapidly changing clinical course. Pain and other symptoms need to be reassessed frequently and treatment adjusted quickly. Finding an effective treatment regimen promptly is particularly critical for patients with a limited life expectancy.

The simplest route of administration, typically oral, should be used. Route of medication may need to be altered as the patient's condition worsens over time. Patients often ultimately become unable to swallow; therefore, rectal, vaginal, transdermal, sublingual, or parenteral administration of medications may become necessary in the final stages of disease. Epidural or intrathecal administration of medications can be used for pain that is difficult to control or when side effects have been problematic with other routes of delivery.

With careful assessment, reassessment, and optimal management, pain and many other symptoms can be controlled throughout the disease course. Pain and other symptoms associated with certain life-threatening illnesses may respond best to the specific treatments described below.

Pain and Symptom Management in Patients with Cancer

Patients with cancer should be evaluated for the role of antineoplastic therapy to improve pain control. Chemotherapy can have an important role in palliating symptoms. For example, gemcitabine has been shown to be more effective for pain management than palliative care alone (Von Hoff & Goodwin, 1998). Radiation therapy is the most effective analgesic modality for treating direct tumor involvement of discrete anatomic sites. Analgesic benefit may be noted within the first few days of treatment but its timing can be quite variable. Common indications for radiation therapy include bone metastases, spinal cord compression, enlarged retroperitoneal lymph nodes, and painful soft tissue metastases. In patients with a very limited life expectancy, the course of radiation can often be markedly shortened.

Various adjuvant medications have roles in the management of specific cancer-related symptoms (Table 11.1). NSAIDs are effective for pain associated with bone metastases and other musculoskeletal pain. Glucocorticoids lessen the pain associated with tumor-associated inflammation or infiltration while enhancing appetite and general sense of well-being. Patients with pain caused by bone metastases may benefit from therapy with bisphosphanates, which inhibit osteoclast activity and reduce bone pain. Typically, an intravenous bisphosphonate is administered on a monthly basis with pain relief occurring after several days and lasting several weeks. Octreotide, a somatostatin-analogue, administered subcutaneously, can control refractory pain and vomiting caused by small-bowel obstruction by nearly completely suppressing gastrointestinal secretions, although its cost is prohibitive.

Several other symptoms common in advanced cancer may affect the experience and management of pain. Fatigue is the symptom most bothersome to patients (Conill et al., 1997). Patients may be reluctant to take opioid analgesics because of concern about worsening fatigue. Pharmacologic therapies that may combat fatigue include glucocorticoids and psychostimulants. Dexamethasone in doses of 2–20 mg per day may result in increased energy and feeling of well-being; however, the effect may wane after 4 to 6 weeks. Psychostimulants, such as methylphenidate (Ritalin), increase energy as well as combat opioid-induced sedation. Starting doses of methylphenidate are 2.5–5 mg dosed in the early morning and midday with dose titration until maximal effect is observed. Methylphenidate can be used safely even in debilitated patients and older adults. Side effects are rare but include insomnia, anxiety, and tremulousness, with tachycardia, arrhythmias, and cardiac ischemia occurring even less frequently.

Noncancer Pain and Symptom Management at the End of Life

End-Stage Heart and Lung Disease

Patients dying of end-stage heart and lung disease often fear and experience respiratory symptoms in addition to pain. The management of dyspnea (and other distressing nonpain symptoms) relies on many of the same principles described for pain management. Accurate assessment relies on asking patients about their symptoms. Dyspnea, nausea, and fatigue are subjective symptoms that are best addressed by asking the patient. Efforts to identify the underlying cause of dyspnea can guide management. For example, bronchospasm can be treated with inhaled bronchodilators and pulmonary edema with diuretics. When the underlying cause of dyspnea is not amenable to treatment or if such treatment is not consistent with the overall goals of care, opioids are the mainstay of therapy. The general principles of opioid use outlined for pain (see

TABLE 11.1 Treatment of Specific Cancer Pain Syndromes and Associated Symptoms

Syndrome	Drugs	Dose range	Comments
Tumor-associated inflammation or infiltration	Corticosteroids Prednisone Decadron	20–80 mg/day 2–16 mg/day	Monitor for side effects with long-term use. May also improve appetite, energy, sense of well-being.
	NSAIDS Ibuprofen	600–800 mg tid–qid	Use with caution in patients with hepatic or renal dysfunction. Consider COX-2 inhibitors for patients at increased risk for bleeding.
Bone metastases	Pamidronate NSAIDS	60–90 mg iv q 2–4 wks	Analgesic effect may take 2 weeks to occur.
Small-bowel obstruction	Octreotide	150–600 mcg/day sc	Cost is substantial.
Fatigue	Psychostimulants Methylphenidate Dextroamphetamine	2.5–10 mg q AM & q Noon 5–10 mg q AM & q Noon	Rare side effects include insomnia, tremor, tachycardia, hypertension. Often controlled with dose adjustment.

chapter 6) also apply to the management of dyspnea, including scheduled dosing of long-acting opioids with short-acting opioids available for
episodic symptoms. Starting doses for an opioid-naïve patient are morphine 5–10 mg given orally or 2–5 mg intravenously (or equivalent doses
of an alternate opioid), repeated until symptoms improve. For frail older
adults, a starting dose of 2.5 mg would be appropriate. Dosages for patients
already on opioid therapy should be titrated based on their previous opioid use and current symptoms. Benzodiazepines can be used to manage
the anxiety associated with dyspnea. Lorazepam 0.5–1 mg or diazepam
2–5 mg orally or parentally can be used safely in combination with a carefully titrated opioid regimen to control the distress associated with dyspnea. Oxygen may provide symptomatic relief whether or not a patient
is hypoxic. In patients who are not hypoxic this improvement may reflect
oxygen's activity at airway receptors or may simply represent a placebo
effect (Luce & Luce, 2001). In either case, a therapeutic trial is generally warranted. Oxygen should be titrated to symptom relief rather than
to a specific oxygen saturation. Similar to pain management, nonpharmacologic interventions, including relaxation techniques and guided
imagery, have an important role in the management of dyspnea (Jacox
et al., 1994). See chapter 3 for further discussion. Simple interventions,
such as a fan blowing across the patient or repositioning, may also provide symptomatic relief.

Dementia

Physical symptoms are common during the last year of life of patients with
dementia, with as many as 60% experiencing persistent pain (McCarthy
et al., 2000). Other common symptoms include constipation, anorexia,
and urinary incontinence. Patients with advanced dementia suffering from
acute medical complications (pneumonia, urosepsis, hip fracture) often
do not receive adequate symptom management compared with patients
with other terminal conditions despite a very poor prognosis for recovery
(Morrison & Siu, 2000). These acute medical complications should prompt
a discussion of goals of care, limiting burdensome interventions, and developing a plan for palliative or hospice care because these events typically
signal a prognosis measured in months. Explicit discussions with a patient's
proxy decision-maker should take place to determine the most appropriate management of acute illnesses in the setting of dementia. Often, treating the symptoms associated with the acute process in the patient's usual
setting (home or nursing home) rather than pursuing hospitalization and
more aggressive care is more consistent with the overall goals and medical situation.

Management of Pain and Symptoms During the Dying Process

Unrelieved pain in the final days of life can leave a patient's family and loved ones with a memory of a death filled with suffering rather than the peaceful end most people hope for. Ongoing attention to the basic principles of pain management can ensure adequate pain control until death. Even when a patient is very close to death, a thorough assessment should occur if the patient appears to be in pain. As many as half of patients experiencing pain in the last 48 hours of life experience a new pain that was not previously present that will require prompt assessment and management (Lynn et al., 1997). A careful history (often obtained from family and caregivers) and physical examination may reveal reversible causes of pain even at this late stage (such as bladder distention, rectal impaction, bedsores) for which simple interventions may provide significant relief. If pain has been well controlled throughout the course of the illness, it is unlikely to become more troublesome in the final stages. However, analgesic requirements in the last 48 hours of life can remain steady, increase, or decrease. Therefore, continued monitoring of pain and dose titration should occur throughout the dying process.

Patients near the end of life often become unable to swallow, and pain medications may need to be administered by a route other than oral. Table 11.2 gives examples of opioid formulations useful for managing pain during the dying process. Doses should be based on a patient's previous opioid use and current symptoms. Skilled use of equianalgesic conversions facilitates appropriate dosing as routes are changed to maintain adequate pain relief (see chapter 6). Morphine and oxycodone are available in concentrated elixirs that can be administered sublingually. Morphine and hydromorphone are available as rectal suppositories. A transdermal fentanyl patch can be substituted for long-acting oral opioids. Intravenous and subcutaneous opioids can be used if other routes are impractical. A continuous opioid infusion may be appropriate if a patient is requiring frequent doses (> every 1–2 hours) of opioids to provide steady pain relief. The starting infusion rate should be based on an approximation of the patient's recent hourly opioid requirements. Bolus doses can continue to be given as often as every 15–30 minutes as needed for signs of ongoing discomfort including grimacing, moaning, and restlessness. The continuous infusion rate can be increased (by approximately 50%) if the patient continues to require frequent bolus doses.

Other features of the dying process must be distinguished from pain and treated accordingly. Terminal delirium presents as agitation, restlessness, and moaning and may be interpreted as pain by family and other caregivers. Unfortunately, these symptoms may actually worsen with increased doses of opioids. Treatment consists of sedating psychotropics

TABLE 11.2 Examples of Useful Drugs for Pain and Symptom Management During the Dying Process

Drug	Formulation	Strength	Route	Typical dose range	Comments
Analgesics					
Morphine	Liquid (Roxanol) Suppository	20 mg/mL 5, 10, 20, 30 mg	SL PR	2.5–20 mg q 1–4 hr prn	Determine starting dose based on previous opioid use. Titrate dose and frequency until effective.
Oxycodone	Liquid (Oxyfast)	20 mg/mL	SL	5–20 mg q 1–4 hr prn	
Hydromorphone (Dilaudid)	Suppository	3 mg	PR	3–6 mg pr q 3 hr prn	
Fentanyl	Transdermal patch	25, 50, 75, 100 mcg/hr	TD	25–300 mcg q 72 hrs	Base initial dose on previous use of opioids. Slow onset of action, not effective for acute pain.
Anxiolytics and Psychotropics					
Lorazepam (Ativan) Diazepam (Valium)	Concentrated elixir Rectal gel	2 mg/mL 5 mg, 10 mg	SL PR	0.5–2.0 mg q 4–6 hrs prn 5–10 mg q 6 hrs prn	Benzodiazepines can cause paradoxical agitation in individual patients and may potentiate falls
Haloperidol (Haldol)	Concentrated elixir	2 mg/mL	SL	0.5–2.0 mg q 4–6 hrs prn	Risk of extrapyramidal side effects and QTc prolongation
Chlorpromazine (Thorazine)	Concentrated elixir Suppository	25 mg/mL 25 mg	SL PR	25–50 mg q 6 hrs prn	More sedating than haloperidol
Antisecretory					
Scopolamine Hyoscyamine (Levsin)	Patch Drops	1.25 mg 0.125 mg/mL	TD SL	1–3 patches q 3 days 0.125–0.250 mg q 4–8 hrs	Slower onset of action. Can be used in combination with scopolamine.

(haloperidol, chlorpromazine, droperidol) or benzodiazepines (lorazepam, diazepam) administered sublingually, rectally, or intravenously and titrated to effect and sedation. Typical dose ranges are described in Table 11.2. Benzodiazepines can cause a paradoxical reaction with increasing agitation; therefore, psychotropics should be tried first, especially in older adults.

Buildup of oropharyngeal secretions as death approaches may lead to gurgling or rattling with each breath. Caregivers may fear that the patient is choking or suffocating. The first intervention involves explaining these changes as an expected part of the dying process that are not usually distressing to the patient. If the symptom remains distressing after explanation, repositioning the patient may help. Anticholinergic agents also can be used to diminish production of secretions. Scopolamine can be administered transdermally, subcutaneously, or intravenously. Other options include hyoscyamine (Levsin) or atropine administered sublingually (see Table 11.2). Suctioning provides only very short-term relief and can be uncomfortable for patients. Though patients and families greatly fear suffering associated with the dying process, careful management of pain and other symptoms of the dying process can usually ensure a peaceful death.

Management of Existential and Spiritual Suffering

Management of pain and other physical symptoms is the first step in alleviating suffering. Prompt and effective management of the physical symptoms seen in advanced illness allows the patient, family, and health care team to focus on the spiritual and existential concerns (including how people find meaning, purpose, and value in life) that may also be contributing to suffering at the end of life. Patients may not be able to articulate these concerns and these issues may instead present as new or worsening physical symptoms. If existential or spiritual distress is not recognized as contributing to a patient's physical complaints, pharmacological efforts at symptom control may remain unsuccessful. Conversely, spirituality and faith represent a strength that can help reduce the suffering that many patients facing a serious illness experience. Therefore, identifying and exploring a patient's spiritual resources and personal strengths can help maximize the role of these inner resources in relieving physical and psychological suffering.

Persons can be spiritual without being religious. Religion refers to a social and culturally based system of beliefs, often practiced within a faith community. Spirituality refers to a more personal and individual sense of meaning and one's place in the universe. Specific spiritual crises brought on by a life-threatening illness include a sense of abandonment by God, feelings of punishment, and unfairness (Why is this happening to me?), a questioning of faith, and a desire for forgiveness. If these crises go unrecognized, efforts at relieving the associated suffering cannot be instituted. Health care providers need to be able to screen for unaddressed spiritual concerns and to take a spiritual history. Instruments can facilitate taking and documenting a spiritual history (Maugans, 1996). Screening questions to explore a person's spirituality include (Lo, Quill, & Tulsky, 1999; Quill, 2000):

- "Is faith or spirituality important to you in this illness?"
- "Are there any spiritual issues you are concerned about at this point?"
- "Has faith or spirituality been important to you at other times in your life?"
- "Would you like to explore religious or spiritual matters with someone?"
- "What is your understanding about what happens after you die?"
- "What are some of the things that give you a sense of hope?"
- "How have you tried to make sense of what is happening to you?"

Primary care providers can explore these issues fully, depending on their interest, comfort, and skill or involve other members of an interdisciplinary team including nurses, social workers, psychologists, and chaplains.

Facilitating a process of life review offers the patient the opportunity to reexamine his or her life and to make sense of it, to resolve old problems, to make amends, and to restore harmony with friends and relatives. Life review can help patients cope with physical symptoms and other aspects of a serious illness (Lohmann et al., 1998). Health care providers and others interacting with patients can facilitate this process by encouraging patients to share stories perhaps triggered by looking at old photos, letters, and other documents. Patients can be encouraged to record important memories in writing or on video- or audiotape as a legacy for current and future generations of family and friends. Asking patients open-ended questions may further facilitate life review and help identify tasks that can still be completed to give the patient a sense of accomplishment and life closure. Such tasks might include tidying legal and financial matters, discussing funeral and burial plans, closure of family and social relationships including expressions of regret, forgiveness, appreciation, and saying goodbye. Helpful questions to initiate discussion might include (Lo et al., 1999; Quill, 2000):

- "Given the severity of your illness, what is most important for you to achieve?"
- "What are your most important hopes?"

- "What are your biggest fears?"
- "As you look back on your life, what has given your life the most meaning?"
- "If you were to die sooner rather than later, what would be left undone?"
- "What do you want your loved ones to remember about you?"

Resources exist that provide just such practical guidance for patients and families facing a serious illness (Lynn & Harrold, 1999). Helping patients to address these tasks may allow them to regain a sense of control and feel less fear and powerlessness about the future, thus reducing their suffering.

Clinicians often feel uneasy when faced with patients who appear to be in denial about the seriousness of their medical condition or who prefer to avoid receiving detailed information about their disease status. Patients in denial may not even acknowledge having a serious illness despite having received the information. Other patients may acknowledge their diagnosis but prefer not to think about it or talk about it and appear to minimize the seriousness of the situation. Both of these strategies are coping mechanisms that can be adaptive in dealing with a distressing or overwhelming situation. Patients deserve to receive only as much information as they want or feel able to handle unless these coping strategies are resulting in dangerous or markedly inappropriate decision making. Clinicians should respect these individual differences and titrate information to the needs of the individual. Patients can be asked in a straightforward manner if they are the kind of person who wants all the information, both good and bad, or if they would rather have the details of their care discussed with their surrogate rather than with them. Providers should remain available and open to further discussion as patients and families come to terms with what they are facing. Over time, most people can accept more of the reality of a difficult situation at their own pace within in the context of trusting, supportive relationships with family, friends, and health care providers.

Addressing Family, Practical, and Financial Needs

Practical and financial concerns also contribute greatly to the suffering experienced by patients approaching the end of life. Patients often require substantial nursing and personal care to be able to continue to live at home. Transportation and homemaking needs, including shopping, cooking, cleaning and banking become greater as disease progresses. Most patients rely completely on family and friends for assistance. Older adults, especially women, may have limited local family or surviving friends to call upon for help. Reliable paid assistance is costly and often difficult to find. Significant economic hardship can result from a family member's advanced illness. As many as 30% of families with a seriously ill loved one will spend all or most of their life savings as well as experience loss of current income in providing for the care of the patient (Covinsky et al., 1994). Patients experience significant shame and suffering by feeling that they have become a financial burden to loved ones. Savings that were planned as a legacy to surviving family members may be spent on uncovered medical costs and are experienced as a significant loss by patients and families. Even if all of a patient's basic needs are met and financial resources are adequate, patients are often distressed by seeing the impact of their illness on their families and loved ones. The increasing dependency that accompanies advanced illness may bring about feelings of hopelessness and worthlessness. Patients may feel that their continued existence only burdens the family. Involvement of a social worker may help the family understand this concern and manage their financial situation more efficiently.

Members of the health care team should participate in assessing the caregiving needs and availability of appropriate caregivers. Even if there are willing family caregivers, unmet needs are still common and become greater as death approaches. Asking about such basic issues as food, safe housing, heat, and light is appropriate. Resources may be available in the community and should be explored. Church, school, work, and neighborhood members are often eager to offer help if they are approached and informed about what needs exist. All members of the health care team should be attentive to the presence of financial and caregiving stress among patients and families.

As noted above, facing a life-threatening illness affects not only the patient but also family and loved ones. Family members often experience altered roles and lifestyles, physical demands, uncertainty about the future, and fear of losing the patient to death. To fully meet the needs of the patient, the health care team should also assess the family's coping and needs for information and support. Social workers are specifically trained to assess and assist both patients and their families and should routinely be part of the health care team caring for patients with serious or progressive illnesses.

Of particular concern is the impact of the serious illness and ultimate death of an older adult on grandchildren and great-grandchildren. Families are often unsure of how to deal with children when faced with the terminal illness of a loved one. Members of the health care team should ask about children in the family, what they know about the illness, and what concerns they have about the children and where they can go for resources. Several books and brochures (McCue & Bonn, 1996) are available that can provide additional information and guidance for families with children.

SETTING-SPECIFIC CONSIDERATIONS

Home

Patients with progressive and life-threatening illnesses who wish to continue to live at home can often benefit from hospice services for both ongoing symptom management and psychosocial support. Eligibility for home hospice coverage under the Medicare Hospice Benefit (and most private insurers) requires a physician-certified prognosis of less than 6 months if the disease runs its normal course and palliative rather than curative treatment goals. Patients can continue in hospice if they survive longer than 6 months if they continue to meet eligibility criteria. Published clinical guidelines (Stuart et al., 1996) assist clinicians in estimating prognosis for the most common noncancer diagnoses.

Hospice services include

- Skilled nursing visits for physical assessment and management of pain and other symptoms
- Home health aide visits to assist with physical needs such as bathing, dressing, feeding
- Coverage for medications to control symptoms
- Short-term inpatient care for symptom management or respite for caregivers
- Social worker services to provide counseling for patients and family as well as preparing for death, including assisting with funeral arrangements, wills
- Pastoral care services to meet the spiritual needs of patients and families
- Volunteer services to assist patient and family
- Bereavement program for family for 1 year after the patient's death

A skilled hospice team provides ongoing assessment of pain and other physical symptoms to ensure that comfort is maintained until death. Ideally, the health care providers who have cared for the patient throughout the disease course interact actively with the hospice team in managing the final phase of the disease. Earlier referral to hospice allows the patient and family to build a relationship with the hospice team and to benefit maximally from the available services.

Nursing Home

Most patients who reside in a nursing home for more than a few months ultimately die in the facility or are transferred to an acute care hospital to die. Currently, 17% of all patients die in nursing homes and the number is growing. While many nursing home facilities have a low threshold for transferring residents to an acute care hospital for treatment of acute illnesses such as pneumonia, urosepsis, and dehydration, the symptoms of these acute medical complications can be effectively managed in the nursing home setting. However, inflexible physician orders and misinterpretation of nursing home regulations may result in inadequate use of medications to control pain, delirium, and agitation in dying patients. For example, escalating doses of psychotropics may be necessary to control intermittent delirium, agitation, and nausea of a dying patient, but use of these medications is restricted in the nursing home setting and such policies may prohibit appropriate efforts at symptom control. Nursing home staff may not be adequately trained in caring for dying patients and may not provide adequate palliative care. Education for staff on issues specific to the care of dying patients is essential. Educational programs for nursing home staff caring for dying patients are being developed (Steele et al., 1999). Use of hospice care in the nursing home setting can provide skilled symptom management and psychosocial support for patients as well as education and support for nursing home staff. Nursing home residents who are no longer relying on Medicare to cover the cost of nursing home care can receive all the benefits of the Medicare Hospice Benefit in the nursing home setting without any additional cost. Residents who are using their Medicare benefits to cover nursing home care would have to pay separately for the addition of hospice care.

Hospital

Most deaths occur in hospitals. However, widespread deficits in the care of dying patients in hospitals include poorly controlled pain and other physical symptoms, limited documentation of preferences for care, and continued intensive diagnostic interventions in the days before death (Field & Cassel, 1997). When death is finally recognized as inevitable, patients are often discharged because of financial incentives for the institution rather than because of patient or family wishes, frequently without home care or adequate supports (Field & Cassel, 1997). Many hospitals are developing systems to improve the care of dying patients. Palliative care consultation services represent one model for improving end-of-life care in the acute care setting. These interdisciplinary services can be used throughout the course of a serious illness to assist with symptom management, advanced care planning, and transitioning to home or other settings. Patients can be seen in the acute setting in consultation with the treating team and followed longitudinally. Individuals with expertise in palliative care can also help ICU staff and specialty services develop skill in attending to pain and symptom management while pursuing curative goals.

Office

Clinicians in the office setting need to recognize when patients might be approaching the end of life—often with the diagnosis of a new life-threatening illness or the progression of multiple chronic conditions. The process of determining a seriously ill patient's goals and values, as well as whom they would like to make decisions for them if they are unable to themselves, ideally begins in the office setting and continues throughout the disease course. Open-ended questions can facilitate a discussion of a patient's understanding and goals including (Lo et al., 1999; Quill, 2000):

- "What makes life worth living for you?"
- "What concerns you most about your illness?"
- "How is treatment going for you?"
- "Would there be any circumstances under which you would find life not worth living?"
- "What do you consider your quality of life to be like now?"
- "If with future progression of your disease you are not able to speak for yourself, who would be best able to represent your views and values?"

Once goals and values are explored and preferences established, they can be discussed with the patient's proxy and health care providers and entered into the medical record. The patient's advanced directive should be reviewed and updated on a periodic basis in response to changes in the patient's medical and life circumstances.

SUMMARY/RECOMMENDATIONS

1. Identify specific patient, family, and caregiver barriers to achieving effective pain and symptom management near the end of life.
2. Understand the principle of double effect as it applies to pain and symptom management at the end of life.
3. Recognize and assess the multiple pains and other physical symptoms experienced by patients with life-threatening illness.
4. Treat distressing symptoms that stem not only from the life-threatening diagnosis, but also from painful comorbid conditions and treatments.
5. Consider the role of antineoplastic therapies, especially radiation therapy, in patients with cancer pain.
6. Address comorbid symptoms such as fatigue and depression that may impact on the experience of pain.

7. Aggressively manage dyspnea in patients with end-stage heart and lung disease using the same principles that guide pain management.
8. Recognize that distressing physical symptoms occur commonly in patients with advanced dementia and actively assess and manage the symptoms identified.
9. Eliminate burdensome interventions and unnecessary medications for patients in the last days of life.
10. Recognize terminal agitation and treat it aggressively with sedating psychotropics and benzodiazepines.
11. Encourage patients to perform a process of life review, to leave a legacy for family and loved ones, and to achieve life closure.
12. Perform a spiritual history and screen for existential concerns and involve social workers, chaplains, and psychologists as appropriate.
13. If appropriate, consider hospice referral to optimize symptom management and offer psychosocial support to patients with terminal illness who hope to remain at home or who reside in a nursing home.
14. Explore patient goals and values in the office setting once the presence of a serious, life-threatening diagnosis is recognized.

CASE STUDIES

Case 1

Mrs. Richards is an 82-year-old woman with metastatic gastric cancer. She recently presented with worsening left hip pain requiring more frequent use of Percocet. After a bone scan revealed a femoral metastasis, she began a 10-day course of radiation therapy and was started on oxycontin and ibuprofen on a scheduled basis with oxycodone as needed for breakthrough pain. Despite careful titration of her opioid pain medications over the course of 7 days, Mrs. Richards continued to have poorly controlled pain and was bothered by sedation from the medications. A trial of methylphenidate was well tolerated and resulted in decreased sedation, an increased energy level, and improved mood. About a week after completing her radiation therapy, she noted decreasing need to use breakthrough pain medicine and her oxycontin does was lowered while maintaining excellent pain relief. Her pain remained well controlled on this regimen until she developed a gastric obstruction that prevented her from taking oral medications and resulted in an exacerbation of her pain. Her opioid regimen was transitioned to a transdermal fentanyl patch applied every 3 days with a sublingual oxycodone concentrated elixir as needed for breakthrough pain. This new regimen was well tolerated and provided adequate pain relief.

Discussion

This case highlights several points in the management of cancer pain. Tumor-directed therapy, specifically radiation therapy, can provide the most effective pain relief, though often with a lag time before taking effect. Psychostimulants can be used safely and effectively for opioid-induced sedation. Maintaining optimal pain relief as disease progresses requires anticipating probable events and complications, continuing ongoing symptom assessment, and adjusting pain regimen, including route of administration, as needed.

Case 2

Mr. Silver is a 71-year-old retired policeman who has lived with a dilated cardiomyopathy and inoperable coronary artery disease for 5 years. He experiences daily angina, dyspnea at night and with exertion, uncomfortable lower extremity edema, anxiety, mild confusion, and abdominal pain, despite a carefully titrated cardiac regimen, regular visits by the visiting nurse, and a salt- and fluid-restricted diet. He has had seven hospitalizations in the last 12 months for refractory angina and congestive heart failure. During his most recent hospitalization, a palliative care consultant met at length with Mr. Silver to discuss his current status, quality of life, physical and psychological symptoms, and expectations for the future. Together with his family and physicians, Mr. Silver decided to transition to care focused on comfort and maximizing his quality of life rather than continued efforts to prolong it. He continued on his regimen of oral cardiac medications but liberalized his diet and fluid restrictions. He took morphine sulfate 5 mg sublingually several times a day as needed for episodes of dyspnea or chest pain with good relief. He received a mild anxiolytic (Klonopin 0.5 mg bid) with relief of his baseline anxiety. He was discharged home with hospice services. Despite his increasing weakness and overall debility, his symptoms are generally better controlled and he is pleased to be at home.

Discussion

This case highlights that management of the multiple symptoms associated with the advanced stages of a chronic disease, such as heart failure, can improve quality of life. Clarifying patient and family goals, by the primary medical team or with the help of a palliative care consultant, guides the appropriate treatment and location of care. Opioids can be used to effectively manage both pain and dyspnea. Management of anxiety with benzodiazepines can also improve the patient's experience of dyspnea and pain. The often-feared risk of respiratory depression is extremely low with careful dose titration even in the setting of severe pulmonary or cardiac disease. Fear of causing side effects such as sedation, respiratory depression, or even death, does not justify withholding of these medications if needed for optimal symptom relief.

REFERENCES

American Geriatrics Society Ethics Committee (1998). The care of dying patients: A position statement. *JAGS, 43*, 577–578. (Also available online: <http://www.americangeriatrics.org/products/positionpapers/careofd.shtml>)

Baer, W., & Hanson, L. (2000). Families' perception of the added value of hospice in the nursing home. *JAGS, 48*, 879–882.

Bernabei, R., Gambassi, G., et al. (1998). Management of pain in elderly patients with cancer. *JAMA, 279*, 1877–1882.

Bruera, E., Kuehn, N., Miller, M., Selmser, P., & MacMillian, K. (1991). The Edmonton Symptom Assessment System (ESAS): A simple method for the assessment of palliative care patients. *Journal of Palliative Care, 7*, 6–9.

Cassell, E. (1982). The nature of suffering and the goals of medicine. *N Engl J Med, 306*, 639–645.

Cleeland, C., Gonin, R., Hatfield, A., et al. (1994). Pain and its treatment in outpatients with metastatic cancer. *N Engl J Med, 330*, 592–596.

Conill, C., Verger, E., Henriquez, I., et al. (1997). Symptom prevalence in the last week of life. *J Pain Symptom Manage, 14*, 328–331.

Covinsky, K. E., Goldman, L., et al. (1994). The impact of serious illness on patients' families. *JAMA, 272*, 1839–1844.

Field, M., & Cassel, C. (Eds.). (1997). Approaching death, improving care at the end of life. Committee on Care at the End of Life. *Institute of Medicine.* Washington, DC: National Academy Press.

Goodlin, S., Winzelberg, G., Teno, J., et al. (1998). Death in the hospital. *Arch Intern Med, 158*, 1570–1572.

Jacox, A., Carr, D., Payne, R., et al. (1994, March). *Management of cancer pain.* (Clinical Practice Guideline No. 9. AHCPR Publication No. 94-0592). Rockville, MD. Agency for Health Care Policy and Research, U.S. Department of Health and Human Services, Public Health Services.

Levenson, J., McCarthy, E., Lynn, J., Davis, R., & Phillips, R. (2000). The last six months of life for patients with congestive heart failure. *JAGS, 48,* S101–S109.

Lo, B., Quill, T., & Tulsky, J. (1999). Discussing palliative care with patients. *Annals of Internal Medicine, 130,* 744–749.

Lohmann, R., et al. (1998). Pain, coping, and psychological well-being in late life. *Eur J Pain, 2,* 43–52.

Luce, J. M., & Luce, J. A. (2001). Management of dyspnea in patients with far-advanced lung disease. *JAMA, 285,* 1331–1337.

Lynn, J., Ely, E. W., Zhong, Z., McNiff, K. L., Dawson, N. V., Connors, A., Desbiens, N. A., Claessens, M., & McCarthy, E. P. (2000). Living and dying with chronic obstructive pulmonary disease. *J Am Geriatr Soc, 48*(Suppl. 5), S91–S100.

Lynn, J., & Harrold, J. (1999). *Handbook for mortals: Guidance for people facing serious illness.* New York: Oxford University Press.

Lynn, J., Teno, J., et al. (1997). Perceptions by family members of the dying experience of older and seriously ill patients. *Ann Intern Med, 126,* 97–106.

Maugans, T. (1996). The SPIRITual history. *Arch Fam Med, 5,* 11–16.

McCarthy, E., Phillips, R., Zhong, Z., Drews, R., & Lynn, J. (2000). Dying with cancer: Patients' function, symptoms, and care preferences as death approaches. *JAGS, 48,* S110–S121.

McCue, K., & Bonn, R. (1996). How to help children through a parent's serious illness. New York: St. Martin's Press.

Morrison, R. S., & Siu, A. L. (2000). Survival in end-stage dementia following acute illness. *JAMA, 284*(1), 47–52.

Portenoy, R., Thaler, H., Kornblith, A., et al. (1994). The memorial symptom assessment scale: An instrument for the evaluation of symptom prevalence, characteristics and distress. *European Journal of Cancer, 30,* 1326–1336.

Quill, T. (2000). Initiating end-of-life discussions with seriously ill patients: Addressing the "elephant in the room." *JAMA, 284,* 2502–2507.

Steele, K., et al. (1999). Incorporating education on palliative care into the long-term care setting: National consensus conference on medical education for care near the end of life. *JAGS, 47,* 904–907.

Stuart, B., Alexander, C., et al. (1996). *Medical guidelines for determining prognosis in selected non-cancer diagnoses* (2nd ed.). Washington, DC: National Hospice and Palliative Care Organization.

Sulmasy, D. (1999). The rule of double effect: Clearing up the double talk. *Arch Intern Med, 159,* 545–550.

SUPPORT Principal Investigators. (1995). A controlled trial to improve care for seriously ill hospitalized patients: The study to understand prognoses and preferences for outcomes and risks of treatments (SUPPORT). *JAMA, 274,* 1591–1598.

Von Hoff, D., & Goodwin, A. (1998). Advances in the treatment of patients with pancreatic cancer: Improvement in symptoms and survival time. San Antonio Drug Development Team. *Br J Cancer, 78*(Suppl. 3), 9–13. Review.

The Ethics of Pain Management

12

Gary Kochersberger

This chapter examines the ethical issues that arise in the treatment of pain in older adults. A review of ethical theories and principles is first presented to provide a foundation for discussion of some of the dilemmas that may present to the clinician. Specific clinical situations that present ethical challenges are reviewed and a series of cases is presented that illustrate the more common ethical quandaries that physicians, nurses, and other health care providers will likely encounter. Where appropriate, discussion of legislation has been included that may complement or perhaps frustrate ethical behavior. For additional reading on ethical issues surrounding pain management, the reader is referred to a recent publication in *Pain Medicine* (2001), "Ethical Issues and Dilemmas Faced by Today's Pain Practitioner: A Bioethical Primer" (Volume 2, Number 2).

EVIDENCE AND PRINCIPLES FOR PRACTICE

Pain is necessary for our survival. It is a universal occurrence in organisms with integrated nervous systems. It causes us to immediately withdraw from potentially injurious stimuli, and through its experience we learn to avoid dangerous situations. But any benefit of pain is lost when the experience becomes chronic. Persistent pain appears to serve no purpose, but human evolution has not yet produced individuals incapable of such suffering. It is left to health care providers to deal with this symptom, and because pain is subjective we have only the reports of our patients and our observations of their behaviors to guide us in determining the extent of their suffering. It is this imprecision in our assessment that most often leads to ethical dilemmas in pain management.

This book is replete with references to the fact that pain is often unrecognized, underevaluated, or undertreated in the older adult. The actions (or inactions) of providers in dealing with this prevalent problem have their basis in training, experience and input from peers, other members of the health care team, and interaction with patients and patients' significant others. The alleviation of suffering is a fundamental responsibility of health care workers. So why is there a perception that such a poor job is being done in meeting this need, especially when it comes to treating persistent pain? Dealing exclusively with chronic illness without chance of cure can frustrate both patient and provider and is in opposition to the curative model of medical care that still predominates in our society (Fox, 1997). Accusations of provider undertreatment and patient overtreatment can occur. Allegations of patient malingering and drug-seeking may develop.

Ethical Guidelines

Ethical principles provide a touchstone with which providers negotiate medical knowledge, societal influences, and desires of patient and family to arrive at a pain treatment plan. Various clinical situations give rise to ethical dilemmas in the treatment of persistent pain. An understanding of basic ethical theory can help the practitioner to appropriately weigh treatment options. Autonomy, beneficence, nonmaleficence, and justice remain fundamental concepts in bioethics review practiced in this country. These principles apply equally to the treatment of pain. For well over half of the twentieth century, paternalism dictated which treatments physicians prescribed for their patients. Over time patients became more assertive and physicians and other health care providers more open to patients' involvement in medical decision-making. Medical information, particularly that available on the Internet, is widely consumed now and has empowered patients to participate in and challenge the care being proffered.

Patients are empowered, through the principle of *autonomy* and through the process of informed consent, to accept or reject treatments offered by their health care provider. To participate in this process the patient must possess decision-making capacity—that is, they must understand their treatment options, weigh the risks and benefits of those options, and communicate their choices. Decisions should be made independently, but the true autonomy of the suffering patient seeking relief from pain may always be questioned. As will be discussed later, this has particular significance when considering agreements, formalized as "pain contracts," between patients and their health care providers.

Another significant impediment to promoting autonomy in older adults is the high prevalence of cognitive impairment in this population. When confronted with a demented or delirious patient in pain, the health care provider must work with a representative of the patient who will provide substituted judgment in reviewing treatment options. The goals of pain treatment are not typically affected by cognitive status, but a risk-benefit analysis of optional interventions will often be affected by an individual's unique set of values. The ideal surrogate decision-maker is one whom the patient has especially appointed for this purpose and in whom the patient has confided his or her health care wishes and personal values. As an example, this health care proxy may be able to offer guidance as to whether increased sedation or worsened cognition would be an acceptable trade-off for the patient's being 100% pain free at all times.

While patients or their surrogates may decide to accept or reject care suggested by the physician, it is not their right to dictate specific treatment. It is in this realm of pain management that the patient-physician relationship is often strained. A patient with a history of persistent pain may express unhappiness with treatment and demand stronger medication. Physicians may learn early on to assume a defensive posture when so confronted. Often they have received their training in large city hospitals and had, as their outpatient experience, service to patients who are often indigent and at high risk of substance abuse. Young physicians may be preyed upon by opioid-seeking patients and not surprisingly, these physicians may develop a defensive posture (Taverner, Dodding, & White, 2000). The physician needs to overcome this bias in order to maintain objectivity and exercise beneficence. *Beneficence* is the state or quality of being kind, charitable, and beneficial.

Gaining personal satisfaction through exercising beneficence is the reason many individuals choose to go into the health care profession. Clearly, the alleviation of pain and suffering is beneficent and a desired goal of the provider-patient relationship. But health care providers are also taught first to do no harm, *primum non nocere*, and here again providers often become uncomfortable when treating pain. The cure of a disease will lead to an alleviation of associated symptoms, but palliation is not cure. Interventions identified as palliative most often have no ameliorating effect on the underlying condition responsible for the symptoms that are being treated.

In treating pain, these interventions may, in fact, further compromise homeostatic reserve and hasten the progress of the disease responsible for the target symptoms. Pain medication can cause renal or liver damage, induce gastrointestinal hemorrhage, impair cognition, exacerbate depression, and lead to falls. In extreme cases it can cause respiratory depression and death. To alleviate suffering, the principle of *nonmaleficence* may need to be interpreted loosely and balanced with the beneficence of the act that led to the desired outcome. Beauchamp and Childress (1994) describe rules of beneficence as presenting positive requirements of action, not needing to be obeyed impartially, and rarely providing reasons for legal punishment. In contrast, nonmaleficence establishes negative prohibitions of action that must be obeyed impartially for all persons. Nonmaleficence is reinforced by legal prohibitions of certain conduct. Intentionally causing the death of a patient is an extreme case of maleficence; yet some will argue that assisted suicide, when it relieves unremitting suffering, is a just act.

Various theories are employed in arguing ethical dilemmas, such as the one presented by assisted suicide. Those believing that the outcome of a particular act determines its moral value subscribe to utilitarianism. Under this theory, no act is good or bad in itself; each affected party is given equal weight and the action chosen should be based on its intended consequences and result in the greatest good. Jeremy Bentham and John Stuart Mill were early nineteenth-century philosophers and champions of utilitarianism. Bentham held that actions were right if they tended to produce the greatest happiness for the greatest number of people. He equated happiness with pleasure, and in the context of pain management his philosophy would support interventions that resulted in pain-free states regardless of the action taken. The only caveat would be that any other consequences of the pain-reducing intervention were not of such significance so as to overshadow the original intent.

Utilitarianism contrasts sharply with another major theory frequently referred to in ethical analysis. In the late 1800s, Immanuel Kant was the first great philosopher to define principles of deontology (Greek *deon*, "duty," and *logos*, "science"). In deontological ethics, an action is considered morally good because of some characteristic of the action itself, not because its end result is good. Clearly, under this principle, intentionally assisting in a suicide could never be justified despite the alleviation of extreme suffering. Similarly, the prescribing of increasing doses of opioids to a terminally ill patient, while effective in relieving pain, would be suspect if it caused respiratory depression and hastened death.

In evaluating cases presenting ethical dilemmas, classic theory is complemented by an examination of paradigmatic clinical/legal cases, such as the Quinlan, Cruzan, and Quill cases. These precedents allow the clinician to examine similarities with real-time cases he is confronted with. Rather than going from the general to the specific in deducing decisions with traditional ethical theory, this practical case-based approach allows for concrete comparisons with similar cases that have already undergone rigorous review. The weakness in this approach is found in the nuances evident in each new situation that arises—certain factors leading to recommendations may be preferentially weighted more heavily than others. Dramatic ethical and medicolegal cases have had the added effect of prompting people to think about and discuss their own preferences related to medical interventions.

Ethical and Legal Considerations Pertaining to Pain Treatment

Both Bentham and Kant survived into their 80s, which was no mean feat in the early nineteenth century. They suffered from various infirmities in their later years and no doubt received limited benefit from the health care profession of that era. What they did have access to were opioid-containing tonics. Preparations such as laudanum were readily available to the consumer with or without prescription. In 1914, the Harrison Act was passed by congress and effectively removed higher potency opioids, including morphine, from over-the-counter distribution and placed the first of many restrictions on the prescribing powers of physicians. In denying addicts supplies of opioids previously available through physicians' offices, this act is credited with the creation of much of the illegal trade of opioids.

Many believe that regulation and the surveillance of prescribing patterns of individual practitioners have had a chilling effect on the adequate treatment of pain. In 1984 Congress gave the Drug Enforcement Agency's Office of Diversion Control discretionary power to revoke a physician's registration to prescribe controlled medications. This legislation enabled the government to invalidate this registration if a physician commits "such acts as would render his registration . . . inconsistent with the public interest." Before 1984, the agency could revoke a physician's registration for only three reasons: if he had falsified a prescription; was convicted of a felony relating to controlled substances; or had his state medical license revoked, denied, or suspended. With the passage of the act, enforcers were given increased discretion in reviewing prescribing concerns, and prescribing that was determined to be against the "public interest" could be used as prima facie evidence of diversion.

Over the past two decades cases have appeared in which physicians have lost their licenses because of prescribing patterns determined to be against the "public interest." There have been, and will continue to be, practitioners who misuse their opioid prescribing powers, but some of those prosecuted were specialists in pain management, whose vindication required considerable time and legal expense. Although the physicians who actually lost their licenses were few, a ripple effect altered prescribing habits of many others, at times leaving patients lacking effective pain control.

It is not only physicians who are affected by federal and state laws, but also nurses who are held to increasingly stringent scrutiny of their documentation of opioid medication administration in hospitals and nursing homes. Pharmacists also play a critical role in drug distribution, acting as gatekeepers who are obliged to determine whether the opioids they are dispensing have a legitimate purpose. A study by Joranson (Joranson & Gilson, 2001) of the University of Wisconsin Pain and Policy Study Group (www.medsch.wisc.edu/painpolicy) suggests that the pharmacist could prove to be a weak link in getting pain medication to the patient in need. Surveys have shown that pharmacies often do not stock morphine and other opioids. A third of pharmacists expressed that they would discourage the use of opioids for the treatment of persistent nonmalignant pain, and a similar number reported that it was illegal to prescribe opioids to a patient with persistent pain and a history of drug addiction and that such an activity should be investigated. It was the authors' conclusion that pharmacists' confusion over state and federal regulations and the accepted use of opioids in different clinical situations could impede the delivery of pain medication to patients in need (Joranson & Gilson, 2001).

Fortunately, in recent years there has also been an increased appreciation among health care providers that pain is often undertreated and that all modalities, including opioid medication, need to be available to the treating provider. In fact, physicians have now been disciplined by medical boards for "grossly undertreating" pain, and in North Carolina and Texas, multimillion-dollar settlements have resulted from suits brought against nursing homes that failed to recognize pain in their residents and offer appropriate treatment. Empirical research into pain and the publication of pain management guidelines, such as those of the American Geriatrics Society (AGS Panel, 1998), have led to greater acceptance of opioids used continuously and safely. Many states have now come forward with their own legislative initiatives to balance aspects of DEA regulation some consider draconian. These laws protect physicians from prosecution by state and local law-enforcement agencies for overprescribing analgesics as long as the medications are needed to treat pain caused by medical disorders. Recently, however, Congress has considered new legislation, The Pain Relief Promotion Act, which many providers fear could have a chilling effect on opioid prescription at the end of life. As originally proposed, this bill has as its basis the rule of double effect.

The Rule of Double Effect

In the use of opioid medication for treatment of persistent pain, side effects such as impaired consciousness and hypoxia occur rarely. Persistent pain management typically involves lower doses and slow titration of opioids that allow for the development of tolerance to these untoward effects.

Higher doses prescribed over shorter periods of time have the potential for causing significant sedation and occasionally respiratory depression and even death.

It is this latter scenario that relates to the concept of "double effect," where an unintended consequence (death) occurs as the result of pursuing a beneficial outcome for the patient (pain relief). The rule of double effect has its origins in thirteenth-century theology. As applied to end-of-life care, it requires that the act not be morally wrong (e.g., intended to kill an innocent person). The prescriber must believe that certain actions are absolutely morally prohibited, or at least that consequences are not the sole determinants of the morality of an action.

The intention must be to do good, even if the undesirable/unintended outcome is not, and the bad effect (death) must not be a means to the good effect (pain relief). Although recent interest in the rule of double effect has been prompted by discussions of physician-assisted suicide, the rule applies to other less dramatic, everyday clinical situations. Each time a physician prescribes a medication, there comes with it a risk of unintended consequences—an allergic reaction to an antibiotic, renal impairment from NSAIDs prescribed for degenerative joint disease pain. Providers may or may not be aware of all the possible consequences of their actions, but if their intent is good, the acts are considered morally just. Under this rule, intentionally killing a patient to end his suffering is never justifiable. But it is the definition of intent that has led to controversy as this rule relates to assisted suicide. Some have suggested that a physician may prescribe a potentially lethal dose of medication to ease the patient's mind by providing a potential escape from suffering. The physician hopes or expects that other measures to alleviate suffering will be successful and that the prescription will not actually be used for lethal purpose. Regardless of the intent of the physician in this case, the patient's intent—to commit suicide with the prescribed lethal dose—stretches the applicability of the rule (Sulmasy & Pellegrino, 1999).

Recently, the United States Congress, in response to individual state initiatives on physician-assisted suicide, as well as the aforementioned legislation on opioid prescribing, has considered the Pain Relief Promotion Act. This legislation is generally based on the rule of double effect but its critics believe the title is malapropos (Angell, 1999). It states that physicians have the right "to dispense or distribute certain controlled substances for the purpose of relieving pain and discomfort even if it increases the risk of death." It goes on to forbid the "intentional dispensing, distributing, or administering of a controlled substance for the purpose of causing death or assisting another person in causing death." It is this latter section that gives pause to practitioners who have long dispensed opioids for pain relief without having to worry about the unintended consequences of their administration. This proposed legislation, actively supported by right-to-life groups and the American Medical Association, would give more attention to the perceived intent of physicians. Medical ethicist Arthur L. Caplan appeared before the Senate Judiciary Committee considering this legislation and testified that "Physicians and nurses may not always fully understand what the law permits or does not, but when the issue requires an assessment of intent in an area as fraught with nuances and pitfalls as end of life care then I believe that this legislation will scare many physicians and nurses and administrators into inaction in the face of pain" (Orentlicher & Caplan, 2000, p. 257).

The Use of Placebo Medication

As has been demonstrated in countless drug studies, placebo medication can produce a significant clinical response. Placebos are capable of reducing pain through a poorly understood but likely complicated interplay of expectancy and suggestibility. Factors such as confidence in the anticipated treatment and confidence in the prescriber are also important determinants of the magnitude of the placebo effect. Our knowledge of the impact of placebos and purported mechanisms of action comes largely from observations in randomized controlled trials.

A placebo is an inert substance or a subtherapeutic dose of a medication that has no remedial value and is deliberately prescribed for its psychological benefit. Prior to the past decade, placebos were routinely administered to patients and sometimes given exotic Latin names to strengthen the deception. With a few notable exceptions, the practice of medicine prior to the twentieth century dealt exclusively with the prescription of various placebo concoctions. In more recent years, the prescription of these substances was justified on the basis that they served a diagnostic and therapeutic role. A response to placebo medication could be helpful to the practitioner in distinguishing between physical and functional conditions. It could reveal malingering behavior or be used to prove to a patient that a condition was psychologically based. More often, placebos were prescribed to patients deemed to be drug seekers or hypochondriacs when the physician felt justified in appeasing patients' need for medication with an agent without potential for addiction or other harm. These all appear to be reasonable justifications, many consistent with utilitarian ethical theory, so why is the use of placebos condemned by bioethicists?

The problem with placebos is not in their effectiveness or the justification in their administration, but in the deception accompanying their use. Such deception undermines the relationship between the physician who prescribes the placebo, the nurse who administers it, and the patient who receives it. Many professional health care organizations have taken a stand against the use of placebos. An example is the American Society of Pain Management Nurses (ASPMN) that has taken the stand that placebos should not be used by any route of administration in the assessment or management of pain in any patient regardless of age or diagnosis. They hold that inappropriate placebo use is one of many ways that pain may be undertreated as well as erroneously assessed. In its position paper on placebo use, ASPMN (1998) cites the ethical tenets of the American Nurses Association that include truth telling, fidelity, trust, and respectful care, all of which are challenged when a placebo is administered to a patient without his or her knowledge. Nonetheless, it is difficult to ignore the fact that 35% to 70% of patients may respond to placebos with symptom reduction.

Largely anecdotal research has suggested that patients may still benefit when the placebo's identity is revealed and such openness could ameliorate ethical concerns. The *New York Times Magazine* examined the placebo phenomena in depth (Talbot, 2000) and queried, "what if (physicians) started thinking of placebos as a way of bridging the gap between the magnificent but sometimes cold efficiency of modern medicine and the unproven but evidently comforting remedies prescribed by homeopaths and herbalists?" (p. 24). The advent of nontraditional and complementary medical practice has indeed provided another opportunity to prescribe or recommend interventions that may be viewed by the practitioner as ineffective but that the patient may be totally committed to. In such cases it is still incumbent upon physicians to share their views of the intervention with the patient even if it may result in a diminution of any placebo effect.

Pain Medication Contracts

Health care providers may view the use of placebos as a means to avoid or limit the prescription of pain medication they view as unnecessary or dangerous. Another attempt at curbing medication use, which may be more palatable to some but ethically dubious to others, is the writing of contracts to manage opioid prescription for persistent pain management. A physician may view a contract as a means of establishing conditions that will provide a basis for the therapeutic relationship with the patient. It can stimulate reflection by both parties on expectations and responsibilities, and its mere presence demonstrates that the decision to prescribe opioids for persistent pain was not made lightly. For physicians it may provide some solace, probably unjustified, that if there is an undesirable outcome from the opioid prescription, they will be protected from liability. Unfortunately, such contracts cannot be truly informed and guaranteed voluntary. A patient with persistent pain who is seeking relief of his symptoms may feel he has no alternative but to sign a contract. Perhaps the biggest downside of the opioid contract is the explicit loss of control experienced by the patient. The locus of control has already shifted away from the patient with persistent pain, and his or her feeling forced into a contract may add to feelings of hopelessness (Biller & Caudill, 1999).

Chronic Opioid Analgesic Therapy

Many providers will never prescribe opioid medication for persistent nonmalignant pain. The specter of the DEA and its state counterparts scrutinizing prescription writing doubtlessly contributes to this behavior, but a fear of maleficence—creating or aiding an addict—appears a more powerful deterrent. These concerns are probably unfounded in the vast majority of cases, and by not considering a class of medication for a group of patients, the provider may still be guilty of wrongdoing.

There are no statistics on the number of older adults who abuse opioids, but the number is likely very small. Fewer than 1% of patients enrolled in methadone treatment programs are 60 years of age or older and drug-related criminal offenses in this age group are extremely rare (Hanlon, Nurco, Kinlock, & Duszynski, 1990). Substance abuse rarely has its onset in advanced age and those with lifelong patterns of opioid misuse will be readily identifiable to most providers (Dhossche & Rubinstein, 1996). Studies of the population in general have not shown correlation between recent trends towards increased medical use of opioids and an increase in health consequences associated with opioid analgesic abuse (Joranson, Ryan, & Gilson, 2000). Concerns about the risk of opioid therapy center on the development of addiction, impairment of cognition, alterations in physical functioning, and depression. For the most part, these fears have not been substantiated in studies of patients with cancer and noncancer pain. For further discussion of opioid therapy, the reader is referred to chapter 6.

The chronic use of opioid medication may lead to tolerance, with increased doses required to achieve the same level of pain relief. Physical dependence is said to be present if sudden cessation of the opioid medication leads to withdrawal symptoms. This phenomenon can occur in individuals receiving chronic opioid pain medication, but such symptoms are generally mild. These characteristics of opioid usage (tolerance and physical dependence) do not imply the existence of substance abuse or psychological dependence. *DSM-IV* criteria for the diagnosis of drug abuse require recurrent, compulsive use in spite of negative effects on life roles, and use in hazardous situations or in spite of legal or relationship problems. The older patient with persistent pain may be more vulnerable to side effects of medications, including opioids, but is unlikely to develop a new onset substance abuse related to prescribed pain medication. Given the demonstrated efficacy and safety of opioid medications in treating persistent pain conditions, various organizations have developed clinical guidelines for their use. The American Pain Society (APS) and the American Academy of Pain Medicine (AAPM) have endorsed the use of opioids for persistent pain in a joint consensus statement (APS, 1996). Suggestions set forth to address specific concerns of health care providers include the following:

- Attention to patterns of prescription requests and the prescribing of opioids as part of an ongoing relationship between a patient and a health care provider can decrease the risk of diversion.
- Emphasis is placed on the promulgation of guidelines for chronic opioid therapy to standardize quality care, as well as to provide regulators with a means of distinguishing legitimate medical practice from questionable practice. This permits the provider to concentrate on investigative, educational, and disciplinary efforts, while not interfering with legitimate medical care.
- Opioids should not be prescribed in the absence of a complete assessment of the pain complaint. Consideration should be given to different treatment modalities, such as a formal pain rehabilitation program, the use of behavioral strategies, the use of noninvasive techniques, or the use of medications, depending on the physical and psychosocial impairment related to the pain. If a trial of opioids is selected, the physician should ensure that the patient or the patient's guardian is informed of the risks and benefits of opioid use and the conditions under which opioids will be prescribed. Some practitioners find a written agreement specifying these conditions to be useful.
- Review of treatment efficacy should occur periodically in order to assess the functional status of the patient, nature of the pain complaint, continued analgesia, opioid side effects, quality of life, and indications of medication misuse. Attention should be given to the possibility of a decrease in global function or quality of life as a result of opioid use.

This last guideline deserves further attention. The effect of opioids on the functional status of older adults, particularly on detailed tasks such as driving, has not been exhaustively studied. Does the physician prescribing opioid medication need to consider its potential impact on the safety of people other than the patient? Although epidemiological evidence suggests that nonalcohol substance abuse may be an important contributor to automobile accidents, studies of persistent pain sufferers taking opioids suggest that impairment of reaction times are likely due to the pain itself (Sjogren, Olsen, Thomsen, & Dalberg, 2000). One recent pilot study examined the driving abilities of chronic opioid users with driving simulator evaluation and other testing (Galski, Williams, & Ehle, 2000). The investigators noted some difficulties in following directions and impulsivity, but in general found no significant impairment in ability. There is increasing interest in the driving abilities of older adults, and the subpopulation of those using chronic opioid therapy deserves further study. For additional discussion of the effects of medications and pain itself on neuropsychological function, the reader is referred to chapter 10.

Prescription of Opioids for the Patient With a History of Substance Abuse

The APS guidelines for opioid usage also include the statement that the management of pain in patients with a history of addiction "requires special consideration, but does not necessarily contraindicate the use of opioids." This clinical situation understandably raises practitioner concerns about violating basic ethical tenets and causing more harm than good. Recent study of the increased use of opioids for the treatment of persistent nonmalignant pain has not provided evidence that this practice has contributed to increases in the health consequences of opioid analgesic abuse (Joranson et al., 2000). Nonetheless, studies of persistent pain clinics suggest that between one in ten and one in four of their patients meet diagnostic criteria for substance abuse, and workers attending compensation clinics have been found to have significant rates of opioid addiction (Chabal, Erjavec, Jacobson, Mariano, & Chaney, 1997). Data specific to older adults is lacking.

As has been pointed out by Portenoy, the specialties of addiction medicine and pain medicine have developed largely in isolation and this separation has "hurt patients, clinicians, investigators, and society as a whole. It has encouraged the undertreatment of patients with pain and contributed to the stigmatization of opioid therapy for pain management and addiction" (Portenoy, 1997). Studies of cancer patients and HIV patients have demonstrated that those individuals with a history of substance abuse are at great risk of having their pain undertreated.

Recommendations suggested by Pappagallo and Heinberg (1997) for managing such patients may be helpful in reducing risk of relapse; these include the following:

- The patient should be encouraged to join or increase involvement in a recovery program or in individual psychological care in order to garner support and develop and bolster relapse-prevention strategies.

- A behavioral contract would provide the patient with a clear definition of problematic use, misuse, and abuse behaviors.
- Close supervision should be provided by the physician, including frequent follow-up appointments and the use of only one prescribing physician and one dispensing pharmacy. Long-acting opioids will help avoid reinforcing/euphoria-generating properties of the opioids.

The provider should have a low threshold for referring such patients to pain specialists who are experienced in working with this subgroup of patients with substance-abuse history.

SETTING-SPECIFIC CONSIDERATIONS

The approach to the treatment of pain and the ethical issues that arise differ, depending upon the clinical setting. Among older adults living independently in the community, concerns over the impact of opioids on functional status and the development of addiction may arise. In the nursing home, questions about over- or undertreatment of pain and issues of substituted judgment will be more commonplace. The prevalence of pain in the nursing home is significant: 45–80%, with analgesia being provided to 40–50% (AGS Panel, 1998). The majority of nursing home residents suffer from some degree of cognitive impairment. What is needed to alleviate suffering and be beneficent is often viewed very differently by family members, the practitioner, and other members of the health care team. The placement of a loved one into a nursing home is often accompanied by great guilt, and this emotion can cloud a family member's objectivity in participating in medical decision making. The impact of dementia on pain assessment is discussed in chapter 2. It presents significant challenges to care providers who need to be as objective as possible but who are also obliged to give the patient any benefit of the doubt with regard to the existence of pain and suffering.

The need to rely on substituted judgment does not apply to nursing home residents only. Older adults entering the hospital have a significant chance of losing their decision-making ability. Studies have demonstrated that among this population, 25–60% will develop evidence of delirium during their acute stay. This has serious significance when one considers that the need for informed consent for medical intervention is never greater than during an acute illness. Pain is also commonplace during hospitalizations, and although it is typically transient, the same concerns about potential for undertreatment or overtreatment exist. Physicians and nurses are not only obligated to assess and treat pain, but also to educate patients on the fact that effective pain management will speed their recovery. Patients concerned about addiction or untoward effects of medication may decline analgesia. We know that older adults respond differently to different types of pain medication; the surgeon choosing to medicate his patients with meperidine may be precipitating more confusion and less effective pain control. There is an ethical imperative not only to treat pain effectively, but also to avoid harming the patient in the process.

SUMMARY/RECOMMENDATIONS

1. Ethical issues commonly arise in the treatment of pain in the older adult and are most often related to concerns of overtreatment, undertreatment, or untoward effects of the intervention.
2. The principles of autonomy, beneficence, and nonmaleficence guide the health care worker in assessing and treating pain. Ethical theories such as utilitarianism and deontology offer contrasting views of dilemmas presenting with end-of-life care, but clinical cases presenting ethical concerns are also evaluated in the context of historical paradigmatic cases that have previously undergone rigorous ethical and legal review.
3. Opioids have proven effectiveness in the management of acute and persistent pain, and yet their prescription remains associated with many ethical concerns. Physicians cannot be compelled to prescribe these medications, but their use in nonterminal care is supported by ethical principles and scientific study. Legislation on federal and state levels has attempted to regulate physician opioid-prescribing patterns. Concern exists that in their effort to control diversion and assisted suicide, legislators have created an atmosphere where decision making may be neither clinically nor ethically sound.
4. Persistent pain is common in the nursing home setting. The mental and physical dependency of nursing home residents makes it incumbent upon staff to be proficient in pain assessment and management. Arguably, the admission of a patient into any setting that cannot provide this expertise violates the fiduciary relationship between the patient, the physician, and the facility.
5. The prescribing of placebos for pain management is an ethically dubious practice. It is contrary to the basic ethical tenet of truth telling and threatens the health care worker's relationship with the patient. Various organizations of health care professionals have criticized this practice. Although possibly effective in individual cases, the writing of "pain contracts" to control opioid usage also violates patient trust and obfuscates the informed-consent process.

6. The rule of double effect is often cited as justification for increasing opioid doses for end-of-life pain control even though respiratory depression and death may be unintended consequences. Many argue that this rule is an oversimplification and the intent to alleviate suffering may blur with a less obvious intent to cause an earlier death to allow escape from suffering.

7. Patients with a history of substance abuse should not be summarily rejected from consideration for opioid pain control. Risks and benefits need to be carefully reviewed with the patient and quasipaternalistic interventions to monitor usage and effect may be employed if agreed to by the patient.

8. The health care worker's moral imperative to alleviate suffering should give rise to beneficent treatment choices for the patient in pain. The practitioner must ensure that these choices are consistent with societal values and laws, but it is ultimately left to patients (or surrogates) to decide if the proposed action is consistent with their values.

CASE STUDIES

Case 1

Opioid administration for persistent, nonmalignant pain

Mrs. Johnson is a 72-year-old patient with a medical history of degenerative joint disease that has affected her knees and shoulders. She also has a history of peptic ulcer disease that became manifest during treatment with nonsteroidal anti-inflammatory medication. As a result, she was initially prescribed acetaminophen with codeine and was subsequently advanced to oxycodone. Her physician of 20 years retired and her new physician is presented with a request to refill a prescription for the six oxycodone per day she is taking. Her new physician refuses to write the prescription, informing her that he fears she has become addicted to opioids. He expresses particular concern over her continuing to drive while on this medication and believes that she is not only placing herself at risk but also others on the road with her. He asks her about her lifelong response to pain and shares with her that he had just seen a man in the office with similar arthritic symptoms who was doing very well without having to resort to using opioids.

Discussion

This patient's treatment options are limited and the provider must weigh the risks of alternative treatments. Mrs. Johnson's driving is cited as a special concern for her physician, and although the judicious use of opioids is not an absolute prohibition, these safety concerns need to be reviewed with her. The patient's right of autonomy must be balanced with that of the physician's. The right to refuse unwanted interventions is well established, but is different than the right of patients to receive any intervention they request. Physicians may contend that they are exercising their autonomy, but unless there are clear challenges to personal religious or moral beliefs (as with a Catholic physician who will not perform abortions), physicians' decisions to deny requested treatment should be supported by expert opinion.

Many practitioners still hold to a belief that opioids should only be utilized for acute pain and for finite periods of time. As evidenced in this chapter and elsewhere in this book, Mrs. Johnson's use of opioid analgesia can be considered consistent with the standard of care for persistent pain management. The stability of her symptoms and the opioid usage that allows her to maintain functional independence speak against addiction. A change in her established treatment regimen must, like every medical decision, be based on a careful analysis of benefits and risks for the patient. If there is evidence of neurologic or psychological dysfunction such as sedation, decreased concentration, or impaired ability to drive, her physician's case against prescribing opioids is certainly strengthened. But this evidence should be found in his interview and examination of Mrs. Johnson and not be based on any preconception. His questions regarding her prior pain threshold and his comparison of her with a male patient with similar pain raise concerns of underlying gender bias, which has been associated with a discounting of chest pain symptoms in women (Schulman, Berlin, & Harless, 1999).

Mrs. Johnson's physician should explore with her the potential risks and benefits of opioid therapy for her pain. Her new physician has the right (actually the obligation) to explore other potentially more effective pain treatment modalities that may not have been tried previously or may not have been available at the time she was prescribed the oxycodone.

Case 2

*The cognitively impaired older adult in need of pain medication—
substituted judgment*

> Mrs. Smith is an 84-year-old nursing home resident with end-stage
> dementia who has recently developed a swallowing disorder. Her other
> medical history is remarkable for degenerative joint disease and osteo-
> porosis with compression fractures. Despite a perception on the part
> of nursing staff that she appears comfortable, her family is request-
> ing increasing doses of opioid pain medication. "How can she possi-
> bly be comfortable?" her adult children question, pointing out her
> bedridden status and her deformity from longstanding osteoporosis
> and advancing neurologic disease. They also relate that their mother
> was an active person who "would never want to live like this." To them,
> mere existence in the state she is in constitutes suffering for her.

Discussion

Twenty percent of Americans over the age of 80 suffer from dementing
illness. In the nursing home population, this number reaches 70%.
Dementia affects patients' clinical expression of pain, as well as their ability to participate in pain management. Mrs. Smith's dementia has left her
unable to comprehend the benefits and risks of medical interventions and
to express her wishes freely regarding such treatments. There is, prima
facie, an obligation to treat pain when it exists. Individuals receiving palliative care may choose to endure some pain to maintain sentience and
cognition, which may suffer with increased doses of opioids, but is this
ever a desired option for the individual who has lost the ability to perceive
and communicate?

  In the case presented, this patient is incapable of offering any real-time
guidance to the health care team regarding her wishes. In such cases the
relief of pain should always be the default goal of treatment. Mrs. Smith's
children's surrogate role has gone beyond medical decision makers to
advocate for a particular course of treatment for their mother—increased
doses of opioid medication. As has already been discussed, practitioners
can claim professional autonomy and not feel compelled to provide care
they believe is not indicated or is substandard. An exploration of what
Mrs. Smith's children's goals are is in order. Their comment that their
mother "would never want to live like this" suggests that pain relief alone
may not be the ultimate objective of the request to increase her opioid
dosing. Opioids prescribed to relieve the patient's suffering from pain are

morally just and good medical practice, and to this end, her symptoms should be interpreted liberally. However, increased pain medication would not ordinarily be prescribed to address the possible suffering of psyche that the family finds deplorable.

In situations such as this, particularly in the nursing home setting, where multiple persons are involved in assessment and care delivery, it is sometimes difficult to maintain objectivity. In such situations it is helpful to invite someone from outside the treatment team to provide an unbiased assessment of the patient's symptoms and treatment plan. Fresh insight could help guide future management and allow the team to reach compromise with the family.

Case 3

Use of placebo medication

> Mr. Felcher is a 74-year-old resident of a nursing home with long-standing opioid usage for hip pain, which followed failure of a hip replacement for degenerative joint disease. The nursing staff has relayed to the physician the patient's increasing demands for pain medication. The physician has been hesitant to increase opioid treatment based on his belief that there is no apparent evidence of worsening disease to explain increasing symptoms. He has shared his assessment with the patient's family, who in turn request that a placebo be prescribed, citing concerns that Mr. Felcher is becoming addicted to opioids. The nursing staff, who have followed the patient serially with pain assessments, believe he is suffering and express discomfort with the placebo prescription.

Discussion

The resident of a nursing home is dependent upon the facility staff to assess his symptoms, weigh their severity, and determine whether his practitioner needs to be contacted to initiate or modify a treatment regimen. Persistent pain is found in a majority of nursing home residents and the quality of its assessment is as varied as the facilities themselves. The undertreatment of pain in this setting has led to multimillion-dollar settlements. Mr. Felcher's nurses are wise in taking his symptoms seriously.

As detailed earlier in this chapter, the use of placebo medication has received mostly condemnation by pain experts and organizations. The prescription of placebo in the case presented understandably has caused angst among the patient's caregivers with its violation of nursing's ethical tenets of truth telling, fidelity, trust, and respectful care. The nursing staff should not feel compelled to participate with the physicians in the deception of Mr. Felcher. In such situations, nurses should apprise the physician of their discomfort with this intervention. They would be morally justified (and supported by their profession) to refuse to administer the placebo.

Nursing homes have an organizational structure that allows for review of medical care delivered. Many facilities have ethics committees to provide such case review. A situation such as this should be brought to the attention of the facility's director of nursing and medical director. It is incumbent upon them to review the patient's medical history and documentation of his symptoms and discuss with the attending physician the nurses' (and facility's) concerns regarding placebo use.

Case 4

Treatment of pain in terminal illness

> Mr. Vasquez was diagnosed with metastatic prostate cancer 4 years ago. He initially responded to hormonal therapy, but developed bony pain approximately 3 months ago. Localized radiation therapy was only minimally successful in alleviating his symptoms and he was enrolled in an outpatient hospice program. He was placed on sustained-release morphine twice per day and immediate-release morphine every 2 hours for breakthrough pain. His dose of morphine has been doubled three times over the past two weeks. Although his pain has become reasonably well-controlled, he spends most of the day sleeping. His wife appears satisfied with his treatment and the resultant control of his symptoms, but his sister has expressed concerns to the home-care nurse that he is being overmedicated and his death is being hastened.

Discussion

For Mr. Vasquez, his pain medication has been appropriately adjusted to alleviate his suffering. The higher dose of the opioid may shorten his life expectancy, but this is by no means certain. The positive effect of reducing or alleviating his suffering was considered of proportionately greater value than the suffering he would otherwise have to endure without opioid intervention.

In the absence of directives from the patient to pursue a different course of action (such as withholding pain medication to allow more time awake to interact with family), his providers are appropriately beneficent in their actions. The sister's comments should be taken seriously and her feelings further explored, preferably in the presence of the wife. The goals of his hospice program must be reviewed and the need to alleviate suffering emphasized. The sister's comments may reflect denial of the terminal nature of her brother's condition rather than an assault on his pain treatment per se.

Occasionally, the endpoint of pain management in such cases may blur with terminal sedation and challenge the double effect rule. Myoclonic movements in the moribund patient related to hyperosmolar states, hypercapnia, or opioids are at times interpreted by those tending the dying patient as an indication of unrelieved pain. Such reflex movements may be responded to with increasing doses of opioids or benzodiazepines. The good effect of these terminal interventions may be found in allaying the personal anguish of distraught survivors witnessing apparent pain, but hastening the already imminent death of the nonsentient patient would violate a strictly interpreted rule of double effect. For further discussion of issues surrounding the patient who is terminally ill, the reader is referred to chapter 11.

Case 5

Pain medication for the patient with prior history of opioid abuse

Mr. Crandall is a 65-year-old patient with a history of spinal stenosis, which has resulted in continuous lower back and leg pain. He has been tried on various analgesics and nonpharmacologic interventions, but continues to report his pain at a level of 8 out of 10. Because of prior unsuccessful laminectomies, he is not a candidate for future attempted surgical correction. He has lost weight and reports not sleeping well as a result of his persistent pain. His primary care provider has contemplated prescribing opioids for Mr. Crandall, but she is aware of his 20+ year past history of opioid abuse, including heroin addiction. Although he has been abstinent for 10 years, both the patient and his physicians express trepidation over advancing his pain medication regimen at this time even though his functional status could improve significantly with better pain relief.

Discussion

For a patient like Mr. Crandall, with an established history of opioid abuse, the risk of relapse is real and a decision to prescribe opioids for such a patient cannot be made lightly. His long period of abstinence perhaps suggests a better prognosis, but there exists a risk of substituting an old problem for his more recent affliction.

Guidelines for prescription of opioids in such situations were reviewed earlier in this chapter. Several of these interventions, particularly the use of behavioral contracts, represent a paternalistic approach to such patients. As described previously, such actions may challenge the health provider–recipient relationship and the suffering patient may think that his physicians don't trust him and feel coerced into an agreement to find relief. This patient's concerns about opioid use suggest that he could participate freely in an informed consent process and enter into a workable agreement with his physician for a trial of opioid therapy.

Fearing relapse, patients with a history of substance abuse may refuse to take opioids suggested by their providers. This refusal of therapy after a review of potential risks and benefits should certainly be respected and efforts should be made at optimizing nonopioid treatment for the patient. If the patient and the provider are willing to undertake a trial of opioid therapy, consideration should be given to referring to a pain specialist experienced in dealing with this clinical situation.

REFERENCES

American Geriatrics Society Panel on Chronic Pain in Older Persons. (1998). The management of chronic pain in older persons. *Journal of the American Geriatrics Society, 46*(5), 635–651.

American Pain Society. (1996). The use of opioids for the treatment of chronic pain: A consensus statement from the American Academy of Pain Medicine and the American Pain Society. [On-line]. http://www.ampainsoc.org/advocacy/opioids.htm

American Society of Pain Management Nurses. (1998). ASPMN position statement: Use of placebos for pain management. [On-line]. http://www.edu.org/PainLink/ placebo.html

Angell, M. (1999). Caring for the dying—congressional mischief. *New England Journal of Medicine, 341,* 1923–1925.

Beauchamp, T., & Childress, J. (1994). *Principles of biomedical ethics* (4th ed.). Oxford, England: Oxford University Press.

Biller, N., & Caudill, M. (1999). Commentary: Contracts, opioids, and the management of chronic nonmalignant pain. *Journal of Pain and Symptom Management, 17,* 144–145.

Chabal, C., Erjavec, M., Jacobson, L., Mariano, A., & Chaney, E. (1997). Prescription opiate abuse in persistent pain patients: Clinical criteria, incidence, and predictors. *Clinical Journal of Pain, 13*(2), 150–155.

Dhossche, D., & Rubinstein, J. (1996). Drug detection in a suburban psychiatric emergency room. *Annals of Clinical Psychiatry, 8*(2), 59–69.

Fox, E. (1997). Predominance of the curative models of medical care: A residual problem. *JAMA, 278*, 761–763.

Galski, T., Williams, J., & Ehle, H. (2000). Effects of opioids on driving ability. *J Pain Symptom Manage, 19*, 200–208.

Hanlon, T. E., Nurco, D. N., Kinlock, T. W., & Duszynski, K. R. (1990). Trends in criminal activity and drug use over an addiction career. *American Journal of Drug & Alcohol Abuse, 16*, 223–238.

Joranson, D., & Gilson, A. (2001). Pharmacist's knowledge of and attitudes toward opioid medications in relation to federal and state policies. *J Amer Pharm Assoc, 41*, 213–220.

Joranson, D., Ryan, K., & Gilson, A. (2000). Trends in medical use and abuse of opioid analgesics. *JAMA, 283*, 1710–1714.

Orentlicher, D., & Caplan, A. (2000). The Pain Relief Promotion Act of 1999: A serious threat to palliative care. *JAMA, 283*(2), 255–258.

Pappagallo, M., & Heinberg, L. (1997). Ethical issues in the management of chronic nonmalignant pain. *Seminars in Neurology, 17*(3), 203–211.

Portenoy, R. (1997). Pain management and chemical dependency: Evolving perspectives. *JAMA, 278*(7), 592–593.

Schulman, K., Berlin, J., & Harless, W. (1999). The effect of race and sex on physicians' recommendations for cardiac catheterization. *N Engl J Med, 340*, 618–626.

Sjogren, P., Olsen, A. K., Thomsen, A. B., & Dalberg, J. (2000). Neuropsychological performance in cancer patients: The role of oral opioids, pain and performance status. *Pain, 86*(3), 237–245.

Sulmasy, D., & Pellegrino, E. (1999). The rule of double effect: Clearing up the double talk [Commentary]. *Archives of Internal Medicine, 159*(6), 545–550.

Talbot, M. (2000, January). The placebo prescription. *New York Times Magazine*, pp. 21–30.

Taverner, D., Dodding, C. J., & White, J. M. (2000). Comparison of methods for teaching clinical skills in assessing and managing drug-seeking patients. *Medical Education, 34*(4), 285–291.

Educating Practitioners About Managing Pain in Older Adults

13

John G. Hennon and
Debra K. Weiner

It has practically become a cliché that undertreatment of pain is related to lack of education of health care professionals about pain management (American Pain Society, 1995; Max, 1990; McCaffery & Ferrell, 1997). The American Academy of Pain Medicine (AAPM) has recently issued a position statement emphasizing the need to educate medical students broadly about pain management early in their careers (Chang et al., 2000). Because management of persistent pain in older adults requires the combined expertise of a variety of health care professionals, pain-care provider education must be designed to reach not only physicians and physicians-in-training, but all critical members of the pain management team including nurses, nurse aides, pharmacists, and occupational and physical therapists. The purpose of this chapter is to serve as a guide for those who wish to design a pain education program for health care providers. Although a large body of literature exists describing the content of pain curricula for health care professionals, none exists specifically with regard to the population on which this book focuses, that is, older adults with persistent pain. Because of the lack of specific educational literature in this area, we draw from a wide variety of resources, including (1) literature on the management of cancer-associated pain, (2) literature on general educational principles for teaching adult learners and the relative efficacy of different educational models, (3) specific educational products on pain management, and (4) our own clinical experience in working with health care professionals who struggle to optimize pain management for the older adult persistent pain sufferer.

EVIDENCE AND PRINCIPLES FOR PRACTICE

Content of Pain Education Programs

Although a variety of pain education programs have been developed for different professional audiences, many contain overlapping elements. Education programs should teach knowledge, attitudes, and skills; correction of knowledge deficiencies alone may not lead to changes in attitudes and skills. Similarly, it is possible that attitudes and skills may improve disproportionately to changes in knowledge.

Knowledge

Each health care profession that treats pain patients brings a unique background, vocabulary, and set of interests to bear on a patient's problem. Even so, the assessment of the pain education needs of various health professions indicates that there are many common areas on which educational programs should focus. These include pain assessment, opioid addiction/dependence/tolerance, proper dosage of medications and dose conversion principles, pain physiology, and nonpharmacological techniques for relieving pain. The International Association for the Study of Pain's Task Force on Professional Education in Pain has proposed a core of common knowledge necessary to best serve the patient and to communicate across disciplinary lines (Fields, 1995). This basic knowledge includes

- Anatomy and Physiology
- Pharmacology of Pain Transmission and Modulation
- Pain Measurement in Humans
- Psychosocial Aspects of Pain
- General Principles of Pain Evaluation and Management
- Designing, Reporting, and Interpreting Clinical Trials of Treatments for Pain
- Drug Treatment I: Opioids
- Drug Treatment II: Antipyretic Analgesics, i.e., Nonsteroidals, Acetaminophen, and Phenazone Derivatives
- Drug Treatment III: Antidepressants, Anticonvulsants, and Miscellaneous Agents
- Physical Medicine and Rehabilitation
- Nonsurgical Peripherally Applied Neuroaugmentative and Counterirritation Techniques
- Surgical Approaches
- Nerve Blocks

- Psychiatric Evaluation and Treatment; Psychological Treatments (Behavioral Interventions)
- Multidisciplinary Pain Management
- Taxonomy of Pain Syndromes
- Low Back Pain
- Myofascial Pain
- Neuropathic Pain
- Headache
- Rheumatological Aspects of Pain
- Cancer Pain
- Postoperative Pain
- Compensation, Disability Assessment, Pain in the Workplace
- Orofacial Pain, Including Temporomandibular Disorders
- Animal Models of Pain, Ethics of Animal Experimentation
- Pain in Children
- Ethical Standards in Pain Management and Research

Attitudes

Based upon a comprehensive review of the literature and our clinical experience, we have identified a core set of persistent pain-related attitudes that all health care professionals who treat older adults with persistent pain should adopt. These include

1. Recognition that persistent pain is prevalent among older adults, but it is not a normal part of aging
2. Awareness of the heterogeneity of underlying disorders that contribute to persistent pain in older adults
3. Openness and awareness of the roles of interdisciplinary team members in the management of older adults with persistent pain
4. Awareness that opioid addiction is rare and should not influence the practitioner's decision to treat the older adult persistent-pain sufferer with opioid analgesics
5. Appreciation of gender and cultural differences in pain reporting
6. Understanding and appreciation of the need for the health care professional to play an active role in eliciting pain complaints from the older adult with persistent pain
7. Awareness that persistent pain is not curable, but that it is eminently treatable
8. Awareness that pain without identifiable organic pathology should not be equated with psychopathology, and that such pain still requires treatment

9. Awareness that pain self-report is reliable, even in many older adults with dementia
10. Awareness that severe dementia may make pain evaluation and management challenging, but that persistence, creativity, and careful observation are necessary in order to alleviate the suffering of this vulnerable population
11. Awareness of the need to routinely evaluate the older adult for pain in the primary-care setting
12. Awareness that comprehensive assessment is the key to effective management of persistent pain in the older adult

Skills

Though all health care professionals should have an appreciation of the core knowledge and attitudes outlined above, some will need to emphasize certain pain assessment and management skills more than others. For example, physicians should be very well versed in the performance of a physical examination geared toward the detection of myofascial pain and other musculoskeletal pathology, whereas this skill is not of critical importance for the pharmacist. The nurse aide, as the primary caregiver for the nursing home resident, should be extremely well versed in behavioral manifestations of pain (e.g., grimacing, rubbing, sighing) that may be exhibited during normal caregiving activities (e.g., A.M. care) because many nursing home residents may be unable to express their pain verbally. Other examples of unique, persistent-pain-related skills appropriate for different professional audiences are provided in Table 13.1.

How to Develop an Educational Program

A systematic way of developing formal courses, continuing-education workshops, or other educational interventions is often referred to as the instructional design or instructional systems development process. A variety of instructional design models have been created that emphasize different aspects of the process, but they are all based on theories of learning and are all oriented to determining what knowledge the students (adults or children) should gain as a result of their experience, and then deciding how the learning experience should be structured and presented in order to achieve this learning outcome. An influential instructional design model used by educators at all levels and for many subjects is the Dick and Carey model. This model includes the phases of analysis, design, development, implementation, and evaluation (Dick, Carey, & Carey, 2001). It can be

TABLE 13.1 Persistent Pain-related Assessment and Management Skills for Different Professional Audiences

Discipline of learners	Areas of skills emphasis
Primary care physicians and physician extenders	Prescription of analgesic medications at all four levels of the WHO ladder (WHO, 1996) Prescription of stimulant laxatives for the opioid user Medication costs and side effects, and how to appropriately counsel patients Specific history and physical examination techniques (e.g., assessment of pain using appropriate instruments, pain interference with ADLs, IADLs, AADLs, performance of musculoskeletal exam including evaluation of soft tissue abnormalities, mobility [gait and balance], depression, dementia) Psychiatric/behavioral manifestations of pain and their treatment When to refer to pain specialists, including alternative medicine practitioners Construction of differential diagnosis for causes of persistent generalized pain
Nurses	Comprehensive pain assessment (e.g., proper use of pain intensity scales, behavioral indicators of pain) Barrier identification and patient advocacy Use of analgesics and side effect management Nonpharmacological management techniques (e.g., massage, simple cognitive-behavioral techniques such as distraction and relaxation) Patient and family education
Nurse aides	Behavioral indicators of pain Techniques that encourage open communication regarding pain and the need for treatment Safe transfer techniques for the pain patient
Physical and occupational therapists	Behavioral indicators of pain Signs of depression that may interfere with rehabilitation Appropriate rehabilitation techniques for the older adult with persistent pain (including need to modify intensity of therapy) Application of appropriate outcome measures to determine success of treatment (chapter 5)
Pharmacists	In-depth knowledge of pharmacokinetics, pharmacodynamics, drug-drug and drug-disease interactions (chapter 6) Analgesics and other pain-alleviating medications on Beer's list (chapter 6; Beers, 1997)

used as a framework for developing instruction in pain management for any group of health professionals. The stages of the process are as follows:

1. *Assess needs to identify instructional goals*—Determine what the learners should *know* or *understand* after they have completed your instruction. This can be determined through such methods as observation of deficits in on-the-job skills or behaviors, formal educational needs assessments, and/or review of practice standards (such as the JCAHO Pain Management Standards), to name a few. A survey of a panel of experts may also be useful at this stage.

2. *Conduct instructional analysis*—Identify the skills, attitudes, and knowledge that should be included in the instruction. Determine what the learners should be able to *do* after they have completed your instruction. Instructional goals should be determined that relate to such elements as intellectual skills, verbal information, psychomotor skills, or attitudes.

3. *Analyze learners and contexts*—Learn as much as possible about the people being educated in order to design instruction that is appropriate. Determine their current skills, attitudes, and preferences, as well as the context in which they will be learning (individually, in a group, etc.) and especially the context in which they will be using what they learn (hospital, home care, nursing home, etc.).

4. *Write performance objectives*—This is an important step and is especially critical if an application for continuing-education credits will be submitted. These performance objectives are sometimes called *learning outcomes*, and should include statements of the specific skills to be learned, the conditions under which the skills will be performed, and the criteria used to assess successful learner performance.

5. *Develop assessment instruments*—Based on the performance objectives, develop assessment tools such as pretests and posttests to measure changes in knowledge or attitudes, and other tools that measure learners' abilities to perform the specified behaviors. These assessments should be both *learner-centered* and *criterion-referenced* (that is, linked to both the instructional goals and the learning outcomes).

6. *Develop instructional strategy*—Take into account learners' ability levels and type of learning outcome desired; determine preinstructional activities; format for presenting information and program content, amount and form of learner participation, assessment approach, and follow-through activities. Select media format for each component or subtopic of the program; determine appro-

priateness of such activities as group discussions, independent reading, case studies, lectures, computer simulations, worksheets, cooperative group projects, and so on.

7. *Develop and/or select instructional materials*—Either produce or select appropriate instructor's materials, learner's materials, and assessment materials. This may include printed, audiovisual, and/or computer-based information.

8. *Design and conduct the formative evaluation of instruction*—Either pretest the completed instructional program with a sample audience similar to the target audience, or gather data and information from participants in initial offerings (if the instruction is to be offered more than once) in order to continuously improve the program.

9. *Revise instruction*—Use evaluation data to review the performance objectives, the instructional strategy, and so on, and make changes in order to make the instruction more effective.

10. *Design and conduct summative evaluation*—Change in knowledge or attitudes may be easy to assess immediately following the educational program, but change in skills may not be. It may take several years before change in skills and improved patient outcomes are demonstrable following change in knowledge and attitudes (cf. Rogers, 1995). Nevertheless, efforts should be made to evaluate the efficacy of the educational program in order to determine if its objectives were met and if its impacts are great enough to warrant continuation.

Aside from determining instructional objectives, content, and formats, attention needs to be given to some practical issues of educational program administration. If the education is to be provided in an interactive in-person format, decisions need to be made about such things as *location* (Where and when will the program be held? Will there be a cost for using the facility? Will anyone need overnight accommodations?), *recruitment and/or program marketing* (How do I advertise the educational opportunity? How do I ensure that people attend the program? Will there be a tuition fee?), *hospitality* (If the program is longer than a half day, will a luncheon be provided? If so, who will provide the food? Will there be coffee breaks, snacks, etc.?), and *record-keeping* (Who will register attendees? Will continuing-education credits be offered? If so, who will submit the CE application, certify participation, and issue certificates? How will bills be paid for program expenses such as copies of instructional materials or instructors' fees?). For overviews of the continuing-education process and advice on developing, conducting, and evaluating effective continuing education programs, see Davis and Fox (1994), Green, et al. (1984), and Rosof and Felch (1992).

Additional Considerations

The preceding process can be used to design traditional classroom-style instruction, as well as instruction presented in alternative formats such as self-study materials, videotapes, teleconferences, or computer-based educational modules. Attention should be given to these modes of presentation during the "Develop instructional strategy" phase. The workshop or seminar format for continuing education of health professionals is familiar and often-used, but it is sometimes inconvenient for busy practitioners. Hence, alternative distance-learning methods using videotapes or computer-based modules should be considered in order to facilitate learner convenience. Also, it should be kept in mind that traditional continuing education workshops are generally rather ineffective in facilitating change in practice behavior. Strategies that appear to be more effective include community-based approaches such as academic detailing and opinion leaders, practice-based approaches such as reminders and patient-mediated strategies, and multiple interventions (Davis, 1998; Davis, Thomson, Oxman, & Haynes, 1995). Traditional workshops usually result in improvements in knowledge and attitudes; improvements in skills are more likely if the workshop contains some sort of hands-on activity in addition to didactic lectures. But other approaches should be considered in order to increase the likelihood that the learners will actually implement what they have learned with their patients. Current reviews of effective CE strategies include Davis et al. (1992, 1995) and Lewis (1998).

No matter what format is chosen, serious consideration should be given to designing educational programs for health practitioners in accordance with principles of adult learning preferences. There have been many efforts to redesign continuing education offerings along these lines. Most contemporary efforts are derived from the adult learning theory articulated by Malcolm Knowles (1980; Knowles, Holton, & Swanson, 1998) which is based on these principles:

1. Adults need to know why they should learn something.
2. Adults are self-directing and prefer to decide for themselves what they want to learn.
3. Adults connect their learning experiences with previous life experiences.
4. Adults become ready to learn something in order to deal with some real life situation.
5. Adults are task oriented in their learning.
6. Adults are motivated to learn mainly in response to internal factors.

In essence, adult learning theory shifts the locus from a teacher-centered model to a student-centered model of education. The role of the instructor changes from that of the expert imparting knowledge to that of the facilitator of individual learning. Instead of lectures, other more hands-on strategies, such as case studies, role playing, simulations, and self-evaluation, are more useful teaching techniques. There is as yet little empirical proof that Knowles's theory of andragogy is superior to education based on pedagogy. However, the fact that lectures to passive audiences (i.e., the pedagogical approach) have little effect on behavior change and on subsequent application of the information received in the lectures has led to the thought that greater attention to adult learning preferences (i.e., the andragogical approach) might result in better outcomes.

Even though undertreatment of pain is widely recognized to be related to a lack of education about pain diagnosis and treatment, education should not be seen as a panacea. Max (1990) was one of the first to point out that although improvements in pain education and changes in practitioner attitudes are the two most common remedies for poor pain management, these approaches rarely result in changes in behavior and practice as far as treatment of pain is concerned. The American Pain Society (1995, p. 1875) recognizes the necessity to rely not solely upon education to improve the treatment of pain: ". . . traditional educational approaches must be complemented by interventions in health care systems that more directly influence the routine behaviors of clinicians and patients, a perspective that has long been advocated by the quality improvement (QI) movement." Some model programs approach pain education in a more holistic way, including education as a key component of a larger process to influence institutional change and improvement in pain management practices (Blau, Dalton, & Lindley, 1999; Bookbinder et al., 1996; Ferrell, Dean, Grant, & Coluzzi, 1995; Grant, Rivera, Alisangco, & Francisco, 1999; Weissman, Griffie, Gordon, & Dahl, 1997).

Some of the noteworthy outcomes of pain education programs are summarized in Table 13.2. As this table illustrates, improvements in health care professionals' knowledge and attitudes about pain and its management are the most common outcomes of pain education initiatives, regardless of the approach used. Changes in behaviors (skills) are less common, and improvements in patients' pain management are even less likely. To a certain extent, this is because the effectiveness of efforts to facilitate practice change or to improve patient outcomes via continuing education in pain assessment and treatment is difficult to measure. Part of the problem is the time required to show changes in practice and any resultant changes in patient health status. Providers of continuing education programs need to lengthen the time they take for program evaluation and to find better ways for measuring positive outcomes that can be attributed to the effects of the educational intervention rather than to some other factor. In addition, developers of pain education programs need to devote more attention to defining appropriate outcome measures so that comparisons of alternative approaches can be evaluated more uniformly.

Theory has advanced since the days when continuing education consisted mainly of formal group lectures or individuals reading journal articles in their spare time. It is increasingly being recognized that the objective of CE is not simply to impart new information or knowledge to practitioners, but rather to attempt to affect changes in practice that result in improved patient outcomes (Davis et al., 1992, 1995; Czurylo, Gattuso, Epsom, Ryan, & Stark, 1999). Because most continuing education (CE) as currently structured falls short of the goal of changing practice behaviors, new learning methods and approaches need to be considered. Davis et al. (1999) reviewed studies that were randomized controlled trials of formal didactic and/or interactive CE interventions (conferences, courses, rounds, meetings, symposia, lectures, and other formats) and found that interactive CE sessions that enhance participant activity and provide the opportunity to practice skills can effect change in professional practice and, on occasion, health care outcomes. A great deal of work remains to be done, however, in order to better understand which formats and instructional strategies are most conducive to promoting learning outcomes that lead to practitioner behavior change and, in turn, to improved patient outcomes.

SETTING-SPECIFIC CONSIDERATIONS

Different settings may lend themselves better to certain educational formats than others. It may be impractical, for example, to implement classroom-based, interactive educational programs in nursing homes that are typically characterized by very high staff turnover rates (Schnelle & Reuben, 1999). Such settings might be better served by self-study materials such as CD-ROMs and videotapes. These standardized materials might also serve as the core educational content in classroom settings, supplemented by interactive learning. Educational symposia, on the other hand, should be driven by live large-group presentations as well as small-group sessions that allow ample opportunity for questions and answers, as some learners may be intimidated by larger settings.

When choosing and/or preparing educational materials, it is critical that the educator consider the level of education of the target audience. The level of nonhealth-care related background education of certified nursing assistants (CNAs), for example, is typically far below that of other health care professionals (Tellis-Nayak & Tellis-Nayak, 1989). In addition to using appropriate language, it may be helpful to supplement written material with ample visual aids.

As with other health care professionals, the education of physicians in

TABLE 13.2 Benefits of Pain Education Programs: Existing Evidence

Target audience	Educational format	Outcomes
4th year medical students	Traditional lectures, problem-based learning tutorials, demonstrations, small-group learning	Improvements in knowledge and attitudes (Sloan, Montgomery, & Musick, 1998)
Physicians	3–day lecture series plus hands-on patient techniques	Lectures improved deficiencies in knowledge and hands-on techniques & hands-on techniques maintained knowledge over time. (von Gunten, von Roenn, & Weitzman, 1994
	Academic detailing	Improvements in knowledge (Hines et al., 1998)
	CD-ROM multimedia module	Improvements in knowledge (Thompson et al., 1999)
Physicians, nurses, pharmacists	Lectures, case studies, role modeling	Improvements in knowledge & attitudes; improvements sustained at 4-month & 12-month follow-up (Janjan et al., 1996)
Nurses	Lectures, role modeling	Lectures & role modeling both improved pain knowledge, but role modeling resulted in a greater increase in retention (Driggers, Nussbaum, & Haddock, 1993)
	Lectures, videotapes	Videotapes may have influenced nurse views on validity of patient pain reports (Dols et al., 1995)
	Didactic workshops, hands-on patient techniques	Both methods equally effective in improving knowledge & attitudes (Lasch et al., 2000)
	5-day course plus clinical practice sessions, homework, group exercises, discussion	Improved knowledge & attitudes (Ferrell et al., 1993)

TABLE 13.2 *(continued)*

Nurses (cont.)	3-day course based on performance improvement principles	Changes in institutional pain management practices (Grant et al., 1999)
	8-hour workshop	Improved knowledge & attitudes; changes in pain assessment & management practice (Howell et al., 2000)
	3-hour lecture & discussion	Improved knowledge (deRond et al., 2000)
	8 weekly 3-hour lectures	Improvements in knowledge & attitudes; positive changes in nurses' behaviors regarding pain assessment & management; decreases in patient pain intensity (Francke et al., 1997a, 1997b)
	Lecture & collaboration with pain management experts	Improvements in knowledge and attitudes, but changes in practice slow to occur (Dalton et al., 1996)
	Lecture	Practice changes (Czurylo et al., 1999)
	Videotaped role play	Practice changes (Daroszewski & Meehan, 1997)
	Letters, personal contact, posters, & videotapes	Videotapes influenced changes in nurse behavior more than other techniques (McNaull et al., 1992)
	Videotapes, pain management game, focus groups, pain rounds, nurse liaisons	Changes in practice; improvements in patient satisfaction with pain treatment (Bookbinder et al., 1996)
	Self-study module, 1-hour seminar, case studies, critical-thinking exercises	More consistent patterns of pain management practice; improved patient outcomes related to pain management (Barnason et al., 1998)

private practice settings should be geared toward changing practice behavior. As noted above, traditional continuing education workshops for this group of practitioners are generally ineffective. Busy practitioners may need to be presented with new information repeatedly before this information is incorporated into their practices. Thus educational efforts should be multipronged and mutually reinforcing, such as academic detailing and opinion leaders, reminders (e.g., periodic mailings) and patient-mediated strategies (Davis, 1998; Davis et al., 1995).

SUMMARY/RECOMMENDATIONS

1. Undertreatment and inappropriate treatment of persistent pain in older adults is related to undereducation of health care professionals.
2. The ultimate goal of pain education programs is change in practice behaviors and improved patient care.
3. At the core of educating health care professionals about evaluation and management of pain in older adults is a combination of knowledge, attitudes, and skills.
4. The development of a pain education program for adult learners requires that the educator proceed through a series of rigorous steps, beginning with the assessment of the learning needs and education level of the audience, and ending with an assessment of the efficacy of the educational program.
5. Passive modes of learning do little to change behavior; interactive learning based in andragogy should be employed in developing pain-education programs.
6. Change in practice behaviors may take several years after correction of deficits in knowledge, attitudes, and skills; long-term learner follow-up is critical in determining the true benefits of educational programs.
7. A variety of adjunctive learning tools are available, such as videotapes, CD-ROMs, and on-line self-study programs. No one of these has been shown to be advantageous over any other. Their use should be dictated by learner preference.
8. There is no shortage of pain education programs. Educational programs based upon rigorous methodology with proven efficacy are scarce, however, and efforts to more effectively educate current and future health care professionals who care for older adults are needed.

MODEL PAIN EDUCATION PROGRAMS

Instruction in the effective assessment and management of pain can be found at many locations (medical schools, hospitals, etc.) and is provided through numerous methods (classroom instruction and clinical instruction for health science students, a variety of continuing education approaches for practitioners, Internet-based programs, etc.). These offerings are directed to a variety of target audiences and some are of uncertain quality and effectiveness. Evidence of the efficacy of some of these initiatives is lacking in many cases. Most of the existing pain education programs are relatively small in relation to the overall objectives of the organizations that have developed these programs, but there are some noteworthy efforts that could serve as models for others. These efforts include the following resources.

Tufts University School of Medicine

Tufts offers a master of science degree in pain research, education, and policy (PREP) intended for physicians, nurses, dentists, physical therapists, occupational therapists, hospice and palliative care providers, psychologists, social workers, health educators and advocates, and other health professionals. This program is the first of its kind and is built on the premise that pain control is influenced by factors ranging from molecules to social and economic issues, including basic science research, government regulation, policies of particular health facilities, and the education and beliefs of professionals, patients, and families. Students must complete 48 credits of course work, including core and elective courses. Required courses include

- Neuroanatomy, Neurochemistry, and Pharmacology of Pain
- Introduction to Clinical Pain Problems
- Ethical and Sociocultural Aspects of Pain
- Psychometrics and Outcomes Measurement
- Principles of Biostatistics
- Principles of Epidemiology
- Pharmacoeconomics
- Regulatory and Policy Issues
- Principles of Change and Education Applied to Pain Management
- Evaluation and Treatment of Pain: Psychological Approaches
- Palliative Care and End-of-Life Issues
- Internship in Clinical or Research Setting

Medical College of Wisconsin

The Wisconsin Cancer Pain Initiative (WPCI) has been a leader in establishing and testing innovative approaches to pain education (Weissman, 1996; Weissman et al., 1997, 2000). The WPCI proposed a model for cancer pain education for physicians in 1987 that stressed three components necessary to bring improvements in clinical practice:

1. dissemination of information about pain assessment and treatment;
2. prioritization of pain management in clinical practice settings;
3. creation of role models.

A pilot Cancer Pain Role Model Program was established to train physicians, together with their nurses and pharmacists, to become role models for better pain management in their clinical practice settings. A combination of lectures and case-based workshops was used to provide participants in 1-day conferences with information about cancer pain assessment and treatment and techniques for instituting changes in their clinical settings. Follow-up studies found that participants reported an impressive number of educational activities that led to clinical practice changes. This led to further expansion of the Role Model Program to include acute pain in addition to cancer pain and to add new features that focused on nurses as the key agents in effecting or facilitating institutional change. Most recently, efforts have addressed the pain management needs of long-term-care settings through the implementation of an educational intervention for improving the institutional commitment towards pain management through adoption of national practice standards.

National Cancer Institute

The WPCI is one of the projects supported by the National Cancer Institute's Cancer Education grant program. The National Cancer Institute has also funded other training and educational programs developed to further cancer-pain education and improve clinical practice. What is noteworthy about many of these projects is the integration of education, that is, the transmission or dissemination of information, with strategies for effecting institutional change, which in many cases are part of institutional continuous quality improvement (CQI) efforts. Results of some of these projects have been reported for the City of Hope National Medical Center (Ferrell et al., 1995; Ferrell, Grant, Ritchie, Ropchan, & Rivera, 1993; Ferrell, Rhiner, & Ferrell, 1993; Grant, et al., 1999); for the Duluth Clinic, University of Minnesota (Elliott et al., 1995, 1997); for the School of

Nursing, University of North Carolina (Blau et al., 1999; Dalton et al., 1995, 1996, 1999); and for the Memorial Sloan-Kettering Cancer Center (Brietbart, Rosenfeld, & Passik, 1998). A 5-year project conducted by the University of Pennsylvania with similar aims of integrating a multidisciplinary cancer-pain education program with efforts to foster innovation and effect institutional change in community hospitals has also reported positive outcomes (McMenamin, McCorkle, Barg, Abrahm, & Jepson, 1995).

Pain: The Fifth Vital Sign

The American Pain Society (APS) has created the phrase "Pain: The Fifth Vital Sign" to elevate awareness of pain treatment among health care professionals. Health care professionals are urged to assess patients for pain in the same way as they routinely assess blood pressure, pulse, temperature, and respiration. Hospitals, health centers, professional associations, and numerous individual physicians and nurses around the nation have reported their efforts to implement this philosophy since the APS first proposed the idea in 1995 (Merboth & Barnason, 2000; Sayers et al., 2000). Perhaps no one has approached this initiative with more zest than the U.S. Department of Veterans Affairs (VA). The VA network of health facilities treats 3.4 million patients at 1,100 sites, and it is now VA policy that clinicians assess, record, and treat pain as routinely as the other vital signs. Toward this end, the Veterans Health Administration has initiated a comprehensive National Pain Management Strategy in order to prevent suffering from pain in persons receiving care in the veterans health care system. One element of this strategy is establishing the concept of Pain as the Fifth Vital Sign for routine assessment and documenting of pain throughout the veterans health care system. Strategies for implementation of this policy include providing education for physicians, nurses, therapists, and other appropriate staff about how to use the 0–10 pain-rating scale, how to document procedures, and how to interpret results. A tool kit has been created to aid individual VA facilities in this effort, as well as in developing the implementation plan, establishing procedures for pain assessment and documentation of pain scores, and coordinating patient and family education activities (U.S. Veterans Health Administration, 1999). Each site is expected to develop an educational plan that is relevant to its local needs. It is too soon to determine the results of this initiative, but it is anticipated that this program will influence broader health care practice in the treatment of pain because about half of all medical students rotate through VA facilities.

PAIN EDUCATION RESOURCES

A great deal of CME is self-directed, independent learning, but there is some evidence that CME is most likely to affect outcomes when problem content is discussed and reinforced in a group (Abrahamson et al., 1999; Davis et al., 1999). The application of new technologies (e.g., computer-based educational programs, CD-ROMs) designed to make learning more accessible, affordable, convenient, and efficient for individuals may inadvertently result in solitary learning experiences that result in less impact than more traditional face-to-face instruction or group discussion and problem solving. Abrahamson et al. (1999) note that the effectiveness of various computer-learning applications is still being weighed, and that computer-driven learning packages for individuals may have minimal impact if they fail to instill collegiality, interaction, and collaboration into the learning process. At any rate, there is a great deal of interest in alternatives to face-to-face instruction in classrooms, workshops, and seminars. These alternative approaches have been applied to pain education as well as to many other areas of the health sciences. With few exceptions (McNaull, McLees, Belyea, & Clipp, 1992; Thompson, Savidge, Fulper-Smith, & Strode, 1999) there is very little indication that any of these types of materials have contributed to significant advances in knowledge, attitudes, or skills regarding pain management.

Studies that have examined how differing types of media compare to traditional approaches have shown mixed results. In general, it seems that instructional technologies or computer-based techniques in themselves are no more effective than traditional, classroom-style, face-to-face instruction in affecting learning (Phipps & Merisotis, 1999; Russell, 1999). However, these distance-learning technologies generally compare favorably with classroom-based instruction as demonstrated by learning gains measured through testing. They typically result in high student satisfaction, and they have an important role to play in reaching busy professionals who may not be able to participate in more traditional learning experiences. Numerous pain-management education products have been developed using a variety of instructional media and the number of these resources is rapidly expanding. A representative, though by no means exhaustive list of these products is shown in Table 13.3. Pain educators may find such resources useful in structuring their own unique educational programs. Media products are constantly changing, however, and new educational products are regularly released. The resources listed in Table 13.3 are representative of the types of pain education resources currently available, but their future availability—especially the Internet-based resources—cannot be guaranteed.

TABLE 13.3 Pain Education Resources

Title	Medium	Source	Description
Use of Opioids in Chronic Noncancer Pain	Self-study module	Power-Pak Communications, New York, NY	Includes a posttest; continuing education credits available
The Impact of Chronic Pain: An Interdisciplinary Perspective	Self-study module	Power-Pak Communications, New York, NY	Includes a posttest; continuing education credits available
Overcoming Barriers to Effective Pain Management	Audiotape	Solutions Unlimited, Rochester, NY	One-hour tape; includes a posttest; continuing education credits available
Chronic Pain in Geriatrics: Assessment	Videotape	Geriatric Video Productions, Shaverstown, PA	25-minute tape; includes a pretest & posttest; continuing education credits available
Chronic Pain in Geriatrics: Management	Videotape	Geriatric Video Productions, Shaverstown, PA	25-minute tape; includes a pretest & posttest; continuing education credits available
Pain Management: An Interactive CD-ROM for Clinical Staff Development	CD-ROM	Aspen Publishers, Gaithersburg, MD	Includes continuing education credits for nurses, physicians, and pharmacists
Management of Chronic Pain in the Elderly	CD-ROM	Medical Communications Media, Wrightstown, PA	1-credit-hour self-study CME program
Pain Management	CD-ROM	Graphic Education Corporation, Columbia, MO	7-credit-hour course
Pain.com	On-line modules	Dannemiller Memorial Educational Foundation, San Antonio, TX http://www.pain.com	3 modules of 10 abstracted articles offered each month; includes posttests & evaluation; continuing education credits available
Chronic Pain Management in the Elderly	On-line module	University of Florida Geriatric Education Center, Gainesville, FL http://www.medinfo.ufl.edu/cme/hmoa2	Slides accompanied by an audio-based lecture; posttest & evaluation must be completed to receive continuing education credits

355

FUTURE DIRECTIONS

Davis et al. (1999) reviewed studies that were randomized, controlled trials of formal didactic and/or interactive CME interventions (conferences, courses, rounds, meetings, symposia, lectures, and other formats) and found that interactive CME sessions that enhance participant activity and provide the opportunity to practice skills can effect change in professional practice and, on occasion, health care outcomes. A great deal of work remains to be done, however, in order to better understand which formats and instructional strategies are most conducive for promoting learning outcomes that lead to practitioner behavior change and, in turn, to improved patient outcomes. In addition, much more effort by educators in undergraduate and graduate health-sciences degree programs and by instructors of continuing-education programs must be given to finding improved methods and techniques for measuring the impacts of knowledge and attitudes on health professionals' practice behaviors and on their patients' health status.

REFERENCES

Abrahamson, S., et al. (1999). Continuing medical education for life: Eight principles. *Academic Medicine, 74*(12), 1288–1294.

American Pain Society Quality of Care Committee. (1995). Quality improvement guidelines for the treatment of acute pain and cancer pain. *JAMA, 274*(23), 1874–1880.

Barnason, S., Merboth, M., Pozehl, B., & Tietjen, M. J. (1998). Utilizing an outcomes approach to improve pain management by nurses: A pilot study. *Clinical Nurse Specialist, 12*(1), 28–36.

Beers, M. H. (1997). Explicit criteria for determining potentially inappropriate medication use by the elderly: An update. *Archives of Internal Medicine, 157*, 1531–1536.

Blau, W. S., Dalton, J. A. B., & Lindley, C. (1999). Organization of hospital-based acute pain management programs. *Southern Medical Journal, 92*(5), 465–471.

Bookbinder, M., et al. (1996). Implementing national standards for cancer pain management: Program model and evaluation. *Journal of Pain and Symptom Management, 12*(6), 334–347.

Breitbart, W., Rosenfeld, B., & Passik, S. D. (1998). The Network Project: A multidisciplinary cancer education and training program in pain management, rehabilitation, and psychosocial issues. *Journal of Pain and Symptom Management, 15*(1), 18–26.

Chang, H. M., Gallagher, R., Vaillancourt, P. D., Balter, K., Cohen, M., Garvin, B., Charibo, C., King, S. A., Workman, E. A., McClain, B., Ellenberg, M., & Chiang, J. S. (2000). Undergraduate medical education in pain medicine, end-of-life care, and palliative care—a position statement from the American Academy of Pain Medicine undergraduate education committee. *Pain Medicine, 1*(3), 224.

Czurylo, K., Gattuso, M., Epsom, R., Ryan, C., & Stark, B. (1999). Continuing education outcomes related to pain management practice. *Journal of Continuing Education in Nursing, 30*(2), 84–87.

Dalton, J. A., et al. (1995). Managing cancer pain: Content and scope of an educational program for nurses who work in predominately rural areas. *Journal of Pain and Symptom Management, 10*(3), 214–223.

Dalton, J. A., et al. (1996). Changing the relationship among nurses' knowledge, self-reported behavior, and documented behavior in pain management: Does education make a difference? *Journal of Pain and Symptom Management, 12*(5), 308–319.

Dalton, J. A., Blau, W., Lindley, C., Carlson, J., Youngblood, R., & Greer, S. M. (1999). Changing acute pain management to improve patient outcomes: An educational approach. *Journal of Pain and Symptom Management, 17*(4), 277–287.

Daroszewski, E. B., & Meehan, D. A. (1997). Pain, role play, and videotape: Pain management staff development in a community hospital. *Journal of Nursing Staff Development, 13*(3), 119–124.

Davis, D. (1998). Does CME work?: An analysis of the effect of educational activities on physician performance of health care outcomes. *International Journal of Psychiatry in Medicine, 28*(1), 21–39.

Davis, D. A., & Fox, R. D. (Eds.). (1994). *The physician as learner: Linking research to practice.* Chicago: American Medical Association.

Davis, D., O'Brien, M. A., Freemantle, N., Wolf, F. M., Mazmanian, P., & Taylor-Vaisey, A. (1999). Impact of formal continuing medical education: Do conferences, workshops, rounds, and other traditional continuing education activities change physician behavior or health care outcomes? *JAMA, 282*(9), 867–874.

Davis, D. A., Thomson, M. A., Oxman, A. D., & Haynes, R. B. (1992). Evidence for the effectiveness of CME: A review of 50 randomized controlled trials. *JAMA, 268*(9), 1111–1117.

Davis, D. A., Thomson, M. A., Oxman, A. D., & Haynes, R. B. (1995). Changing physician performance: A systematic review of the effect of continuing medical education strategies. *JAMA, 274*(9), 700–705.

de Rond, M. E. J., de Wit, R., van Dam, F. S. A. M., van Campen, B. Th. M., den Hartog, Y. M., & Klievink, R. M. A. (2000). A pain monitoring program for nurses: Effects on nurses' pain knowledge and attitude. *Journal of Pain and Symptom Management, 19*(6), 457–467.

Dick, W., Carey, L., & Carey, J. O. (2001). *The systematic design of instruction* (5th ed.). New York: Longman.

Dols, C., et al. (1995). Enhancing nurses' reliance on patients' perception of pain during pain assessment: A comparison of two educational methods. *Journal of Continuing Education in Nursing, 26*(5), 209–213.

Driggers, D. L., Nussbaum, J. S., & Haddock, K. S. (1993). Role modeling: An educational strategy to promote effective cancer pain management. *Oncology Nursing Forum, 20*(6), 959–962.

Elliott, T. E., et al. (1997). Improving cancer pain management in communities:

Main results from a randomized controlled trial. *Journal of Pain and Symptom Management, 13*(4), 191–203.

Elliott, T. E., Murray, D. M., Oken, M. M., Johnson, K. M., Elliott, B. A., & Post-White, J. (1995). The Minnesota Cancer Pain Project: Design, methods, and education strategies. *Journal of Cancer Education, 10*(2), 102–112.

Ferrell, B. R., Dean, G. E., Grant, M., & Coluzzi, P. (1995). An institutional commitment to pain management. *Journal of Clinical Oncology, 13*(9), 2158–2165.

Ferrell, B. R., Grant, M., Ritchey, K. J., Ropchan, R., & Rivera, L. M. (1993). The Pain Resource Nurse Training Program: A unique approach to pain management. *Journal of Pain and Symptom Management, 8*(8), 549–556.

Ferrell, B. R., Rhiner, M., & Ferrell, B. A. (1993). Development and implementation of a pain education program. *Cancer, 72*(Suppl. 11), 3426–3432.

Fields, H. L. (1995). *Core curriculum for professional education in pain* (2nd ed.). Seattle, WA: International Association for the Study of Pain.

Francke, A. L., Garssen, B., Luiken, J. B., de Schepper, A. M. E., Grypdonck, M., & Abu-Saad, H. H. (1997a). Effects of a nursing pain programme on patient outcomes. *Psycho-Oncology, 6*(4), 302–310.

Francke, A. L., Luiken, J. B., de Schepper, A. M. E., Abu-Saad, H. H., & Grypdonck, M. (1997b). Effects of a continuing education program on nurses' pain assessment practices. *Journal of Pain and Symptom Management, 13*(2), 90–97.

Grant, M., Rivera, L. M., Alisangco, J., & Francisco, L. (1999). Improving cancer pain management using a performance improvement framework. *Journal of Nursing Care Quality, 13*(4), 60–72.

Green, J.S., Grosswald, S. J., Suter, E., & Walthall, D. B. (Eds.). (1984). *Continuing education for the health professions.* San Francisco: Jossey-Bass.

Hines, C., Bingham, J., Muirden, N., & Beavis, M. (1998). Evaluation of a cancer pain education program for general practitioners. *Australian Family Physician, 27*(Suppl. 2), S70–S72.

Howell, D., Butler, L., Vincent, L., Watt-Watson, J., & Stearns, N. (2000). Influencing nurses' knowledge, attitudes, and practice in cancer pain management. *Cancer Nursing, 23*(1), 55–63.

Janjan, N. A., Martin, C. G., Payne, R., Dahl, J. L., Weissman, D. E., & Hill, C. S. (1996). Teaching cancer pain management: Durability of educational effects of a role model program. *Cancer, 77*(5), 996–1001.

Knowles, M. S. (1980). *The modern practice of adult education: From pedagogy to andragogy* (Rev. ed.). Wilton, CT: Association Press.

Knowles, M. S., Holton, E. F., & Swanson, R. A. (1998). *The adult learner* (5th ed.). Houston, TX: Gulf.

Lasch, K. E., Wilkes, G., Lee, J., & Blanchard, R. (2000). Is hands-on experience more effective than didactic workshops in postgraduate pain education? *Journal of Cancer Education, 15*(4), 218–222.

Lewis, C. E. (1998). Continuing medical education: Past, present, future. *Western Journal of Medicine, 168*(5), 334–340.

Max, M. B. (1990). Improving outcomes of analgesic treatment: Is education enough? *Annals of Internal Medicine, 113*(11), 885–889.

McCaffery, M., & Ferrell, B. R. (1997). Nurses' knowledge of pain assessment and management: How much progress have we made? *Journal of Pain and Symptom Management, 14*(3), 175–188.

McMenamin, E., McCorkle, R., Barg, F., Abrahm, J., & Jepson, C. (1995). Implementing a multidisciplinary cancer pain education program. *Cancer Practice, 3*(5), 303–309.

McNaull, F. W., McLees, J. P., Belyea, M. J., & Clipp, E. C. (1992). A comparison of educational methods to enhance nursing performance in pain assessment. *Journal of Continuing Education in Nursing, 23*(6), 267–271.

Merboth, M. K., & Barnason, S. (2000). Managing pain: The fifth vital sign. *Nursing Clinics of North America, 35*(2), 375–383.

Phipps, R., & Merisotis, J. (1999). *What's the difference: A review of contemporary research on the effectiveness of distance learning in higher education.* Washington, DC: Institute for Higher Education Policy.

Rogers, E. M. (1995). *Diffusion of innovations* (4th ed.). New York: Free Press.

Rosof, A. B., & Felch, W. C. (Eds.). (1992). *Continuing medical education: A primer* (2nd ed.). New York: Praeger.

Russell, T. L. (1999). *The no significant difference phenomenon as reported in 355 research reports, summaries, and papers: A comprehensive research annotated bibliography on technology for distance education.* Raleigh: North Carolina State University.

Sayers, M., Marando, R., Fisher, S., Aquila, A., Morrison, B., & Dailey, T. (2000). No need for pain. *Journal of Healthcare Quality, 22*(3), 10–15.

Schnelle, J. F., & Reuben, D. B. (1999). Long-term care in the nursing home. In E. Calkins, C. Boult, E. H. Wagner, & J. T. Pacala (Eds.), *New ways to care for older people: Building systems based on evidence* (pp. 168–181). New York: Springer.

Sloan, P. A., Montgomery, C., & Musick, D. (1998). Medical student knowledge of morphine for the management of cancer pain. *Journal of Pain and Symptom Management, 15*(6), 359–364.

Tellis-Nayak, V., & Tellis-Nayak, M. (1989). Quality of care and burden of two cultures: When the world of the nurse's aide enters the world of the nursing home. *Gerontologist, 29*(3), 307–313.

Thompson, A. R., Savidge, M. A., Fulper-Smith, M., & Strode, S. W. (1999). Testing a multimedia module in cancer pain management. *Journal of Cancer Education, 14*(3), 161–163.

U.S. Veterans Health Administration. (1999). *Pain assessment: The fifth vital sign.* Washington, DC: Author.

von Gunten, C. F., von Roenn, J. H., & Weitzman, S. (1994). Housestaff training in cancer pain education. *Journal of Cancer Education, 9*(4), 230–234.

Weissman, D. E. (1996). Cancer pain education for physicians in practice: Establishing a new paradigm. *Journal of Pain and Symptom Management, 12*(6), 364–371.

Weissman, D. E., Griffie, J., Gordon, D. B., & Dahl, J. L. (1997). A role model program to promote institutional changes for management of acute and cancer pain. *Journal of Pain and Symptom Management, 14*(5), 274–279.

Weissman, D. E., Griffie, J., Muchka, S., & Matson, S. (2000). Building an institutional commitment to pain management in long-term care facilities. *Journal of Pain and Symptom Management, 20*(1), 35–43.

World Health Organization (1996). *Cancer pain relief* (2nd ed.). Geneva, Switzerland: Author.

An Approach to Reimbursement Issues 14

Robb McIlvried and Paula Bonino

The other chapters of this text primarily focus on the relationship between two parties: the practitioner (e.g., physician, physical therapist, or psychologist) and the patient. For many years these two parties were the only ones involved in the clinical interaction. The health care provider would be directly reimbursed with goods or services for the care provided. Currently, however, in the vast majority of cases this interaction now also includes an additional component—the third-party payer. Frequently, patients and their providers give very little consideration to this new element, but increasingly the third party can have influence on the interaction of the other two parties.

When considering the interaction among these three parties one must be aware of the motivating forces for each. For a patient with persistent pain the motivating forces might include relief or palliation of pain, return to work or improved functional status, improvement in emotional or psychological symptoms related to the pain, and improved quality of life. The patient also is concerned with the cost of the service provided because he or she is responsible for payment, whether in the form of direct out-of-pocket payment or indirectly through a third-party payer. For the physician treating a patient with persistent pain, the motivating forces might include a desire to improve the patient's pain and quality of life, improve functional status, alleviate psychological symptoms, and be paid for the service provided. The insurer might be motivated to maintain customer satisfaction by providing the proper treatment to its client, and doing so as cost-effectively as possible. Thus, the insurer is only interested in providing payment for services that are proven to be necessary for treatment and result in positive outcomes.

The insurer may consider a multidisciplinary treatment approach to pain as a costly alternative to other treatments, such as chronic opioids or management by a primary care physician. In the area of pain management, cost-effectiveness can sometimes be hard to assess and prioritize because it is difficult to put a price tag on pain relief (Ferrell & Griffith, 1994). However, evidence exists showing multidisciplinary pain clinics to be more effective in relieving pain and returning the patient to work, and ultimately more cost-effective (Flor, Fydrich, & Turk, 1992; Stieg, Williams, Timmermans-Williams, & Tafuro, 1986). It is important to note, however, that these studies were based on younger pain patients, so whether these findings also would be true for older adults is not known.

A specific description of every insurer and its reimbursement policies on persistent-pain management would be an impossible task. Rapid change and wide geographic variations also would make it difficult to apply to a general readership. Therefore, the goal of this chapter is to provide the clinician with some general background regarding the process of reimbursement, some suggestions on how to receive payment for services provided to patients, and where to look for further information.

EVIDENCE AND PRINCIPLES FOR PRACTICE

General Background and Definitions

The issue of reimbursement and third-party payers can be an incredibly complex and confusing topic for many health care practitioners. The variety of plans can be overwhelming and the multiple codes can seem like an "alphabet soup" of CPTs, ICDs, and DRGs. For this reason it may be helpful to provide a brief history and description of various forms of insurers and some basic definitions.

Definitions (Kovner & Jonas, 1999)

- Fee-for-service (FFS)—A reimbursement system in which a health care provider receives a fee for each service that is provided to the patient. Typically this is done after the service is provided.
- Capitation—A reimbursement system in which the clinician is reimbursed (per set time period) for each patient that he or she is under contract to serve, regardless of the number of visits or services provided to these patients.
- Prospective Payment System (PPS)—A system for reimbursing institutional and individual providers of health services using a predetermined, fixed fee/payment per unit of service.
- Managed Care—A system of health care delivery that influences or controls utilization of services or costs of services.

- Health Maintenance Organization (HMO)—A system where a pre-paid, capitated payment is made on behalf of a beneficiary and all covered services are provided to the beneficiary by a designated group of providers.

Perhaps the insurance most familiar to clinicians, especially those taking care of older adults, is Medicare. The Medicare program was established in 1965 as an amendment (Title XVIII) to the Social Security Act of 1935. It was intended to cover persons over the age of 65, who were the population group most likely to be living in poverty at that time. Medicare was expanded to patients with renal failure and patients with disability in 1972. In 1966, more than 19 million Americans were enrolled in Medicare, and in 2000 more than 39 million seniors and disabled people were served by Medicare. Medicare is a federally funded program managed by the Centers for Medicare and Medicaid Services (CMS). Traditionally, Medicare was a fee-for-service provider; however in 1982 Medicare began contracting with health maintenance organizations on a risk basis.

The 1970s and 1980s saw a dramatic rise in the costs of health care in the United States. Managed care was seen as a method for controlling these costs. Managed care organizations (MCOs), with health maintenance organizations (HMOs) the most common example, typically use a capitated reimbursement system. MCOs have been present in various forms since the 1930s. The federal HMO act in 1973 was passed in order to increase the prevalence of managed care systems. However, it wasn't until the 1980s that MCOs became widespread.

Given the different reimbursement systems, capitated versus fee-for-service, it is important again to note the various motivating forces for the three parties—the patient, the clinician and the insurer—as these motivations may influence the interaction. Under a fee-for-service plan there may be an incentive for the physician to perform an increased number of services in order to receive greater compensation. Under a capitated plan there is fear that the incentive is to provide as little service as possible because the physician payment is not directly related to the number of services provided. In the area of pain this may result in more primary care physicians treating patients with persistent pain themselves rather than referring them to a pain specialist (Kulich & Lande, 1997).

The concern regarding insurers is that they will deny needed care to a patient in order to avoid paying for expensive services, especially given the high costs that can be generated during the treatment of persistent pain. Fishman, Von Korff, Lozana, and Hecht (1997) evaluated costs of a large MCO and found that patients with chronic conditions, including persistent pain, can cause a significant increase in cost to the insurer. For the insurer, the motivation may be to provide the least expensive service possible. This has led to some MCOs encouraging cheaper alternatives to pain treatment centers (Kulich & Lande, 1997). It is not known whether these alternatives would provide the optimal treatment.

The best solution to this problem is an increase in the number of quality outcome studies to evaluate treatments, perhaps even in partnership with MCOs (Turk, 1999). The American Pain Society (APS) has developed a position statement on pain assessment and treatment in the managed care environment (Fox et al., 2000). This position statement outlines recommendations for an effective pain management program in a managed care setting, including assessment and referral, education of primary care providers, provider credentialing, outcomes, and communication.

Principles of Practice: General Considerations

In the simplest individual reimbursement terms, clinicians would like to be paid for the services provided to patients, patients would like the services to be paid for on their behalf by their insurance coverage, and insurers would like to pay for "reasonable and necessary" services to their enrolled members. On a larger scale, clinicians would like fair and equitable reimbursement from multiple insurers in a predictable manner, with the fewest administrative requirements (paperwork burden). Patients would like to have the most helpful and accessible services paid for in a predictable and efficient manner, also with minimal paperwork. Insurers would like to pay for high-quality services at a reasonable and predictable cost, maintain high member and provider satisfaction, and continually expand their businesses.

Although this chapter focuses primarily on how clinicians' and patients' goals can be met with respect to reimbursement, their interdependence with insurers and the fact that insurers would like to have the lowest cost possible to process claims accurately also need to be considered. The more one can help the insurer make a decision on the first submission of a claim by including all requested information, the more likely the insurer is to make a rapid and equitable decision. A proper initial determination is less expensive than multiple appeals and redeterminations, which often involve increasingly higher priced clinicians to review the claim. Thus by considering an insurer's motivation, a clinician can better achieve his or her own goals as well as the patient's goals.

It is important to understand the rules, regulations, eligibility requirements, and coverage policies of the insurers most commonly dealt with in the treatment of older patients with persistent pain. One important point to note is that it is not a common practice to provide an overall fee for a multidisciplinary pain treatment program. Rather, it is more common that each clinical provider is required to file an individual claim for service. This often can lead to problems in providing proper pain management because the vital services of some treatment team members may not be reimbursed by all insurers.

The insurance provider is motivated to provide coverage only for services that are proven to be efficacious. Unfortunately, in the area of pain management, it is often difficult and complex to determine efficacy (Loeser, 1999). To improve the likelihood that the services will be paid for, it is helpful for the clinician to document specific outcomes for the goal of treatment. Whenever feasible, the outcomes should be quantifiable along a standard scale. Useful scales, particularly in a population of older adults, are those that assess function and the functional impact of the service or treatment. Chapter 5 of this volume deals with the many scales that can be used to assess function. The clinician may need to use a combination of scales that fully encompass the pain and functional components of treatment. In addition to functional goals, patients' goals or preferences can be used as meaningful outcomes. These can include return to work, reduction in pain medication usage, or increase in social activities. Once these outcomes are established, it is necessary to relate the assessment and plan to these specific outcomes.

Another area of concern for many patients with persistent pain is the high cost of medication. Most "self-administered" medications, especially those orally administered, are not covered under the traditional Medicare program at present, although a prescription-drug benefit is being debated in Congress. Ironically, the lack of medication coverage may result in increased cost to the insurer when a costlier alternative therapy, such as indwelling epidural catheter or patient-controlled analgesia (PCA), is chosen over oral medications because the insurer will cover these services (Ferrell, 1993; Joranson, 1994). Some older adults have supplemental or secondary insurance that provides medication coverage but frequently requires a copayment, which may be substantial for older adults on multiple medications. For those patients without insurance or with limited coverage, some states have additional special programs such as Pennsylvania's Pharmaceutical Assistance Contract to the Elderly (PACE) program. Furthermore, pharmaceutical companies may provide some assistance for coverage of medications. Chisholm, Reinhardt, Vollenweider, Kendrick, and DiPiro (2000), in the *American Journal of Health System Pharmacy*, list several pharmaceutical companies that provide assistance or free medications. Also, the Pharmaceutical Research and Manufacturers of America publish a directory of pharmaceutical assistance programs that is available via the Internet at *www.phrma.org*.

Another important point is that alternative or nontraditional therapies, despite often providing effective pain relief, are frequently not reimbursed by insurers. The patient usually pays for these services directly, and the number of patients using these services is increasing (Eisenberg et al., 1998). Due to this increased consumer interest and market demand, some insurance carriers have begun to provide coverage for alternative therapies (Pelletier, Marie, Krasner, & Haskell, 1997). Some therapies, such as acupuncture, have received considerable attention recently and more research is being conducted. Clinical trials of alternative therapies actually may be a method of providing a service to a patient without cost, except that frequently insurers need evidence that a treatment is effective *before* they are willing to pay for it.

As outlined above and described by Jost (2000), there are many gaps in the coverage provided by Medicare to older adults with persistent pain. These gaps may require a clinician to be creative in finding a payer for the patient. Besides clinical trials and pharmaceutical companies as potential sources of payment for services and medications that are not covered by insurers, charitable organizations or support groups may be able to provide some assistance to the patient with persistent pain and limited financial resources. The physician should use all members of the treatment team, including social services, to learn about all the possible options.

Understanding the Practical Matters

Filing Claims for Payment

Claims are filed differently depending on the insurance provider that covers the patient, but most insurers use electronic billing of claims whenever possible. Because most older adults are covered by the traditional fee-for-service Medicare program, and because the practices of Medicare often influence those of other insurers for this population, this section will focus primarily on Medicare reimbursement. In the traditional fee-for-service Medicare program, there is no preauthorization for payment as there frequently is with a MCO. Thus, a claim for payment is submitted after each service is provided.

The claim must pass through several levels of evaluation before payment can be made. First, it must pass through the insurer's database. Here it is screened for basic information, such as whether the patient is actually a participant in the health plan. Second, the claim must be properly billed. This is usually done through the use of various codes. These codes include, but are not limited to, International Classification of Disease (ICD) codes, the American Medical Association's Current Procedural Terminology (CPT) codes, Diagnosis Related Group (DRG) codes, and Resource Utilization Group (RUG) codes. These codes are under continual revision as the payment system changes and new drugs, devices, and procedures are developed and approved. In the management of persistent pain in older adults, it is important to recognize that there is no single specific diagnostic code for the diagnosis of "persistent pain." Nor is there a single procedural code for the assessment or treatment of persistent pain. According to Stieg, Lippe, and Shepard (1999) the current codes frequently do not adequately encompass the complexity of treating patients with persistent pain. It is therefore important to become sufficiently knowledgeable about the coding systems relevant to the claims submitted in order to accurately and as specifically as possible describe in code what occurred in practice. It is necessary for clinicians, unless they do their own billing, to clearly communicate with billing staff to code claims properly. After the claim is submitted with the proper codes, it is then checked to see whether the payment requested is for services that the insurer will reimburse, that is, covered services. For example, under federal law Medicare currently does not reimburse for cosmetic surgery.

Once the above steps are completed, the claim is evaluated to determine if the service provided was "reasonable and necessary" for the patient at that time. For Medicare the pertinent legislation covering this is the Social Security Act, section 1862(a)(1)(A), which defines services as those "reasonable and necessary for the diagnosis or treatment of an injury or illness or to improve the functioning of a malformed body member." The majority of the claims for payment that reach the question of "reasonable and necessary" are still reviewed and paid electronically, based on the codes submitted. Some claims will not complete the process electronically, causing a request for clinical documentation to be sent out.

Documentation

In the *APS Bulletin*, Taricco (1998) urges providers to inform payers "what they need to do, why they need to do it, how they should justify charges" and to make the payer aware of the reason certain treatments are necessary in one case but need modifications in a similar case. Thus, it is vital that the clinician supply the proper records and that the documentation be thorough. The documents needed are records that were used clinically while care was given, such as progress notes from physicians, therapists, and others; discharge summaries; consultations; physical therapy treatment plans; and other pertinent records such as diagnostic study reports. Clinical documentation requested by the insurer also may include the physician's orders for the various treatments and diagnostic studies. The requested clinical documentation includes only records that were generated before the claim for payment was sent.

There are several critical factors in proper documentation.

- All records must be signed, dated and timed.
- All records should be legible.
- The record should state the necessity or rationale for the treatment. This may include
  - previous treatments and the results
  - benefit of one diagnostic test over another
  - benefit of a specific setting over another (e.g., requirement for skilled care or home care services)
  - explanation for what could be considered overlap of services, that is, need for a pain specialist when the patient is already followed by a primary care physician

In some instances there are specific requirements for separate statements, above and beyond the usual notes and orders, which certify that the service is necessary for this patient at this time. For Medicare, these requirements are defined in Title 42 of the Code of Federal Regulations (42CFR 424.10, 424.11, and 424.20). This is particularly important in skilled nursing facilities and for services given in an outpatient setting, such as occupational therapy, physical therapy, and speech therapy. The certification statement establishes the primary role of the physician in the direction of medical care, and in the oversight of interdisciplinary care. The physician must certify that the care is necessary and may need to recertify, depending on the patient's progress and continued need for services. The details of timing, content, and so forth, are described in the legislation referenced above.

It is important that the person receiving the requests from the insurers for clinical documentation understand what is being requested. Again, it is important for clinicians to work closely with the billing and/or medical records staff to clarify any misunderstandings. It is in everyone's best interest that claims for services are paid correctly the first time. When the provider does not submit the proper requested documentation or when it is incomplete or illegible, for example, it is more likely that the claim will not be paid and that the patient and provider will need to appeal the decision of the insurer.

Appealing Decisions

When a claim for services is denied, or partially denied, it is important to review the information the insurer gives as to why this decision was reached. It is also critical to review whether or not the decision is subject to appeal. Once again, because the Medicare program is bound by federal law and regulations, there are rules about the decisions and the appeals process described in the law and regulations. Most denials, full or partial, will be due to issues that are open to appeal; usually the information the insurer had did not support the claim that the services were reasonable and necessary. This may be due to a failure to supply the most accurate codes or the requested clinical documentation. The appeals process is usually straightforward, and it is relatively easy for clinicians to assist with this process. It is not a "second opinion," but rather an opportunity to provide information that was improperly submitted, or not submitted, the first time.

Where To Go for More Information

The Internet is an extremely useful tool for quickly accessing insurance and reimbursement information. Government programs maintain active websites, such as *www.cms.hhs.gov* maintained by the Centers for Medicare and Medicaid Services (CMS) for the Medicare and Medicaid programs. Other insurers, including those who hold contracts with CMS to administer the Medicare program, also have websites. CMS has created a site for accessing all of their contractors' Local Medical Review Policies, which describe local payment guidelines—*www.lmrp.net*. Private insurance companies, both individually and through their organizations (Blue Cross and Blue Shield Association), are accessible electronically. Individual states have their own Web pages that also can be helpful, especially with questions such as scope of practice and details of state Medicaid programs. Pharmaceutical company Web sites are helpful and often include information about their assistance programs for patients with limited finances. Written materials are also available such as the Social Security Act, the Federal Register, the Code of Federal Regulations, Medicare and other insurers' manuals, newsletters, notices, and bulletins. The Code of Federal Regulations and the legislation cited in this chapter can be viewed online at *www.access.gpo.gov/nara*.

SETTING-SPECIFIC CONSIDERATIONS

Some reimbursement aspects of care for patients with persistent pain are consistent throughout settings; others vary. One principle that does not vary across settings is the need for proper documentation. This is an area of rapid change as technology and payment move services to different places (e.g., former inpatient procedures now done in an outpatient setting).

Inpatient Facility

An inpatient, comprehensive, structured, pain management program that meets Medicare guidelines may be reimbursable as a comprehensive program. This is different from the outpatient setting where each individual component of the treatment plan will usually be reimbursed separately. In the inpatient hospital setting, payment is made according to the patient's Diagnosis Related Group (DRG). This is a global, comprehensive payment for services. For those patients who require care exceeding the usual parameters, documentation of those exceptional circumstances is required. As mentioned earlier, clear discussion of the rationale for treatment choices is always helpful.

Home Care

In 1995, the CMS (then known as the Health Care Financing Administration) paid over $28 billion for home health care (CMS, 1996). Medicare coverage was recently changed to a prospective payment system for home health care, using the OASIS assessment as a basis for determining the proper prospective payment. Home health care has its own set of certification and recertification requirements that providers need to become familiar with, as well as the coverage policies regarding the management of persistent pain in older adults in the home setting.

Skilled Nursing Facility

In 1997 there were 1.6 million residents of nursing homes in the United States (National Center for Health Care Statistics, 1998). Pain is a very common condition affecting up to 45–80% of nursing facility residents (Ferrell, 1995). Due to the prevalence of pain in the nursing facility it is important to understand some basic principles of reimbursement regarding nursing facility care. Payment for skilled nursing services can come from a variety of sources. According to the CMS, in 1995 47% of nursing home expenditures were paid for by Medicaid and 9% were paid for by Medicare (CMS, 1996). Unfortunately, the current policies of Medicare and Medicaid may not be favorable to the management of pain in a skilled nursing facility (Jost, 2000). The remainder comes from out-of-pocket expenditures and various other public and private sources. Medicare may pay for skilled nursing services as posthospitalization care following at least a 3-day acute inpatient hospitalization. Physician certification of the necessity for skilled nursing-facility care is critical for reimbursement.

Payment for skilled nursing-facility services also is through a prospective payment system, based on the results of the Minimum Data Set (MDS) assessment, which supports the assignment of a Resource Utilization Group (RUG) code. Accurate and timely completion of the MDS assessments is crucial to proper reimbursement. Further, the clinical record must substantiate what the MDS assessment claims. If a patient, for example, requires a stated level of therapy services for the management of persistent pain, the clinical record should reflect the rationale for the treatment choice, the patient's ability to reasonably tolerate the therapy, and the patient's response and progress.

Outpatient Pain Center

Reimbursement for services provided at a multidisciplinary outpatient pain facility can be a complicated matter. This is primarily due to the fact that the overall service is not reimbursed as a whole, but each individual component is reimbursed separately. Services provided by hospitals to outpatients are reimbursed under a prospective payment system (OPPS), which uses CMS's billing codes (e.g., HCFA Common Procedure Coding system and revenue codes) to assign Ambulatory Patient Classifications (APCs), which dictate payment. The situation for the management of persistent pain in older adults is complicated by the fact that therapy services (e.g., physical and occupational therapy) are currently not under OPPS and remain under a fee-for-service. Thus, patients may have some services provided in the same setting that are reimbursed using different payment methods. Further, patients may receive care at nonhospital outpatient facilities that may submit claims for payment to different Medicare contractors.

SUMMARY/RECOMMENDATIONS

1. Documentation is critical in order to make the reimbursement process as simple and efficient as possible.
   a) All handwritten notes should be legible.
   b) The provider must ensure that all notes are signed and dated.
   c) Notes should be comprehensive and specific in regard to
      i)   Necessity for treatment
      ii) Previous treatment that has failed

      iii) Reason for possible overlap of services (pain specialist and primary care provider)

      iv) Requirement for skilled care or home care when appropriate

2. The clinician should become familiar with the primary insurers that provide coverage for patients with persistent pain.
   a) Many of these companies have Internet sites that provide information on what is covered.
      i)   The Centers for Medicare and Medicaid Services (CMS) maintains a site, *www.cms.hhs.gov*, for government programs.
      ii)   Most private insurance companies have Internet sites.
3. The clinician should be creative about payment and consider alternative payers including
   a) Clinical research studies
   b) Charitable foundations, such as the American Pain Foundation (*www.painfoundation.org*)
   c) Pharmaceutical companies
      i)   Samples may be provided to patients unable to pay for medications.
      ii)   List of companies providing medication assistance is available (Chisholm, 2000).
4. Utilize all available resources to find further information.
   a) The physician should utilize other treatment team members: physical therapy, social worker, psychologist, and so forth, as a source of information about reimbursement.
   b) The clinician should educate billing staff and medical records staff on the proper coding and medical records necessary to achieve accurate and rapid claims processing.
   c) The Internet provides a number of sources regarding pain management reimbursement issues.
      i)   American Pain Society (*www.ampainsoc.org*)
      ii)   American Academy of Pain Medicine (*www.painmed.org*)
      iii) American Academy of Pain Management (*www.aapainmanage.org*)
      iv) National Center for Alternative and Complementary Medicine (*www.nccam.nih.org*)

CASE STUDIES

Case 1

RS is a 92-year-old man who reports overall good health but has been experiencing chronic pain in his lower legs for 3 to 4 years. His pain has been diagnosed as secondary to small fiber neuropathy of unknown etiology. The pain has affected his quality of life by limiting his ability to travel and leave the house. Before being seen by a pain specialist he was seen by his primary care physician and two neurologists. When he was initially seen by the pain specialist he was taking gabapentin at a dose of 400 mg tid, because higher doses resulted in side effects. NSAIDS and acetaminophen had not provided significant relief. After evaluation by the pain treatment team, a course of nortriptyline was prescribed and then discontinued due to side effects. The patient then was treated with acupuncture and had significant improvement in pain and in his ability to participate in activities. The patient must pay $75 out of pocket for each acupuncture treatment. He has private insurance and is generally satisfied with his insurance coverage; however, he does believe that the acupuncture should be covered.

Discussion

There are two main issues pertaining to reimbursement raised by this case. The first is the issue of multiple assessments by similar providers. The patient was seen by the pain treatment team only after being seen previously by his primary care physician and two neurologists. Reimbursement can become problematic when a patient undergoes multiple assessments for the same problem or condition. This is often viewed as duplication of services. Therefore, it is vital that clinicians clearly identify what is unique about their assessment and how it added to the previously known data. This can include the fact that this is a second opinion, even if it is in agreement with other clinicians' assessments. This issue can arise frequently in pain treatment centers because the majority of patients will have already had their problem addressed by a primary care physician and often by other specialists, such as neurologists, orthopedic surgeons, or neurosurgeons.

   The second main issue regarding this case is the use of acupuncture. Though there has been some literature documenting the effectiveness of acupuncture, it is still considered an alternative medicine technique. Therefore, many insurance providers, including Medicare, will not provide coverage for this service. As mentioned previously, some insurance companies will pay for acupuncture. This information can often be obtained from the company's Web page. If the patient's insurance will not cover this service it is important to inform the patient that this treatment will need to be paid for out-of-pocket.

Case 2

GJ is a 58-year-old man who was referred to a pain specialist for pain that had been present for approximately 3 years and, despite extensive evaluation, had not been diagnosed. After evaluation by the pain treatment team the patient was diagnosed with fibromyalgia. His treatment plan included physical therapy, which resulted in improvement in his pain. His insurer paid for a total of 10 sessions but would not cover any further sessions, stating that he had received the maximum benefit. His treatment plan also included psychological services for treatment of depression and anxiety. It was felt that psychological services were necessary for the optimum treatment of the patient's pain. His insurance carrier, however, was unwilling to provide coverage for this service. The patient agreed that these services were necessary and paid out of pocket, but was unable to pay further when he had paid a total of $600. The patient found the whole experience frustrating and anxiety-provoking. He also felt that there was a belief at the insurance company that fibromyalgia "didn't exist," which contributed to their reluctance to provide coverage for services.

Discussion

The first issue of reimbursement related to this case is the coverage for physical therapy or rehabilitative services. Rehabilitative services are generally reimbursable subject to the documented necessity of the frequency, intensity, and duration of services. Patients may have difficulty with reimbursement for prolonged or seemingly repetitive therapy when little or no progress appears to be made. This is another situation where clarity and specificity of documentation is crucial. The documentation needs to describe

- why the therapy needs to continue;
- what is unique about the current therapy compared to previous therapy sessions, that is, physical therapy specifically for pain management when the patient has already received therapy for gait or balance disorders;
- what reasonable and necessary goals are for this person in relation to job, home, or desired activities;
- how progress toward these goals is being measured.

The second main point of discussion in this case is the issue of reimbursement for mental health services. There is a significant number of psychiatric conditions that are found in patients with persistent pain and these patients are probably best treated at pain treatment facilities with a multidisciplinary approach (Fishbain, Rosomoff, Steele-Rosomoff, & Cutler, 1995). The American Pain Society has emphasized the importance of behavioral assessment and therapy when reviewing reimbursement guidelines by Medicare intermediaries (Ashburn, 1997). Unfortunately, psychological services are often not reimbursed by the insurer. Again, the principles previously discussed are critical here, especially thorough clinical documentation. It is important to use all resources to find a potential source of payment. This can include mental-health treatment options through the patient's employer as part of a return-to-work program. The insurance company's Web site may also be useful in providing information about whether mental health services are reimbursed.

The third issue that is involved in this case is the reimbursement for conditions that are relatively new or areas of some controversy. For example, there is no specific diagnostic test for fibromyalgia; rather it is a diagnosis made by overall clinical assessment. Thus, it is critical for clinicians to specifically document their assessment and their rationale supporting the diagnosis and the necessity for specific treatments prescribed. It may also be helpful for the clinician to provide additional educational material about the condition and its management to the insurer.

REFERENCES

Ashburn, M. A. (1997). Medicare guidelines for chronic pain reimbursement. *APS Bulletin, 7*(4). (Also available on-line: *www.ampainsoc.org/pub/bulletin/jul97/policy.htm*)

Chisholm, M. A., Reinhardt, B. O., Vollenweider, L. J., Kendrick, B. D., & DiPiro, J. T. (2000). Medication assistance programs for uninsured and indigent patients. *American Journal Health-Syst Pharm, 57*, 1131–1136.

Eisenberg, D. M., Davis, R. B., Ettner, S. L., Appel, S., Wilkey, S., Van Rompay, M., & Kessler, R. C. (1998). Trends in alternative medicine use in the United States, 1990–1997: Results of a follow-up national survey. *Journal of the American Medical Association, 280*, 1569–1575.

Ferrell, B. (1993). Cost issues surrounding the treatment of cancer related pain. *Journal Pharm Care Pain Symptom Control, 1*, 9–23.

Ferrell, B. (1995). Pain evaluation and management in the nursing home. *Annals of Internal Medicine, 123*, 681–687.

Ferrell, B. R., & Griffith, H. (1994). Cost issues related to pain management: Report from the cancer pain panel of the Agency for Health Care Policy and Research. *Journal of Pain and Symptom Management, 9*, 221–234.

Fishbain, D. A., Rosomoff, H. L., Steele-Rosomoff, R., & Cutler, R. B. (1995). Types of pain treatment facilities and referral selection criteria: A review. *Archives of Family Medicine, 4*, 58–66.

Fishman, P., Von Korff, M., Lozana, P., & Hecht, J. (1997). Chronic care costs in managed care. *Health Affairs, 16*(3), 239–247.

Flor, H., Fydrich, T., & Turk, D. C. (1992). Efficacy of multidisciplinary pain treatment centers: A meta-analytic review. *Pain, 49*, 221–230.

Fox, C. D., Berger, D., Fine, P. G., Gebhart, G. F., Grabois, M., Kulich, R. J., Lande, S. D., McCarberg, B., & Portenoy, R. (2000). Pain assessment and treatment in the managed care environment; A position statement from the American Pain Society. *APS Managed Care Forum on Pain*. [On-line]. www.ampainsoc.org/managedcare/position.htm

Health Care Financing Administration, Office of the Actuary. (1996). Data from the Office of National Health Statistics. *Health Care Financing Review, 18*, 211.

Joranson, D. E. (1994). Are health care reimbursement policies a barrier to acute and cancer pain management? *Journal of Pain and Symptom Management, 9*, 244–253.

Jost, T. S. (2000). Medicare and Medicaid financing of pain management. *Journal of Pain, 1*, 183–194.

Kovner, A. R., & Jonas, S. (1999). Health care delivery in the United States. New York: Springer.

Kulich, R., & Lande, S. D. (1997). Managed care: The past and future of pain treatment. *APS Bulletin, 7*(4). (Also available on-line: *www.ampainsoc.org/pub/bulletin/jul97/clinic.htm*)

Loeser, J. D. (1999). Economic implications of pain management. *Acta Anaesthesiologica Scandinavica, 43*, 957–959.

National Center for Health Care Statistics. [On-line]. *www.cdc.gov/nchs*.

Pelletier, K. R., Marie, A., Krasner, M., & Haskell, W. L. (1997). Current trends in the integration and reimbursement of complementary and alternative medicine by managed care, insurance carriers and hospital providers. *American Journal of Health Promotion, 12*, 112–123.

Stieg, R. L., Lippe, P., & Shepard, T. A. (1999). Roadblocks to effective pain treatment. *Medical Clinics of North America, 83*, 809–821.

Stieg, R. L., Williams, R. C., Timmermans-Williams, G., & Tafuro, F. (1986). Cost benefits of interdisciplinary chronic pain treatment. *Clinical Journal of Pain, 1*, 189–193.

Taricco, A. (1998). Pain centers and the payer industry: Points we should consider. *APS Bulletin, 8*(2). (Also available on-line: *www.ampainsoc.org/pub/bulletin/mar98/clinic.htm*)

Turk, D. C. (1999). Here we go again: Outcomes, outcomes, outcomes. *Clinical Journal of Pain, 15*, 241–243.

Index